Epidemiological Research Applications for Public Health Measurement and Intervention

Simon George Taukeni
University of Namibia, Namibia

A volume in the Advances in Human Services and Public Health (AHSPH) Book Series

IGI Global
PUBLISHER of TIMELY KNOWLEDGE

Published in the United States of America by
IGI Global
Medical Information Science Reference (an imprint of IGI Global)
701 E. Chocolate Avenue
Hershey PA, USA 17033
Tel: 717-533-8845
Fax: 717-533-8661
E-mail: cust@igi-global.com
Web site: http://www.igi-global.com

Library of Congress Cataloging-in-Publication Data

Names: Taukeni, Simon George, 1973- editor.
Title: Epidemiological research applications for public health measurement and intervention / Simon George Taukeni, editor.
Description: Hershey, PA : Medical Information Science Reference, [2021] | Includes bibliographical references and index. | Summary: "This book provides relevant theoretical frameworks and the latest empirical research findings in the field of epidemiology to help professionals improve their knowledge of epidemiological research and measurement to investigate, detect and monitor emerging pathological infections to increase the effectiveness of public health practice"-- Provided by publisher.
Identifiers: LCCN 2020040686 (print) | LCCN 2020040687 (ebook) | ISBN 9781799844143 (hardcover) | ISBN 9781799844150 (ebook)
Subjects: MESH: Epidemiologic Research Design | Public Health Surveillance--methods | Communicable Diseases, Emerging--prevention & control
Classification: LCC RA652.2.P82 (print) | LCC RA652.2.P82 (ebook) | NLM WA 950 | DDC 362.1--dc23
LC record available at https://lccn.loc.gov/2020040686
LC ebook record available at https://lccn.loc.gov/2020040687

This book is published in the IGI Global book series Advances in Human Services and Public Health (AHSPH) (ISSN: 2475-6571; eISSN: 2475-658X)

British Cataloguing in Publication Data
A Cataloguing in Publication record for this book is available from the British Library.

Advances in Human Services and Public Health (AHSPH) Book Series

Jennifer Martin
RMIT University, Australia

ISSN:2475-6571
EISSN:2475-658X

Mission

The well-being of the general public should be a primary concern for any modern civilization. Ongoing research in the field of human services and public healthcare is necessary to evaluate, manage, and respond to the health and social needs of the global population.

The **Advances in Human Services and Public Health (AHSPH)** book series aims to publish high-quality reference publications focused on the latest methodologies, tools, issues, and strategies for managing the health and social welfare of the public. The AHSPH book series will be especially relevant for healthcare professionals, policy makers, government officials, and students seeking the latest research in this field.

Coverage

- Healthcare Reform
- Health Policy
- Social Work
- Medicare and Medicaid
- Public Welfare
- Social Welfare Policy
- Public Funding
- Assistance Programs
- Poverty
- Domestic Violence

IGI Global is currently accepting manuscripts for publication within this series. To submit a proposal for a volume in this series, please contact our Acquisition Editors at Acquisitions@igi-global.com or visit: http://www.igi-global.com/publish/.

The Advances in Human Services and Public Health (AHSPH) Book Series (ISSN 2475-6571) is published by IGI Global, 701 E. Chocolate Avenue, Hershey, PA 17033-1240, USA, www.igi-global.com. This series is composed of titles available for purchase individually; each title is edited to be contextually exclusive from any other title within the series. For pricing and ordering information please visit http://www.igi-global.com/book-series/advances-human-services-public-health/102256. Postmaster: Send all address changes to above address. ©

Titles in this Series

For a list of additional titles in this series, please visit: www.igi-global.com/book-series

Global Issues and Innovative Solutions in Healthcare, Culture, and the Environment
Mika Merviö (Kibi International University, Okayama, Japan)
Information Science Reference • © 2020 • 366pp • H/C (ISBN: 9781799835769) • US $195.00

Handbook of Research on Leadership and Advocacy for Children and Families in Rural Poverty
H. Carol Greene (East Carolina University, USA) Bryan S. Zugelder (James Madison University, USA) and Jane C. Manner (East Carolina University, USA)
Information Science Reference • © 2020 • 525pp • H/C (ISBN: 9781799827870) • US $265.00

Emerging Trends in Indigenous Language Media, Communication, Gender, and Health
Kehinde Opeyemi Oyesomi (Covenant University, Nigeria) and Abiodun Salawu (North-West University, South Africa)
Medical Information Science Reference • © 2020 • 320pp • H/C (ISBN: 9781799820918) • US $285.00

Impact of Textile Dyes on Public Health and the Environment
Khursheed Ahmad Wani (Government Degree College, Bijbehara, India) Nirmala Kumari Jangid (Banasthali Vidyapith, India) and Ajmal Rashid Bhat (Government Degree College, Bijbehara, India)
Information Science Reference • © 2020 • 335pp • H/C (ISBN: 9781799803119) • US $245.00

Handbook of Research on Health Systems and Organizations for an Aging Society
César Fonseca (Universidade de Évora, Portugal) Manuel José Lopes (Universidade de Évora, Portugal) David Mendes (Universidade de Évora, Portugal) Felismina Mendes (Universidade de Évora, Portugal) and José García-Alonso (Universidad de Extremadura, Spain)
Medical Information Science Reference • © 2020 • 323pp • H/C (ISBN: 9781522598183) • US $365.00

Cases on Cross-Cultural Counseling Strategies
Bonnie C. King (Midwestern State University, USA) and Tiffany A. Stewart (Midwestern State University, USA)
Medical Information Science Reference • © 2020 • 380pp • H/C (ISBN: 9781799800224) • US $245.00

Environmental Exposures and Human Health Challenges
Paraskevi Papadopoulou (Deree – The American College of Greece, Greece) Christina Marouli (Deree – The American College of Greece, Greece) and Anastasia Misseyanni (Deree – The American College of Greece, Greece)
Medical Information Science Reference • © 2019 • 449pp • H/C (ISBN: 9781522576358) • US $255.00

IGI Global
PUBLISHER of TIMELY KNOWLEDGE

701 East Chocolate Avenue, Hershey, PA 17033, USA
Tel: 717-533-8845 x100 • Fax: 717-533-8661
E-Mail: cust@igi-global.com • www.igi-global.com

Table of Contents

Detailed Table of Contents

Investigating an outbreak involves naming the cause ofthe disease, the people affected, the facts that surround someone and mode of spread of the disease, and other related factors involved in spreading the disease, and to take effective actions to contain and prevent the spread of the disease. This chapter explores investigating an outbreak.

Epidemiology is the technique used to detect the origins of health outcomes and diseases in inhabitants. In epidemiology, the patient, the individual, and community are viewed mutually. Epidemiology is not only the analysis of health in inhabitants; it also includes applying the information enlarged by the analysis of public-based practice. In case of medicine, the practice of epidemiology is both an art and science. Currently, COVID-19 has spread all around the world. It is basically a severe acute respiratory syndrome coronavirus-2 (SARS-CoV-2). Through the binding of receptor in gene region of its spike protein, ACE2 is bounded by corona virus. In this chapter, the authors summarized the epidemiological characteristics, clinical features, diagnosis, and treatment prognosis of COVID-19. A complete consideration will help to control the disease.

In this chapter, the authors describe the essential need of mental health and psychosocial support for people accommodated in mandatory quarantine and isolation facilities during the outbreak of COVID-19 pandemic in Namibia through a multi-sectoral response. Namibia recorded its first two index cases on 13 March 2020 when a married couple arrived in the Windhoek district in Namibia from Madrid, Spain on 11 March 2020. Namibia has since March 2020 provided supervised quarantine services to 12,128 persons in facilities around the country. The Ministry of Health and Social Services provides mental health and psychosocial support services, which were critical in the short and long-term response to COVID-19 pandemic. Public health measures were developed in line with WHO guidelines to contain the virus. These measures include the need of setting up quarantine and isolation facilities. Recommendations for future research in strengthening mental health and psychosocial support services and coping strategies are provided in the chapter.

Section 3
Measurements and Interventions

In this chapter, the authors present a system that uses smart immunization and develops structures to allow collaboration between parents, healthcare workers, and government agencies to cooperate at a grass-roots level to help spread immunization, collect and upload demographics, and allow for its multi-instance analysis. This system will enhance the spread of vaccination and reduce vaccine hesitancy. Information is coagulated and presented as statistical results that are presented in an engaging visualization form. Further, a reminder system has been set up to enable automated email service for parents by reminding them of proper and timely vaccinations. It collates the immunization data to present usable demographics for timely interventions, as may be necessary. The immunization perspective is retrained by easy storage and retrieval and quick remedial measures to contain the spread of vaccine-preventable diseases and reduction in child mortality. Statistical analysis has been done to predict immunization spread among different regions and detect any possible epidemic.

The disease interactome is a network of genes that are related to each other through some attributes. These genes, being part of various diseases, show a high correlation among many diseases. Genes being a major part of the interactome thus can be used to determine the relationship between various diseases, their symptoms, clinical similarity, and co-morbidity. Subgraphs and similarity factors such as Jaccardian distance, cosine similarities, and others have been exploited to calculate the relationship between two or more diseases. Many diseases that did not show much resemblance on the basis of gene similarity or symptom similarity were seen to be closely related according to network interactome. The quantitative analysis between disease-disease was also done. Clustering algorithms like hierarchical clustering involving single, complete, and average linkage were applied to get a visual representation in the form of a dendrogram. Thus, disease-disease interactome was created, analyzed for finding related secondary diseases, and their basic nature was understood.

Therapeutic decision making is crucial to address any health problems. Household livelihood assets had significant impact on therapeutic decision making in the study village. The researchers administered participant observation, in-depth interview, and FGD for data collection by using purposive sampling during November 2010 to June 2011. Among 250 households, the number of ill persons were 316, of which 297 received treatments from popular, folk, and professional sectors while the rest did not seek any options. The decision makers were varied for newborn, children, adolescent, adult, and aged people, and it depended on the cyclical issues of an illness episode.

The developing countries of the world are still lagging in the implementation of the universal newborn hearing screening (UNHS). In other to eradicate unnecessary earshot impairments via suitable rehabilitation processes, there is need for more studies. Thus, this chapter is channeled to bridge this gap. This study used secondary data by comprehensively reviewing the published researches and other relevant and related works and found that UNHS practices in Malaysia and Nigeria have both differences and similarities. The two countries use AABR and OAE as their protocol, and the newborn hearing screening is not binding on the caregivers in both countries. However, their approaches differ in the area of finance, follow-up intervals, and the years of introduction among others. Nevertheless, there are some challenges impeding the effective implementation of the programme which includes include lack of awareness, death of personnel, inadequate diagnostic centers, among others. Given these findings, this chapter could be said to have practical implications for the stakeholders.

The prevalence of gonorrhea has not discontinued in several countries and still remains as one of the top sexually transmitted diseases (STD) and it's caused by Neisseria gonorrhoeae. This bacterium gains entry into the human host via receptors, and by the usage of several virulence factors, it manages to spread through the cells and leads to severe complications. The study of these bacteria in various in vitro and in vivo models have paved the way for gaining insights on various aspects of bacterial infection, such as the study of pathogenesis of the organism in the host. It also drove the development of more appropriate drugs for the treatment of the gonorrhea illness caused by this 'superbug'. This chapter focuses on providing a concise overview on the general aspects of N. gonorrhoeaeas an update and the in vitro and in vivo models used for understanding this bacterium over the years. Despite gonorrhea not being a rare STD, it is still a big challenge for researchers, healthcare professionals, and communicators with public awareness to communicate effectively with the general community.

Hepatitis E (HEV) remains one of the foremost public health problems globally and it is estimated to have affected one-third of the human population. Usually, symptoms appear 2 to 9 weeks after exposure to the virus and include fever, fatigue, lack of appetite, abdominal pain, and jaundice. While the government has a duty to provide access to clean water, communities, and individuals can equally play an important role in practicing and maintaining good physical and environmental hygiene. In Namibia, the spread of HEV has been a public health concern since it's outbreak in 2017. Before then, the country had two outbreaks in 1983 and 1995-1996 which affected mainly areas lacking potable water and waste disposal facilities in Kavango region. This chapter ought to provide an overview and different prevention measures and supportive management approaches used to contain and prevent the spread of HEV. The above statistic calls for plans and actions from national, regional, district management teams to implement effective active surveillance interventions in place that are geared towards curbing the spread of HEV.

Preface

Epidemiological Research Applications for Public Health Measurement and Intervention provides relevant theoretical frameworks and the latest empirical research findings in the field of epidemiology. The chapters within this essential reference source enhance the knowledge of epidemiological research and measurement to investigate, detect, and monitor emerging pathological infections. While highlighting topics that include the history of epidemiology; the applications of epidemiology; and also the uses, principles, and roles of epidemiology, this book is ideally intended for professionals and researchers working in the field of health sciences in various disciplines and government officials, policymakers, practitioners, stakeholders, researchers, academicians, and students who are interested in epidemiological research and measurement for increasing the effectiveness of public health practice.

INSIDE THIS BOOK

1. Outbreak Investigation: Epidemiology in Search of Communicable Diseases

Investigating an outbreak is a set of ways used to name the cause responsible for the disease, the people affected, the facts that surround someone and mode of spread of the disease, and other related factors involved in spreading the disease, and to take effective actions to contain and prevent the spread of the disease. Manage and do an epidemic of response to ask questions, and try to find the facts about something requires preparation and achieving goals in order to respond to these key questions. In a small geological area an epidemic may occur or may spread to a country or many. A single instance of a contagious infection is long overdue, not present in a population, or brought about by a specialist not before that perceived in that network or region, or focuses on a precedent that unknown disease would lead to a outbreak and something would be carefully considered and checked to find out the reality. Outbreaks could be detected by carefully examining observation facts, detailing by health office, influencing people, local leaders, or holding reports that could be true vault or media.

2. The Study of the Epidemiology and Clinical Feature of Novel Coronavirus (COVID-19)

Epidemiology is the technique used to detect the origins of health outcomes and diseases in inhabitants. In epidemiology, the patient is the individuals and community are viewed mutually. Epidemiology not only the analysis of health in an inhabitants; it also includes applying the information enlarged by the analysis of public based practice. In case of medicine, the practice of epidemiology is both an art and science. Currently, COVID-19 has spread all around the world basically it is a severe acute respiratory syndrome coronavirus-2 (SARS-CoV-2). Through the binding of receptor in gene region of its spike protein,

ACE2 is bounded by Corona virus. In this chapter, we summarized the epidemiological characteristics, clinical features, diagnosis and treatment prognosis of COVID-19. A complete consideration will help to control the disease.

3. Mental Health and Psychosocial Support for Persons in Quarantine and Isolation Facilities During COVID-19 Pandemic in Namibia

In this chapter, the authors describe the essential need of mental health and psychosocial support for people accommodated in mandatory quarantine and isolation facilities during the outbreak of COVID-19 pandemic in Namibia through a multi-sectoral response. Namibia recorded its first two index cases on 13 March 2020 when a married couple arrived in the Windhoek district in Namibia from Madrid, Spain on 11 March 2020. Namibia has since March 2020 provided supervised quarantine services to 12 128 persons in facilities around the country. The Ministry of Health and Social Services provides mental health and psychosocial support services, which were critical in the short and long-term response to COVID-19 pandemic. Public health measures were developed in line with WHO Guidelines to contain the virus. Of these measures, include the need of setting up quarantine and isolation facilities. Recommendations for future research in strengthening mental health and psychosocial support services and coping strategies are provided in the chapter.

4. Towards the Development of IT-Enabled Immunization Monitoring Framework

In this paper, we present a system that uses smart immunization and develops structures to allow collaboration between parents, healthcare workers, and government agencies to cooperate at a grass-roots level to help spread immunization, collect and upload demographics and allow for its multi-instance analysis. This system will enhance the spread of vaccination and reduce vaccine hesitancy. Information is coagulated and presented as statistical results that are presented in an engaging visualization form. Further, a reminder system has been set-up to enable automated email service for parents by reminding them of proper and timely vaccinations. It collates the immunization data to present usable demographics for timely interventions, as may be necessary. The immunization perspective is retrained by easy storage and retrieval, and quick remedial measures to contain the spread of vaccine-preventable diseases and reduction in child mortality. Statistical analysis has been done to predict immunization spread among different regions and detect any possible epidemic.

5. Disease Interactome: An Assessment Case-Study Based on Analysis and Measures to Predict Secondary Diseases

The disease interactome is a network of genes that are related to each other through some attributes. These genes, being part of various diseases, show a high correlation among many diseases. Genes being a major part of the interactome thus can be used to determine the relationship between various diseases, their symptoms, clinical similarity, and co-morbidity. Subgraphs and similarity factors such as Jaccardian distance, cosine similarities, and others have been exploited to calculate the relationship between two or more diseases. Many diseases that did not show much resemblance on the basis of gene similarity or symptom similarity were seen to be closely related according to network interactome. The quantitative analysis between disease-disease was also done. Clustering algorithms like hierarchical clustering involving single, complete, and average linkage were applied to get a visual representation in the form of a dendrogram. Thus, disease-disease interactome was created, analyzed for finding related secondary diseases and their basic nature too was understood.

6. Therapeutic Decision-Making Process: An Anthropological Study on a Disaster-Prone Bangladeshi Village

Therapeutic decision making is crucial to address any health problems. Household livelihood assets had significant impact on therapeutic decision making in the study village. The researchers administered participant observation, in-depth interview and FGD for data collection by using purposive sampling during November 2010 to June 2011. Among 250 households, the number of ill persons were 316 of which 297 received treatments from popular, folk and professional sectors while the rest did not seek any options. The decision makers were varied for newborn, children, adolescent, adult and aged people and it had depended on the cyclical issues of an illness episode.

7. Universal Newborn Hearing Screening Programme in Malaysia and Nigeria: A Comparative Analysis

The developing countries of the world are still lagging in the implementation of the Universal Newborn Hearing Screening (UNHS). In other to eradicate unnecessary earshot impairments via suitable rehabilitation processes, there is need for more studies. Thus, this chapter is channeled to bridge this gap. This study used secondary data by comprehensively reviewing the published researches and other relevant and related works and found that UNHS practices in Malaysia and Nigeria have both differences and similarities. The two –countries use AABR and OAE as their protocol, and the newborn hearing screening is not binding on the caregivers in both countries. However, their approaches differ in the area of finance, follow-up intervals, and the years of introduction among others. Nevertheless, there are some challenges impeding the effective implementation of the programme which includes include lack of awareness, death of personnel, inadequate diagnostic centers among others. Given these findings, this paperwork could be said to have practical implications for the stakeholders.

8. In Vitro and In Vivo Models for Pathogenic *Neisseria gonorrhoeae* Infections: Infection Models for Pathogenic N. Gonorrhoeae

The prevalence of gonorrhea has not discontinued in several countries and still remains as one of the top sexually transmitted diseases (STD) and it is caused by Neisseria gonorrhoeae. This bacterium gains entry into the human host via receptors and by the usage of several virulence factors, it manages to spread through the cells and leads to severe complications. The study of these bacteria in various in vitro and in vivo models have paved way for gaining insights on various aspects of bacterial infection, such as the study of pathogenesis of the organism in the host. It also drove the development of more appropriate drugs for the treatment of the gonorrhea illness caused by this 'superbug'. This chapter focuses on providing a concise overview on the general aspects of N. gonorrhoeae as an update and the in vitro and in vivo models used for understanding this bacterium over the years. Despite gonorrhea not being a rare STD, it is still a big challenge for researchers, health care professionals and communicators with public awareness to communicate effectively with the general community.

9. Hepatitis E-Overview and Management in Namibia

Hepatitis E (HEV) is one of the foremost health problems globally and is estimated that affects one-third of the human population. Usually, symptoms appear 2 to 9 weeks after exposure to the virus and include fever, fatigue, lack of appetite, abdominal pain, and jaundice. While the government has a duty to provide access to clean water, communities and individuals can equally play an important role to improve their own situation. In Namibia, the spread of HEV has been a public health concern since 2017. Before then, the country had two outbreaks in 1983 and 1995-1996 which affected mainly areas lacking potable water and waste disposal facilities in Kavango region. This chapter ought to provide an overview and different prevention measures and supportive management approaches used to contain and prevent the spread of HEV. The above statistic calls for plans and actions from national, regional, district management teams to implement effective active surveillance interventions in place that are geared towards curbing the spread of HEV.

CONCLUSION

We at IGI Global believe without any doubt that this book is best fitting in all health sciences discipline both in undergraduate and postgraduate programs. Different levels in health sciences, in particular public health, have acknowledged the significant role of epidemiology methods for early detection of emerging infections, alert systems, and preparedness interventions. Therefore, it is important to understand how epidemiological research is conducted and how it can be used at various levels to make exposure or incidence data on a general population available. In this, epidemiological research connected to both human and technology interactions is of primary importance.

Finally, this book could not be what it is if it were not for the contributions of all our esteemed authors. We thank them for their hard work and well researched chapters.

Section 1
Outbreak Investigation

Chapter 1
Outbreak Investigation: Epidemiology in Search of Communicable Diseases

Peddarapu Rama Krishna
https://orcid.org/0000-0001-5023-257X
VNR Vignana Jyothi Institute of Engineering and Technology, Hyderabad, India

Pothuraju Rajarajeswari
Koneru Lakshmaiah Education Foundation, Guntur, India

ABSTRACT

Investigating an outbreak involves naming the cause ofthe disease, the people affected, the facts that surround someone and mode of spread of the disease, and other related factors involved in spreading the disease, and to take effective actions to contain and prevent the spread of the disease. This chapter explores investigating an outbreak.

INTRODUCTION

An outbreak or an endemic is the happening of a greater figure of disease cases than expected in a certain region or between a specific gathering of persons over a definite interval frame. For the most part, the cases are hazarded to have a distinctive reason or to recognize with each other somehow or another.

Epidemic disease is normally applied to locations including more quantities of personalities over a wide-ranging land zone. Epidemic disease constrained to just occurring or existing in one little spot increment in the occasions something occurs of disease, (such as, village, town, or closed institution) can be named as outbreak.(Outbreak Investigation: National Health Portal of India, n.d.)

DOI: 10.4018/978-1-7998-4414-3.ch001

The major purpose of conducting outbreak examinations is to recognize the basis to build up mechanism and to start quantifies that will avoid upcoming scenes of illness. They are additionally once in a while embraced to prepare new staff or to get familiar with the illness and its systems for transmission. Epidemic investigation is a lot of methods used to distinguish the reason, such as the infectious agent, liable for the disease. The primary motivation behind epidemic investigation is to control the spread of the infection before it causes more deaths and sickness.

Types of Epidemic

- Point source - An outbreak in which all cases are uniformly disease-ridden, typically from a single source or presentation.
- Continuous source — An epidemic in which the underlying agent (e.g. contaminated water, rotted food) contaminates people who deal with it for a long time.(Communicable Diseases Module: 42. Epidemic Investigation and Management,)

Objectives of outbreak investigation are (i) To control the outbreak! (ii) To avoid future outbreaks, (iii) To give statutory ordered administrations (iv)To strengthen surveillance at local level, (v) To propel information about a sickness, and (vi) To offer training opportunities.

What Is the Justification for Investigating Outbreaks?

Events are taking place on purpose. Hence, outbreaks of infection have instrumental components irrespective of whether they are found. Discovering an explanation makes it possible to organize steps to end the ongoing outbreak and avoid future repetitions. Instead of any disease, an infectious occurrence emulates a change in the normal relation between (i) the host (e.g. immune ability, environment, diet, exposure, etc.), (ii) the agent ("e.g. bacteria, toxin or physical power") and (iii) the earth ("e.g. climate, crowding, pollution, social conditions, etc.").

In this way, so as to carry out suitable control methods for an outbreak, it is important to analyze and recognize each of these three components and their cooperation. On the off-chance that this is not done, the control methods at that stage are not based on the greatest rational facts. Epidemics set up one of a kind environment tests from which the normal history and range of a particular disease, the hidden hazard issues, and the effect of existing general well-being programs on the study of disease transmission can be largely discovered. The investigation of outbreaks is therefore equally important for research and preparation.

BACKGROUND

Many in the pharmaceutical network were certain in the mid-1970s that the war was about to end as opposed to infectious diseases. Irresistible sicknesses were on the melt away, groundbreaking anti-toxins were demonstrated against infectious infection weapons in the armamentarium, smallpox was almost annihilated, and new vaccines were still being developed to combat a variety of diseases. Such environmental advancements be necessary endorsed by community health improvements. The general population was very attentive to these advances but they were not really seen as part of public health by the great findings of medical science. Nonetheless, people's consciousness led patients to have greater expectations of their surgeons and strengthened the entitlement theory that noble administration of quality of access to health care facilities is a social right of every person.

Governments have felt the pressure to popularize the new medicine and listen to the wishes of their people. Chiefs were taken into account by questions about substance abuse, chronic diseases, tobacco use, teenage pregnancy, ecological pollution and geriatric issues. General health care systems were relied upon to discuss these complex, overwhelming, and diverse issues facing people in general, just as they continued to do their traditional work in disease detection, respond to epidemics, and avoid irresistible diseases. Nevertheless, the creation of these new jobs was ineffectively established, not properly protected, and not fully understood.

Today, at a crossroads, the public health system is about how its role can be described and improved. Environmental health's changing complexity presents new obstacles in the identification, treatment and response to infectious diseases. Historically, local public health departments, medical clinics, and hospitals were the main hotspot for identifying and managing outbreaks of infectious diseases. Individuals from regulated health care partnerships and the pace of public health laboratory privatization continue to expand in view of the needs of the networks they represent. At the same time, a much amount of the specific elements of facilities and foundations for public health research that offer epidemiological administrations could be disintegrated. In addition to this disintegration, there may be a reduced ability in the nearby general wellness frameworks to differentiate and respond to infectious diseases. However, the capability of the open solid network can also be adversely affected by the growth of the uninsured population, which has concentrated the greater part of the weight of the assets on the open security net and accessible labs. The challenge for public health research centers will be to carry out cost-movements or to get new funding sources.

Tensions emerge in public health as it moves from its usual emphasis on infectious disease control to addressing the emerging fields of chronic disease and injury prevention. With the general strategic public health, each of these areas is predictable. Sadly, they compete overwhelmingly for the available equivalent capital.

The public health system has been tested for years to respond to a variety of new and reappearing disease threats, ranging from Legionnaires disease to "HIV infections, to Lyme disease", and to the latest reappearing disease attack, such as those caused by life forms impervious to anti-infectious agents. The suffering problems of constant disease and damage, the rising phantom of ecological contamination and the change in the country's medicinal services framework give strong impetus to public health to create inventive systems for the surveillance and reaction of infectious diseases.

ISSUES, CONTROVERSIES, PROBLEMS

The outsourcing of health care and public health labs raises enormous challenges in the usual way that surveillance of diseases is driven. This has ultimately contributed to the transfer of high-volume; slight effort tests to the private sector, while low-volume and large-cost tests stay in the open area. Changes in the health care system raise serious concerns about the usual way in which control of the disease has been carried out. For example, the private insurance industry (most specifically managed care) is now increasingly servicing patients whose health information was once readily available to public health agencies, who may not have similar motivators for sharing information. A re-examination and an elective way to keep up those important components that have been successful and continue to be convincing for the surveillance of infectious diseases are necessary.

For example, Medicaid patients, whose health information was once readily open to public health agencies, are now being served slowly by the private insurance industry (most specifically, managed care), which may not have similar motivators for sharing information. A re-examination and an elective way to support those important components that have been effective and continue to be persuasive for infectious disease surveillance are needed. By the way, the test would be in the public health care system to make a more grounded and increasingly relevant monitoring system work best with the changing health care system. The open door will be to promote public health science and its unique significance in health care.

Rising diseases (Davis & Lederberg, 2000) keep on troubling the health care system and are getting progressively confounded to distinguish and treat effectively. Also, the public health system is consistently helped to remember the difficulties presented by the unforeseen, regardless of whether it is the following flu illness or a Eco terrorists demonstration. "In 1988 the Institute of Medicine (IOM)" suggested that "each general health agency routinely and deliberately collect, assemble, analyze, and make accessible data on the health of the community, remembering insights for health status, community health needs, and epidemiologic and different investigations of medical issues" (Davis & Lederberg, 2000) ("IOM, 1988, p. 141"). In this way, the diagnosis and investigation of health hazards in the community is one of the fundamental public health services. Health departments at government, state, and neighborhood level, regularly with the scholastic network's guide, can play these capabilities off-chance to have the proper degree of resources, adequately prepared faculties, and build up announcement and correspondence frameworks.

Every sector offers new capacities, and each division faces some usual and unusual challenges, but most infectious disease epidemic investigations follow a similar general method:(1) Identifiable proof of the circumstances that show the need for examination (e.g., more than the average number of cases of a specific disease); (2) Inspection; (3) Confirmation of the need for examination; (4) Reaction, typically involving outbreak control, and suggestions and reaction coordination, both open and private, to prevent further illness.

Inside every examination are a few parts which may join, however are not constrained to epidemiological, research center, and natural appraisals. Every part may likewise must coordination at a few levels, from the neighborhood to the state, private, and government. As a rule, government assets, through the "Centers for Disease Control and Prevention (CDC)" and the "U.S. Food and Drug Administration (Davis & Lederberg, 2000) (FDA)", are accessible to aid examinations, yet they possibly do as such if state and local public health agencies have set up the framework to recognize and report unusual disease occurrences. Succinct and auspicious correspondence between every part is basic to a good examination.

Challenges and Options

Epidemic sickness investigations is a hard and fast of methods used to find the motive, in different words the (capable to be without difficulty caught from others) agent, chargeable for the disease. It is also used to pick out the people affected, the data or conditions that surround someone and mode of unfold of the sickness, and other absolutely linked or related elements involved in spreading the Epidemic disease. That is mainly vital if the epidemic disease has uncommon functions, if it provides a huge danger to public health, and it isn't always self-limiting (i.e. it does not end in a surprising and unplanned way without expert (movement that facilitates a terrible scenario).

An epidemic sickness investigation is a difficulty activity for medical experts. The principle purpose of epidemic disease investigations is to govern the spread of the disease before it cases more deaths and infection. As a health official or professional person, the primary movement they need to take is to verify the lifestyles of an epidemic disease.

To do this, they need to recognize the common variety of cases of that sickness all through this unique month in that community in preceding years, so one can test that number with the cutting-edge amount of cases. Is there an extra some cases or deaths from the disease as compared to the standard occasion? If there definitely are excess instances, they ought to document their findings to the District fitness workplace right away. Epidemic disease investigations and management includes team work. Their function as health official or professionals is to record the occasion of an epidemic sickness,

to get ready for action and train the community, and to aid the district health people in charge in wearing out manage and prevention measures was wanted.

Issues and Problems

Wherever a field research is preferred for practice, they need to be well-trained before they leave for the region. The systems can be divided into broad categories: (a) Issues of health and science and (b) Issues of management and service. Good training is essential in both groups for a smooth experience on the field.

Clinical and Research Issues

As a subject researcher, they must have the best medical know-how, supplies and equipment to conduct research earlier than you go to the sector. Discuss the condition with someone who is familiar with the disease and relevant cases, and study the literature. In past comparable outbreaks, what were the causes, transmission pathways and chance factors for the disease? Combine useful references from journal articles and sample questionnaires.

Until leaving for a topic of study, seek advice from the laboratory staff to make sure that they take the right sample material and conduct the right techniques for collection, storage and transport.And also tell them about the outbreak by talking to the laboratory body of workers, and they can count on what kind of laboratory assets might be desired.

Often, they need to know which items or equipment they need to bring to protect themself. Many outbreak investigations do not need special equipment, although work on "SARS or Ebola hemorrhagic fever" may also include private protective devices that include masks, gowns, and gloves.

Finally, before they leave, they must have a course of action. What are the goals of this study, that is to say what are they trying to do? What will they do first, second, and third? Having an action course on which everyone has the same view will allow them to "hit the ground walking" and avoid delays due to misunderstandings.

Management and Working Issues

A good field investigator, as well as a good epidemiologist, must be a good supervisor and collaborator, since most investigations are conducted by a group than just one man or woman. Earlier than departure, the group contributors must be selected and recognize their anticipated disciplinary roles and obligations. Do they need a laboratory professional, veterinarian, translator / interpreter, professional pc, entomologist, or other professional? What is the role of each body? Who is on that rate? When they have been asked to take part but are not working for the local health department now, are they expected to lead the investigation, deliver a session to the study staff's community team, or really give a hand to the staff around? And who are their close-by contacts?

Based on the type of outbreak the some agencies involved may be quite high. In addition, an investigation into an animal source outbreak may include state and federal agriculture agencies, and/or the "Food and Drug Administration (FDA)." If criminal or eco-terrorists intent is suspected, law enforcement agencies and the "Federal Investigation Bureau (FBI)" may be or may at least be interested in the pace. The "Federal Emergency Management Agency (FEMA)" may be the leader in an herbal catastrophe (hurricane or flood). Exclusive business team of staff with one-of - a-kind experiences, approaches and goals to discuss. Of example, while the public health investigation may also be aware of detecting a pathogen, source, and mode of transmission, a criminal investigation may focus on finding the culprit.

To meet the disparate goals of one-of - a-kind corporations, Roles and responsibilities in such multi-enterprise enquiries are important.

A Communications Strategy should be developed. The need to connect with the public health and healthcare community has been discussed for a long time but the need to interact quickly and easily with elected officials and the public became clear through the epidemics of "West Nile Virus Encephalitis, SARS, and Anthrax."

The plan must include how often and when to have conference calls with the relevant agencies, which can be the specific spokesperson, who will prepare health alerts and press releases, and the like. If a federal agency is concerned with 10 or more people in the sample, the records series system must first be approved through the "White House Management and Budget Office (OMB)."

More critical is organizational and logistical awareness. Arrange to carry a PC, mobile phone or smart phone card, digital cam, and other components. If they are going back out of the area, they can set up earlier when and where they will meet local officials and contacts when they are coming into the city. Travel, accommodation, and nearby transportation should be arranged. Most departments and entities have to follow stringent approval policies and budget limits. They will need a passport and often a visa if they are moving to another country. Until they leave, they should also deal with personal matters, particularly if the work is likely to be lengthy.

The role of the department of local public health in an outbreak study is important. It is the corporation most commonly charged with preserving surveillance structures that detect outbreaks and that gets the first call for a response when a virus occurs. During maximum outbreaks, during addition to relevant environmental investigations, the nice potential for collection of epidemiological details and laboratory specimens is within the first few hours to days of the outbreak. Those appear as the local health department's vital roles, as on-web page state and federal participation is often at least 1 to 2 days away.

Despite that there are many barriers to this important public health service being adequately achieved.

Detection and reporting systems in many areas are still insufficient. Most local public health agencies serve small counties (often jurisdictions with populations below 15,000 to 20,000) and are funded through a nurse, a health care provider, a clerk, and a part-time health officer. Consequently, a limited variety of contributors to the workforce be there for outbreak investigations because other critical functions are desirable in the meantime. Furthermore, due to the infrequency of the occurrence of outbreaks, it is very difficult to expand and keep up the skills required to conduct a research.

Generally, outbreak investigations are routinely given a low administrative priority because little money or proposals are dedicated to what is mostly a rare and sporadic occurrence. Local health authorities want basic research expertise in questionnaire layout, interviewing methods, and sequence of environmental and clinical specimens as a bare minimum. They want talents for laptop, internet, communications, and teamwork.

Importantly, they need to extend these talents beyond traditional food-borne outbreak investigations as they are increasingly called upon to investigate respiratory diseases in school systems, occupational exposures, nonsocial infections, mid-stage outbreaks of day care, and so on. Electronic communications systems want to be strengthened so that records can be shared about outbreaks and resources can be acquired during the outbreak. Ultimately, there are many core-potential files, offers, and so on that explicitly define gadget expectations to the most effective state level (or combine state and local expectations). Approximately local health branch resources need to be better established in outbreak investigations.

In short, local health departments, often the primary to be looked to as when an epidemic occurs, are often the least ready to respond. With the help and guidance of national and federal businesses and with stronger collaborations with nearby groups, inadequacies can be conquered today. General principles to be kept in mind when designing solutions to these problems are the following: (1) Local health authorities want and should be informed about outbreaks in their jurisdictions. In most cases, the legal authority for investigating the outbreak is locally based. (2) Training must be designed to support and improve these skills, and training should be accessible from a long distance. (3) Maximum local health departments already have (although they will be administratively independent) working relationships with states. (4) Community health branch workers are open to the direction, route and advancement of the latest skills, but they need clear expectations and enough resources to meet them.(5) Building and maintaining local capacity to detect and react to an outbreak that much enhance the size of the public health system to respond to major epidemics (e.g., a flu pandemic or a ecoterrorists attack).

SOLUTIONS AND RECOMMENDATIONS

Most health departments have specific methods for handling calls from the public about potential communicable disease outbreaks, and some states have guidance on how to respond to cluster reviews of non-infectious diseases (Bender et al., 1990; Fiore et al., 1990; Investigating an Outbreak: Principles of Epidemiology in Public Health Practice, An Introduction to Applied Epidemiology and Biostatistics Lesson 6, 2001). The choice of whether and how an ability outbreak is definitely investigated depends on a variety of factors.

They usually consist of a few health-related elements, some related to health division and some related to external issues. Factors related to the problem itself include the severity of the outbreak, the number of cases, the source, process or ease of transmission, and prevention and exploitation provision. Total local health agencies are more likely to investigate an obvious outbreak, since the number of infected (or uncovered) people is high, where the disease is severe (serious disease with unnecessary risk of hospitalization, complications or loss of life), where powerful control measures are in place, and because the outbreak has the potential to have an effect on others until it is held promptly.

Of example, it is not possible that a single case of gastroenteritis will trigger an investigation into a subject, but a cluster of instances may also prompt.

Nevertheless, only a single case of botulism is likely to be treated to find and get rid of the supply because each is potentially fatal and preventable, and the supply can typically be identified. The unusual occurrence of illness at the state or national level may trigger an investigation. The occurrence of a new or unusual disease or a change in pattern of disease in an area is much more likely to cause research than the amount of a common disease with well-established patterns of transmission and exploitation.

Nonetheless, field investigations are a burden on a health department, so the decision is often dependent on staff availability and resources, and competing priorities. Likewise, some departments of health require the tradition of actively handling outbreaks and thus have ability in doing so, while other departments of health may also lack such experience.

Nonetheless, field investigations are typically justified on one or more of the following grounds: (i) Health problem management or prevention, (ii) Benefit for learning (research opportunity),(iii) Economic, political or legal considerations, (iv) Considerations of the public health plan and (v) Education Management and prevention.

Health Problem Management or Prevention

Helping direct illness is the most important reason an outbreak is inspected. These attempts to handle sickness rely on many factors, including the agent's experience, the outbreak's natural course, the same old sickness transmission process, and available controls.

For instance, If a health department learns of an outbreak of "hepatitis A" (recognized agent) in which one of the patients is a restaurant chef, the division can give immune globulin to restaurant customers to avoid a second wave of instances (degree of control), but most effective if they are within 14 days of exposure (time). However, if an outbreak seems to be almost over, the health agency may not want to carry out control steps, but identifying factors that contributed to the outbreak that will help them to prove strategies that will prevent similar outbreaks in the future might be inquisitive.

The balance between management strategies and further analysis focuses on how much consideration is being delivered to the intent, source, and mode of transmission of the agent. (Goodman et al., 1990) Figure 1 shows how these variables foster focus on public health research versus control. Specifically, if the supply and/or mode of transmission is known, then steps that focus on source or interrupt transmission may be implemented.

Specifically, if the supply and/or mode of transmission is known, then interventions that focus on the source or disrupt the transmission could be implemented. If they don't know the transmission source and/or mode, and they can't recognize what control measures to start, then research takes precedence.

Figure 1. Relative history of research and control efforts during an outbreak based on source, mode of transmission and causative agent understanding.
"Source: Goodman RA, Buehler JW, Koplan JP. The epidemiologic field investigation: science and judgment in public health practice. Am J Epidemiol 1990;132:9–16."

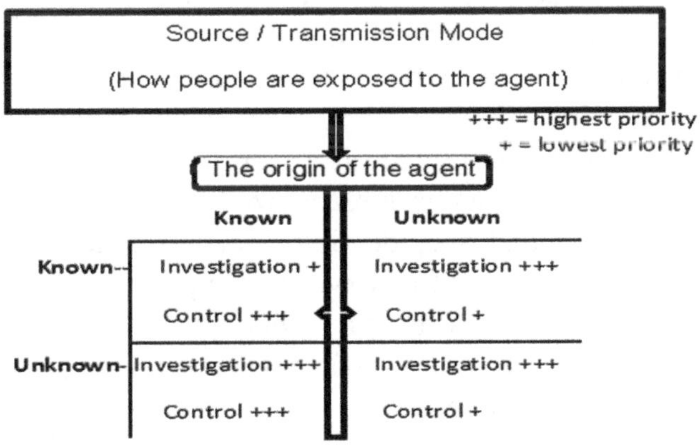

Benefit for Learning (Research Opportunity)

Another critical aim of many investigations about the outbreak is to improve studies. Health officials are not in a place to conduct randomized trials for full public health problems.

They cannot randomized who consumes the undercooked hamburger, or who sits near the ice resurfacing machine releasing carbon monoxide, nor should they randomized who profits from preventive health ("e.g. mammogram screening"). Data, they can exploit and learn from what's already gone. Some see an outbreak as a natural experiment waiting for study and exploitation. For a newly identified illness, subject analysis offers the chance of characterizing the natural records including agent, mode of transmission, and duration of incubation, and the medical disorder continuum.

In addition, researchers are seeking to find the populations at the greatest risk and to discover specific elements of chance.The discovery of such knowledge becomes a critical incentive for researchers to investigate newly identified diseases as "Legionnaires sickness in Philadelphia in 1976, AIDS in the early 1980s, hanta virus in 1993, extreme acute respiratory syndrome (SARS) in 2003, and avian flu in 2005".

Even for well-characterized diseases, by analyzing the effects of intervention approaches and the efficacy of the latest epidemiological and laboratory methods, an outbreak can also give opportunities for further learning. For example, outbreaks of "varicella (chickenpox)" in particularly immunized groups enabled researchers to assess the efficacy of the brand new vaccine and vaccination recommendations (Galil et al., 2002; Tugwell et al., 2004). The giardia outbreak providing an opportunity to look at the appropriateness of a medical case description (Hopkins & Juranek, 1991), even as a virulent Rota virus disease was used to test the effectiveness of a specific diagnostic method (Fischer et al., 2004).

In the 1990s, outbreak investigations were used for increased internet access and e-mail to decide how capacity controls would respond to e-mail requests for involvement.(Kuusi et al., 2004; Pryor et al., 2002; Raupach & Hundy, 2003)

Economic, Political or Legal Considerations

The use of force at the back of the decision to conduct a study can be economic, political, or legal issues. A cluster of most cases of cancer in a community can set up people involved to propose a research. Now and again, the public is aware that the group of diseases is the result of an environmental program involving toxic waste. Such cluster investigations almost never discover a causal link between exposure and disorder.(Caldwell, 1990; Schulte et al., 1987) Despite that many exercise departments have recognized that they must be "responsible" for public issues, although they agree that an epidemiological correlation is unlikely(Bender et al., 1990; Cartwright, 1999; Fiore et al., 1990). However, the public may also be concerned that an outbreak is the result of a deliberate criminal or Eco terrorists act. These concerns can be alleviated by the health department by reporting that the epidemic has transformed into the end result of an inadvertent or clear exposure.

There are many investigations, because they are required by law. "The National Institute for Occupational Safety and Health (NIOSH) of the CDC", such as, is required to decide health and safety hazards in the workplace if requested by a group, three or more workers or a company (Centers for Disease Control and Prevention, 2000).

Considerations of the Public Health Plan

Most health departments have programs for control and prevention of communicable diseases like influenza, hepatitis, vaccine-preventable diseases and sexually transmitted diseases. An outbreak of a disease centered on the public health system that shows a weak spot in that program and an opportunity to change or improve software efforts. Examining the reasons for the outbreak may also find overlooked populations, deficiencies in methods of action, or changes within the agent. Using the outbreak to find the efficacy of the procedure will help program managers improve future guidance and techniques.

Education Management and Prevention

Investigating an outbreak requires a combination of diplomacy, scientific analysis, problem-solving skill, technical competencies, epidemiological know-how, and judgment. Through practice and experience, these abilities are reinforced. Therefore, several research teams are matching a professional epidemiologist with an aspiring epidemiologist. The latter receives treasured education and experience on - the-activity, even as providing help in investigating and managing the outbreak.

EVOLVING CONCEPTS IN THE FIELD OF OUTBREAK INVESTIGATIONS

There has been a change in the response to acute outbreaks in India, as in many international locations. Researcher have gone from the traditional method where the outbreak cause was believed to be anything that was obviously an idea for similar outbreaks in the past (e.g. contaminated water system explains acute outbreaks of diarrhea disease) to systematic, evidence-based, entirely subject epidemiological approaches.(Murhekar et al., 2009)

Modern Approach

Traditionally, disease-specific specialists used counting instances to investigate outbreaks, look at laboratory specimens, and conduct other environmental studies as needed. In the pathogen or toxin that caused the outbreak, these investigations needed subject knowledge. They developed specific prevention measures based primarily on the diagnosis of the case or the mode of transmission defined (Figure 2)(Murhekar et al., 2009). For example, a typical scenario could be a specialist in disease prevention that would conduct an investigation into a cholera outbreak.

The measures may consist of recording the outbreaks, collecting water samples from water sources, examining the water supply, and suggesting chlorination of water sources in the absence of specific proof that the water supply had precipitated the outbreak. No defined, sequential steps or specific method have been detected on this technique.

Systematic, Field Epidemiology Methods

Current areas epidemiological approaches use quantitative data, created from an inspection of the relationship between the host, agent and climate, and analyze exposures within the outbreak instances to right comparative companies to prove primarily dependent findings (Figure.2). The latter are primarily based on epidemiological methods but usually need cooperation with other disciplines (e.g. statisticians, laboratory specialists, environmental professionals, physicians, entomologists, to name a few).(Murhekar et al., 2009)

Figure 2. Modern approaches for investigating outbreaks and field epidemiology.

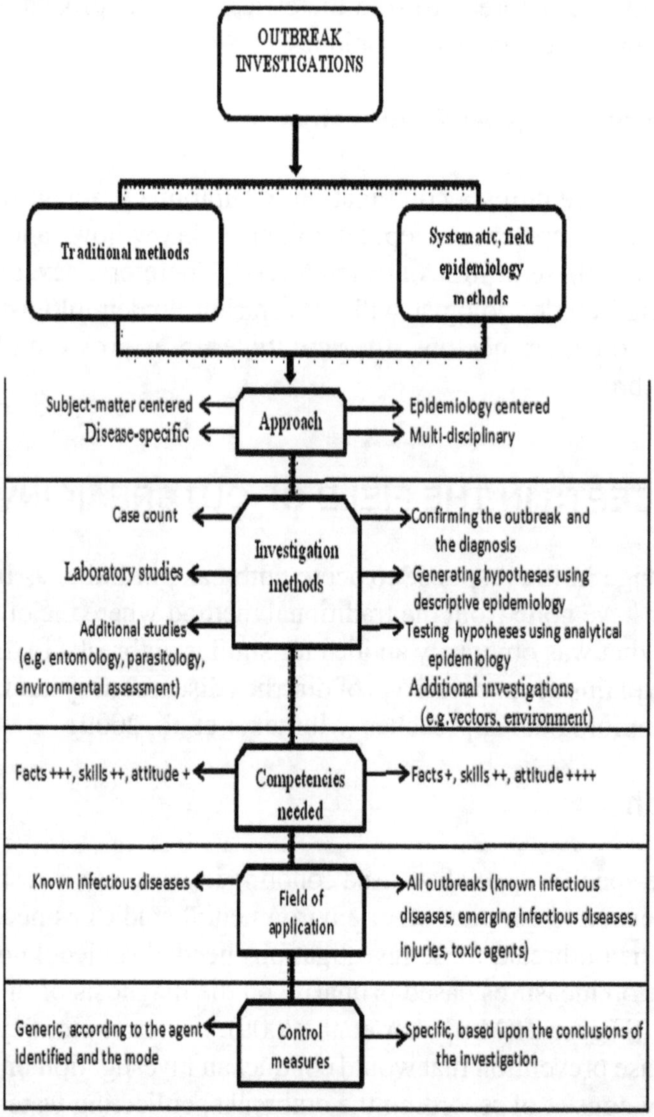

These strategies use a systematic, step-by-step technique consisting of (i) Confirmation of an outbreak and diagnosis, (ii) Hypothesis technology on the concept of descriptive epidemiology and other factors, (iii) Testing the use of analytical epidemiology techniques from those hypotheses, and (iv) Providing evidence-based control measures. Except for knowledge on challenges, the use of these methods requires skills in applied epidemiology and an open-mindedness that could extend ideally from the experience of practice. This method of outbreak research results in suggestions that could be adapted to the real situation of the discipline and based entirely on the results of a specific investigation. These strategies can be applied to any form of outbreak, regardless of the reason (infectious or non-infectious), supply, or mode of transmission.

In "Western Uttar Pradesh," a group led by local pediatricians recently proposed proof of persistent clusters of encephalopathy using surface epidemiology techniques(Vashishtha et al., 2007a; Vashishtha et al., 2007b; Vashishtha et al., 2007). A typical state of affairs is an epidemiologist who investigates a cholera outbreak, confirms diagnosis with rectal swabs, records incidents, tests instances to check for clues after whom. For example, the infection can be food-borne rather than water-borne, and thus controlled by using interventions for improving food hygiene instead of water-borne chlorination. A recent investigation into cholera in India found that the disease could be either water-borne or food-borne, and that a medical, step-by-step, epidemiological method would prefer to distinguish between the two (Das et al., 2009).

How Should Outbreaks Be Investigated?

Once a decision takes to do an acute investigation into the area of outbreaks, it is important to work quickly— as the right solution is obtained. To put it another way, epidemiologists cannot afford to do a "quick and dirty" study. They must carry out "fast and clean" research.(Palmer, 1989) In such situations, epidemiologists find it beneficial to have a systematic procedure to follow, including the choice mentioned in Figure.3. This strategy means that the research goes on without taking significant steps

Figure 3. Epidemiological methods in investigating an outbreak

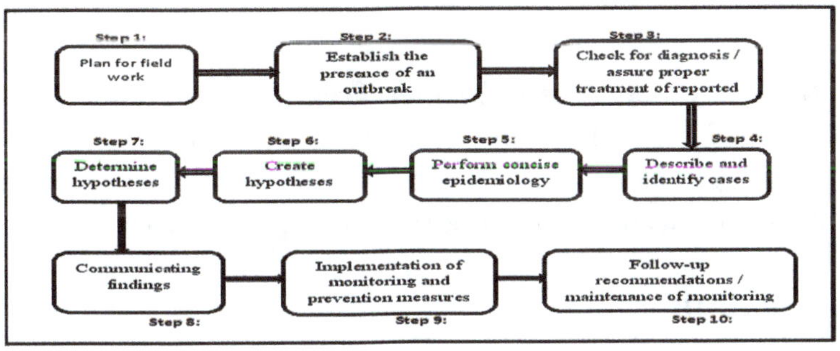

Step 1: Plan for Field Work: The numbering system for this stage is troublesome because it is not always the first step to plan for field work . Public health officials only rarely plan to do a field examination before verifying instance growth and diagnosis verification. More commonly, in the wide variety of instances of a particular disease, officers discover an increase and then decide that a field investigation is justified.

Researchers often collect enough observations to carry out detailed epidemiology without leaving their desks and end that a field study is most successful if they cannot reach a compelling conclusion without one.

They need to be well educated before making the decision to conduct a field investigation before they leave for the industry. The systems could be divided into two broad classes: (a) Science and Research issues; and (b) Management and Operation issues. Top training is required in each group for a smooth experience in the field.

Step 2: Establish the Presence of an Outbreak: An epidemic or a virus is the occurrence of other cases of disorder predicted in a given area or between a specific group of people over a specific time period.

The wide variety expected is usually the amount from the last few weeks or months or from a comparable period over the last few years and can be based primarily on national data such as statistics from outpatient health facility reports, integrated disease surveillance programs, hospital admission / discharge records, mortality statistics or local facts.

The amount of cases reported to decide the presence of an epidemic is in contrast with the number predicted for a certain place or time period.

Even if the number of cases in question exceeds the predicted wide variety, the increase will not necessarily show an epidemic. Check for the various factors that could increase the number of instances along with:

- **Seasonal Variation**: in a few diseases-diarrhea, seasonal boom may occur.
- **Notification Variant**: Due to changes in the local reporting process, changes in case definition, increased interest due to local or national recognition, case reporting may increase. Unanticipated population size shifts including resort areas, college towns and migrant farming regions.
- **Diagnostic Alternative (New Technique)**: Changes or improvements in diagnostic methods can boom cases as well.
- **Diagnostic Error (False Epidemic):** Such Clear increases that result from misdiagnosis or laboratory errors.

Step 3: Check for Diagnosis / Assure Proper Treatment of Reported Cases: Testing for diagnosis is closely related to testing for outbreak. This is crucial: (a) Ensuring that the disease is well diagnosed, on the grounds that it is often disease-specific to manipulate measures; and (b) Remove laboratory error as the basis for growth in reported cases.

Diagnostic Verification

- Researchers should first talk to medical examiners, then analyze scientific findings and laboratory results.
- When laboratory diagnosis is no longer done or there is some uncertainty in the study, team member may also get a sufficient range of proper specimens to confirm the condition in a similar way.
- Visiting one or more patients with the disease is helpful, and talking to some patients immediately can give a better understanding of the clinical function.
- Summarize the frequency distribution scientific findings (number of cases).

Step 4: Describe and Show Cases: For the identity of cases a case description is made. It's miles of a general set of standards to decide whether a person must be classified as having an interest in the health condition. A case description is through clinical conditions (signs and symptoms) and time, place, and distinct constraints. All people under investigation must carry out the guidelines.

Investigators also create specific case description categories that include confirmed, probable, and potential or suspected cases. Usually, a case has to have laboratory testing to be graded as shown. A case typically categorized as likely has normal clinical characteristics of the disease with confirmation from the laboratory. Typically, a case identified as can be done has less traditional clinical characteristics. The case definition should not include exposure or risk factor.

Step 5: Perform Concise Epidemiology (Systematically Show Cases and Record Information): Cases that cause concern in an outbreak situation are often only a few cases and do not represent the full spectrum of cases. Hence, researchers must look for other cases with the aid of public health experts to decide the real geographical measure of the issue and the populations with it.

Both cases must be remembered as reported either by using passive surveillance (patient coming directly to the hospital) or by using vivid surveillance (health worker trying to find the cases).

Line list: statistics are made in a tabular form on paper (hard copy) or on a laptop (digital model) for each person listed with a disorder at some stage of an outbreak.

A line list must be drawn up that includes the following details:

- **Figuring Data**: Name, address with, and telephone number
- **Demographic Facts**: Age, sex, ethnicity, occupation-information on character traits is required to show populations at risk.
- **Health Statistics:** Consist of signs and symptoms, date of onset of infection, more medical statistics along with length of disease and last effects of disease whether hospitalized, advanced or death occurred.
- **Information about the Risk Factor**: This information must be adapted to the particular illness concerned. Of example, since food and water are not uncommon cars of hepatitis A but not hepatitis B, exposure to sources of food and water should be identified in the former but not the latter.
- **Reporter Statistics**: The case file will consist of the report's source, usually a clinical officer, or health professional, clinic, health center, or laboratory. Sometimes the investigator needs to contact the author, either to check for more clinical details or to announce the investigation findings.

After finding out and gathering primary statistics about the people with the disease, the next step is to systematically find some of the key time, place, and person characteristics of those people. This is mentioned to as an epidemiology of classification.

Time: Traditionally, the time period of an outbreak is represented using a unique type of curve or histogram. This model is called an outbreak curve (epi curve). This provides an easy visual display of the importance and time pattern of the outbreak.

In order to draw an epidemic curve, the investigator must recognize the time for each case to start the infection. The date of onset is enough for some diseases. For various sicknesses, especially those with a relatively short incubation period (the period between exposure to an infection and the occurrence of preliminary signs), it may be more right to start an hour.

Epidemic curve provides many data about the outbreak:

- **Magnitude of the Outbreak**: The epi curve shows the size of the epidemic over the years. The shape of the epidemic curve might also give clues about the sample of spread of outbreak within the populace, e.g., point source, intermittent source or propagated outbreak.
- **Outbreak Time Developments:** The curve suggests the exceptional stage of epidemic nonetheless at the upswing, or on the down slope, or after the epidemic when it has ended. The curve might be used for assessment, answering questions like: How lengthy did it take for the health department to name a problem? Are intervention measures running?
- **Outbreak Outliers:** Cases that doesn't suit into the frame of the curve may also provide essential Clues.
- **Exposure date / Incubation Period for the Outbreak:** If the timing of the reported exposure is known, epi curves may be used to measure the incubation period of the disease, which will promote the discovery of the causative agent. Recognizing the disorder and its incubation period, the epi curve can be used to meet a possible exposure time and help increase a questionnaire centered on that term.

Location: Area-based outbreak evaluation provides information about a problem's spatial existence and identifies clusters or patterns that provide useful etiological clues. A spot map is an easy and helpful way to illustrate where live, work, or may have been discovered. Descriptive epidemiology can also provide valuable information that can be converted into hypotheses

Step 6: Create Hypotheses: In an epidemic sense, hypotheses are produced in an expansion of methods. Second, note what about the disease itself is understood: What is the normal reservoir of the agent? How is it distributed often? Normally, what vehicles are involved? What are the risk factors recognized?

Step 7: Determine Hypotheses: The next step is to decide the probability of that hypothesis following a hypothesis that could give a clarification for an outbreak. Usually, the use of a grouping of environmental data, analytical technologies, and epidemiology is inspected in a field investigation. From an epidemiological point of view, hypothesis is tested in one approach in each of two approaches: Either by contrasting the hypotheses with the installed records, or using analytical epidemiology to measure relationships and test the role of chance.

Step 8: Communicating Findings: The main goal is to summarize and effectively communicate the investigation, its findings and its final results in a report. An oral briefing for local authorities and a written report according to the same old professional style of advent, context, practices, observations, discussion and suggestions need to be sent to the authority concerned.

Step 9: Implementation of Monitoring and Prevention Measures: The number one goal of most outbreak investigations is to contain outbreaks and to prevent more incidents. Management and mitigation measures are performed as early as possible in practice.

Step 10: Follow-up Recommendations / Maintenance of Monitoring: As soon as control and preventive steps have been applied, the situation must be monitored. Effective monitoring would be continued as it is necessary for:

- Determining whether epidemic is over and for this surveillance it is possible to support for at least the incubation periods of the disease involved after initiation into the last case

- Documenting the efficacy of control measures

RELATED WORK

Google Search Trends Predicting Disease Outbreaks

One of the works in this field involves Google Search. This timely diagnosis is a pillar of infectious disease control and prevention. India's "Integrated Disease Surveillance Program" detects outbreaks, but it is not anticipating outbreaks specifically now. This research is conducted to assess the temporal link between the data of the "Google Trends and Integrated Disease Surveillance Program (IDSP)" and to find the possibility of using "Google Trends" to forecast outbreaks or epidemics.(Madhur Verma, 2018) Google search queries for "Malaria, Dengue Fever, Chikungunya and Influenza for India from January 2017 to September 2019". Using the Spearman correlation and scatter plots, the statistical link between the two datasets were represented. Time pattern plots were created to look at the relation between Google search patterns and disease detection under the "IDSP." (Madhur Verma, 2018)

"Google Search Trends"

Google is one of the most commonly used search engines, where a whole host of searches are done daily. Google's modern market share is about 97 percent of current search engines such as "Google and Yahoo"(Madhur Verma, 2018). Google responds to requests and keeps records of search queries like this. The documents are collected to mechanically show patterns. A special open get entry to the Google area can be obtained from "Google Trends.(https:/trends.google.com/trends/)"

"Google Trends" is a randomly generated series of real-time (the last 3 years) and non-real-time ("facts from January 2017 to September 2019) Google search queries." That piece of data is labeled and marked with a subject after personal information has been deleted. This record point is split over a time to measure relative awareness through total searches in a particular geographical area.

"Google Trends" refers to the search frequency output as a standardized record collection, and the resulting numbers are scaled to a number of 0 to 100 based on the theme's share of all searches on all subjects (Figure 4 to 7). Numbers are the search value on that time, and the best point in the graph of the locality. A mark of 100 is the peak popularity of a term. A 50 sense means the word is half as popular as it was at its height. Likewise, a score of 0 means that the time period at the height was as normal as it was, much less than 1 percent. They can use the information in a format CSV.

The "Google Trends" implementation excludes searches performed by very few people, frequent searches and searches connected to special characters.

Figure 4. "Google Trends website" screen shot showing the search strategy used to track the trend for dengue-related searches in India produced "from January 2017 to September 2019".
"Data source: Google Trends (https://trends.google.com/trends/explore?q=dengue&geo=IN)."

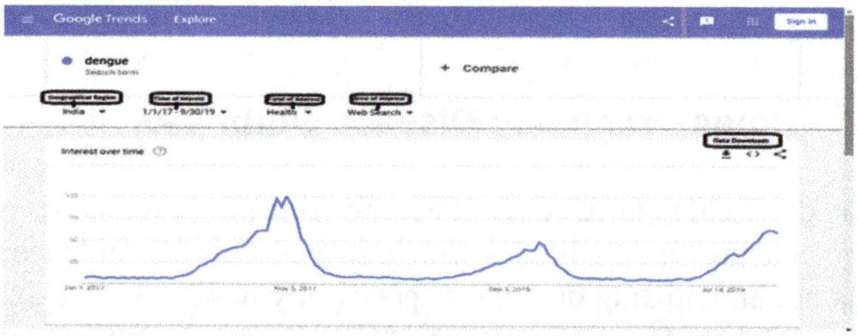

Figure 5. Screenshot of the "Google Trends website" showing the search technique used to track the "January 2017 to September 2019" pattern for chikungunya searches in India.
"Datasource: Google Trends (https://trends.google.com/trends/explore?geo=IN&q=chikungunya)".

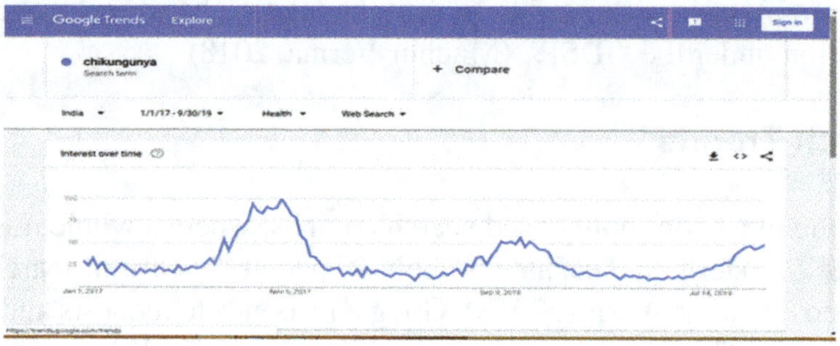

Figure 6. "Google Trends website" screen shot depicting the search strategy used to observe the pattern generated for malaria-related searches in India "from January 2017 to September2019."
"Data source: Google Trends (https://trends.google.com/trends/explore?geo=IN&q=malaria)".

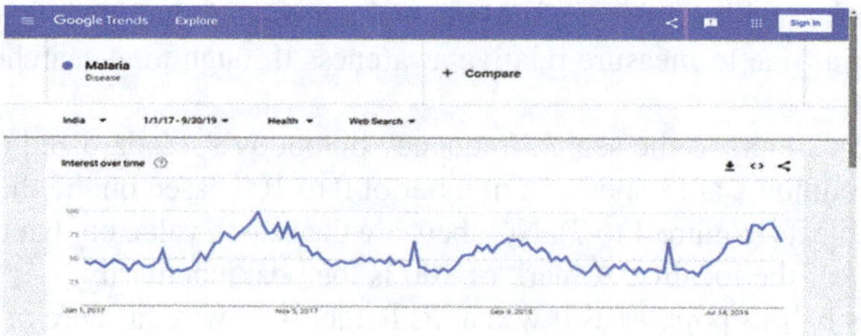

Figure 7. "Google Trends website" screen shot depicting the search strategy used to observe the trend created for influenza-related searches in India "from January 2017 to September 2019."
"Data source: Google Trends (https://trends.google.com/trends/explore?geo=IN&q=influenza)".

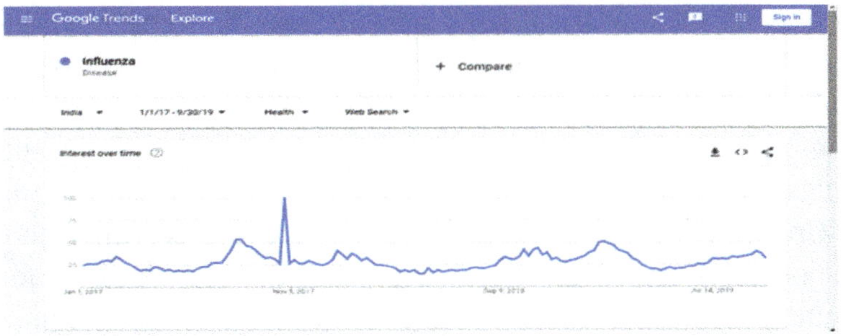

Figure 8. Describes research on infectious diseases using a country-level line map.

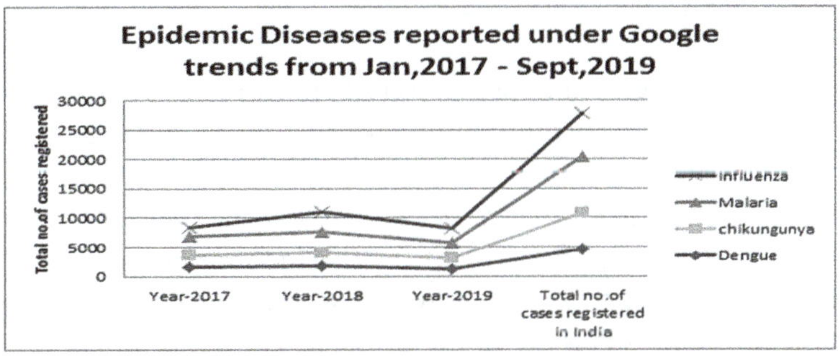

RESULTS

Table 1 shows the total number of cases identified for the four diseases under study via "Google Trends". In India, malaria was the highest number recorded, followed by influenza, chikungunya, and dengue(Madhur Verma, 2018).

Table 1.

Epidemic Diseases reported under Google trends from Jan,2017 - Sept,2019

Disease Name	Year-2017	Year-2018	Year-2019	Total no.of cases registered in India	highest percentage of cases recorded in State/UT
Dengue	1539	1706	1301	4546	Nagaland
chikungunya	2172	2274	1844	6290	Gujarat
Malaria	3219	3723	2554	9496	Arunachal Pradesh
Influenza	1525	3358	2522	7405	Sikkim

The "Google Trends" prediction system is capable of identifying disease outbreaks well in advance for the modest reliability illnesses studied (Cervellin et al., 2017). In the early stages of a disease outbreak, real disease surveillance can also alert the health departments and various stakeholders, encouraging them to trigger appropriate reaction steps, including case detection, sickness control, and accessibility of care, thus reducing the burden of disease(Ferguson et al., 2005; Longini et al., 2005).

In each communicable and non-communicable disease for developing nations, the implementation of sickness surveillance has been tried with effective reporting systems and rapid response teams. "Bragazzi(Bragazzi, 2013)" said that web-based fully monitoring system is possible to check non-suicidal self-injuries. Because of the launch of "Google Flu Trends in 2009", the latest emerging "department of digital epidemiology" has been devoted to a lot of attention and admiration(Ginsberg et al., 2009; Polgreen et al., 2008).

FUTURE RESEARCH DIRECTIONS

Future trends may also include the amalgamation of multiple sources of information to offer a much more accurate model for detecting outbreaks in a particular region, thereby helping to detect and predict future spread of the disease.

"Integrated disease surveillance program," countrywide "Center for Disease Control" under "General Directorate of Health Services, Ministry of Health and Family Welfare (MoHFW), Government of India (GOI)" imposes and monitors the surveillance of disorder in the country. By developing a decentralized state-based surveillance system (completely laboratory-based and IT-enabled) for epidemic susceptible diseases, early warning signals could be identified, so that prompt and effective public health campaigns can be implemented in response to district, regional and world-wide health challenges in the region.

"Integrated Health Information Platform (IHIP)", an internet-enabled, near-real-time digital information system, is also integrated for disease surveillance and disease outbreak management "since November 2018 in selected districts of seven states (Karnataka, Andhra Pradesh, Himachal Pradesh, Orissa, Uttar Pradesh, Telangana & Kerala)" in its first phase.

CONCLUSION

Researcher conclude that there are still active studies in this field. Further approaches and mechanisms can be built to improve the exactness of results that could theoretically be used to predict multiple disease outbreaks for better public health.(Alessa & Faezipour, 2018) Public awareness and interest in public health has grown in the last few years. In addition, health departments have made excellent strides in trying to keep the public informed. Most health departments try to talk without hesitation to the public, usually through the media, each during an investigation and at the inference of the study.

REFERENCES

Alessa, A., & Faezipour, M. (2018). A review of influenza detection and prediction through social networking sites. *Theoretical Biology & Medical Modelling*, *15*(1), 2. doi:10.118612976-017-0074-5 PMID:29386017

Bender, A. P., Williams, A. N., Johnson, R. A., & Jagger, H. G. (1990). Appropriate public health responses to clusters: The art of being responsibly responsive. *American Journal of Epidemiology*, *132*(suppl1), S48–S52. doi:10.1093/oxfordjournals.aje.a115788 PMID:2356835

Bragazzi, N. L. (2013). A Google Trends-based approach for monitoring NSSI. *Psychology Research and Behavior Management*, *7*, 1–8. doi:10.2147/PRBM.S44084 PMID:24376364

Caldwell, G. G. (1990). Twenty-two years of cancer cluster investigations at the Centers for Disease Control. *American Journal of Epidemiology*, *132*(suppl1), S43–S47. doi:10.1093/oxfordjournals.aje.a115787 PMID:2162625

Cartwright, R. A. (1999). Cluster investigations: Are they worth it? *The Medical Journal of Australia*, *171*(4), 172. doi:10.5694/j.1326-5377.1999.tb123590.x PMID:10494229

Centers for Disease Control and Prevention. (2000). *NIOSH health hazard evaluation program.* Cincinnati, OH: Department of Health and Human Services (NIOSH). *Publication No.*, *132*, 3.

Cervellin, G., Comelli, I., & Lippi, G. (2017). Is Google Trends a reliable tool for digital epidemiology? Insights from different clinical settings. *Journal of Epidemiology and Global Health*, *7*(3), 185–189. doi:10.1016/j.jegh.2017.06.001 PMID:28756828

Communicable Diseases Module: 42. Epidemic Investigation and Management. (n.d.). Retrieved from https://www.open.edu/openlearncreatc/mod/oucontent/view.php?id=128&printable=1

Das, A., Manickam, P., Hutin, Y., Pattanaik, B., Pal, B. B., Chhotray, G. P., Kar, S. K., & Gupte, M. D. (2009). Two sequential outbreaks in two villages illustrate the various modes of transmission of cholera. *Epidemiology and Infection*, *137*(6), 906–912. doi:10.1017/S0950268808001611 PMID:19171080

Davis, J. R., & Lederberg, J. (2000). *Public Health Systems and Emerging Infections: Assessing the Capabilities of the Public and Private Sectors.* National Academies Press (US).

Ferguson, N. M., Cummings, D. A., Cauchemez, S., Fraser, C., Riley, S., Meeyai, A., Iamsirithaworn, S., & Burke, D. S. (2005). Strategies for containing an emerging influenza pandemic in Southeast Asia. *Nature*, *437*(7056), 209–214. doi:10.1038/nature04017 PMID:16079797

Fiore, B. J., Hanrahan, L. P., & Anderson, H. A. (1990). State health department response to disease cluster reports: A protocol for investigation. *American Journal of Epidemiology*, *132*(suppl1), S14–S22. doi:10.1093/oxfordjournals.aje.a115776 PMID:2356826

Fischer, T. K., Gentsch, J., & Ashley, D. (2004) *Evaluation and utility of a novel diagnostic method in the investigation of an unusual outbreak of rotavirus diarrhea among children.* Presented at: *53rd Annual EIS Conference*, CDC, Atlanta, GA.

Galil, K., Lee, B., Strine, T., Carraher, C., Baughman, A. L., Eaton, M., Montero, J., & Seward, J. (2002). Outbreak of varicella at a day-care center despite vaccination. *The New England Journal of Medicine*, *347*(24), 1909–1915. doi:10.1056/NEJMoa021662 PMID:12477940

Ginsberg, J., Mohebbi, M. H., Patel, R. S., Brammer, L., Smolinski, M. S., & Brilliant, L. (2009). Detecting influenza epidemics using search engine query data. *Nature*, *457*(7232), 1012–1014. doi:10.1038/nature07634 PMID:19020500

Goodman, R. A., Buehler, J. W., & Koplan, J. P. (1990). The epidemiologic field investigation: Science and judgment in public health practice. *American Journal of Epidemiology*, *132*(1), 9–16. doi:10.1093/oxfordjournals.aje.a115647 PMID:2356818

Hopkins, R. S., & Juranek, D. D. (1991). Acute giardiasis: An improved clinical case definition for epidemiologic studies. *American Journal of Epidemiology*, *133*(4), 402–407. doi:10.1093/oxfordjournals.aje.a115894 PMID:1994703

Investigating an Outbreak: Principles of Epidemiology in Public Health Practice, An Introduction to Applied Epidemiology and Biostatistics Lesson 6. (2001). (3rd ed.). Retrieved from https://www.cdc.gov/csels/dsepd/ss1978/lesson6/section1.html

Kuusi, M., Nuorti, J. P., Maunula, L., Miettinen, I., Pesonen, H., & von Bonsdorff, C.-H. (2004). Internet use and epidemiologic investigation of gastroenteritis outbreak. *Emerging Infectious Diseases*, *10*(3), 447–450. doi:10.3201/eid1003.020607 PMID:15109411

Longini, I. M. Jr, Nizam, A., Xu, S., Ungchusak, K., Hanshaoworakul, W., & Cummings, D. A. (2005). Containing pandemic influenza at the source. *Science*, *309*(5737), 1083–1087. doi:10.1126cience.1115717 PMID:16079251

Madhur Verma, M. D. (2018). Google Search Trends Predicting Disease Outbreaks: An Analysis from India. *Healthcare Informatics Research*, *24*(4), 300–308. doi:10.4258/hir.2018.24.4.300 PMID:30443418

Murhekar, M., Moolenaar, R., Hutin, Y., & Broome, C. (2009). Investigating outbreaks: Practical guidance in the Indian scenario. *The National Medical Journal of India*, *22*(5). PMID:20334049

Outbreak Investigation: National Health Portal of India. (n.d.). Retrieved from https://www.nhp.gov.in/outbreak-investigation_pg

Palmer, S. R. (1989). Epidemiology in search of infectious diseases: Methods in outbreak investigation. *Journal of Epidemiology and Community Health*, *43*(4), 311–314. doi:10.1136/jech.43.4.311 PMID:2693574

Polgreen, P. M., Chen, Y., Pennock, D. M., & Nelson, F. D. (2008). Using internet searches for influenza surveillance. *Clinical Infectious Diseases*, *47*(11), 1443–1448. doi:10.1086/593098 PMID:18954267

Pryor, J. H., Martin, M. T., Whitney, C. G., Turco, J. H., Baumgartner, Y. Y., & Zegans, M. E. (2002). Rapid response to a conjunctivitis outbreak: The use of technology to leverage information. *Journal of American College Health, 50*(6), 267–271. doi:10.1080/07448480209603444 PMID:12701651

Raupach, J. C., & Hundy, R. L. (2003). An outbreak of Campylobacter jejune infection among conference delegates. *Communicable Diseases Intelligence, 27*, 380–383. PMID:14510066

Schulte, P. A., Ehrenberg, R. L., & Singal, M. (1987). Investigation of occupational cancer clusters: Theory and practice. *American Journal of Public Health, 77*(1), 52–56. doi:10.2105/AJPH.77.1.52 PMID:3789238

Tugwell, B. D., Lee, L. E., Gillette, H., Lorber, E. M., Hedberg, K., & Cieslak, P. R. (2004). Chickenpox outbreak in a highly vaccinated school population. *Pediatrics, 113*(3), 455–459. doi:10.1542/peds.113.3.455 PMID:14993534

Vashishtha, V. M., Kumar, A., John, T. J., & Nayak, N. C. (2007a). Cassia occidentalis poisoning as the probable cause of hepatomyoencephalopathy in children in western Uttar Pradesh. *The Indian Journal of Medical Research, 125*, 756–762. PMID:17704552

Vashishtha, V. M., Kumar, A., John, T. J., & Nayak, N. C. (2007b). Cassia occidentalis poisoning causes fatal coma in children in western Uttar Pradesh. *Indian Pediatrics, 44*, 522–525. PMID:17684305

Vashishtha, V. M., Nayak, N. C., John, T. J., & Kumar, A. (2007). Recurrent annual outbreaks of a hepato-myoencephalopathy syndrome in children in western Uttar Pradesh, India. *The Indian Journal of Medical Research, 125*, 523–533. PMID:17598938

KEY TERMS AND DEFINITIONS

Case Definition: It is a set of common criteria for classifying a person with a specific illness, disease, or other health condition.

Endemic: It is the infectious disease present in a certain geographic region, or in a certain race of people.

Epidemic Curve: It is a vertical column bar chart showing the number of new cases of a specific disease that arise over a period of time.

Epidemiology: It is the approach used to classify the causes of illnesses and health outcomes in populations. The patient is the group of epidemiology, and is treated collectively by individuals.

Outbreak: It is exactly the same as an epidemic, i.e., an elevated incidence of a disease in a given population or geographic area above the normal (endemic rate).

Outbreak Investigation: It is a series of techniques used to determine the cause of the disease, the people affected, the circumstances and manner of disease transmission and other relevant factors involved in epidemic propagation.

Pandemic: It refers to epidemics that occur in multiple locations around the globe at the same time.

Section 2

Coronavirus Disease (COVID-19)

Chapter 2
The Study of the Epidemiology and Clinical Features of the Novel Coronavirus (COVID-19)

Ranjit Barua
https://orcid.org/0000-0003-2236-3876
Indian Institute of Engineering Science and Technology, Shibpur, India

Sudipto Datta
Indian Institute of Engineering Science and Technology, Shibpur, India

Amit Roychowdhury
Indian Institute of Engineering Science and Technology, Shibpur, India

Pallab Datta
Indian Institute of Engineering Science and Technology, Shibpur, India

ABSTRACT

Epidemiology is the technique used to detect the origins of health outcomes and diseases in inhabitants. In epidemiology, the patient, the individual, and community are viewed mutually. Epidemiology is not only the analysis of health in inhabitants; it also includes applying the information enlarged by the analysis of public-based practice. In case of medicine, the practice of epidemiology is both an art and science. Currently, COVID-19 has spread all around the world. It is basically a severe acute respiratory syndrome coronavirus-2 (SARS-CoV-2). Through the binding of receptor in gene region of its spike protein, ACE2 is bounded by corona virus. In this chapter, the authors summarized the epidemiological characteristics, clinical features, diagnosis, and treatment prognosis of COVID-19. A complete consideration will help to control the disease.

DOI: 10.4018/978-1-7998-4414-3.ch002

INTRODUCTION

By the late of 2019 a novel virus started spreading in Wuhan city of China from a Seafood market. This virus spread very fast from Wuhan to worldwide within a couple of months (Huang et al; 2020). Very soon it is identified that the virus belongs to a family of virus known as coronavirus like SARS and MERS having spikes on the outer surface of the spherical virus. That spikes acts like a key for specific human lung cells, by lock and key mechanism the virus attaches with the human lung cells and infects the host. This new novel coronavirus was named as SARS-CoV-2 as it is very much similar to SARS-CoV because the new coronavirus also causes severe acute respiratory syndrome and due to high homology i.e. 80% like that of SARS-CoV of 2003 (Zhou et al; 2020). Earlier the novel coronavirus was thought to have been transmitted from seafood animals like zoonotic mode of transmission but this assumption was proved wrong as afterwards it was found out that human transmission also played a important role for the following situation (Lu et al; 2020). WHO i.e. World Health Organization initially named the novel coronavirus as 2019-nCoV on January 12th 2020. Later WHO changed the name to 2019 coronavirus i.e. COVID-19. Meanwhile CSG (Coronavirus Study Group) of the international committee proposed to change the name from COVID-19 to as SARS-CoV-2 from Feb 11th 2020. The researchers of China on 7th January 2020 identified a SARS-CoV-2 virus from an infected patient and studied done the genomic sequencing (Zhou et al; 2020) soon WHO declared the new virus outbreak as a pandemic. SARS-CoV-2 infected approximately 200 countries worldwide (Riou et al; 2020) (WHO, 2020).

EPIDEMIOLOGY OF SARS-CoV-2

The novel coronavirus of unknown type was first spread from the seafood market of Wuhan, China from 12th Dec 2019. Many studies showed that bats can be the main source of this novel coronavirus transmission to the human population (Giovanetti et al; 2020) (Paraskevis et al; 2020). There is lack of evidence to prove that the SAR-CoV-2 spread from the seafood marked presented at Wuhan, China. Which in turn points towards the bats because earlier bats were found out to be a virus carrier of both SARS-CoV and MERS-CoV (Hampton et al; 2005) (Banerjee et al; 2019) (Li et al; 2005). After the genomic sequencing of the virus was done it was found out that genomic sequence identity matched with the Bat CoV RaTG13 with a similarity of 96.2% (Zhou et al; 2020) which showed the scientists that SARS-CoV-2 and Bat CoV RaTG13 originated from the same ancestor but bats are not sold in the seafood market of the Wuhan, China (Wu et al; 2020). COVID-19 has spread worldwide. As per the data till April 2020, COVID-19 has highest number of patients in US followed by Spain, Italy, Germany, France and China, whereas Italy was more significantly affected by COVID-19. Maximum fatality cases were reported in elderly patients. At that time, the fatality rate of Italy was 7.2% (G. Onder et al; 2020) (Livingston et al; 2020). Also the fatality rate in Italy was mainly affected by the patients aged 70 years or more. The fatality rate of Italy was described with the help of demographic features .The data from US and other countries is obtained in the number of resources (Zheng et al; 2020) (Dong et al; 2020). Till the date 28th September, 2020, there are 33,034,598 confirmed cases of COVID-19, including 996,342 deaths (Figure. 1) (WHO; 3:52pm CEST, 28 September 2020).

Figure 1. COVID-19 confirmed cases referred by WHO
(Data last updated: 2020/09/28, 3:52 pm CEST)

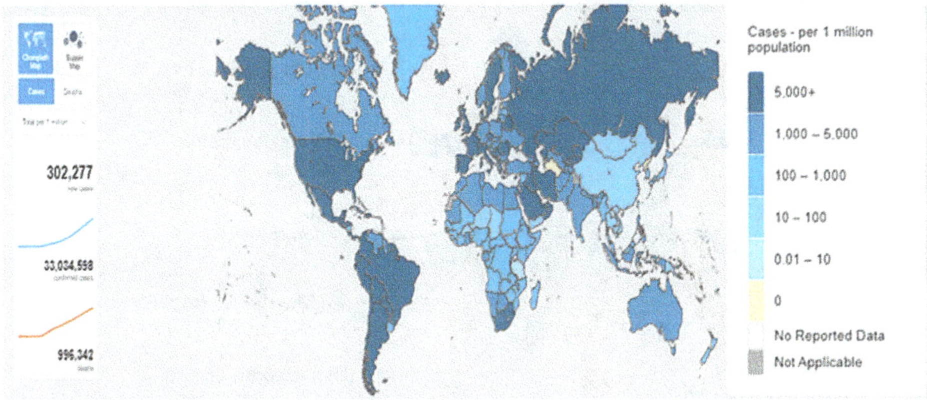

Globally, as of 3:52pm CEST, 28 September 2020, there have been 33,034,598 confirmed cases of COVID-19, including 996,342 deaths, reported to WHO.

SARS-CoV-2: GENOME CHARACTERISTICS

Beta-coronavirus Strains i.e. SARS-CoV, MERS-CoV and SARS-CoV-2 all three causes severe respiratory distress (Zumla et al; 2020). In the current history various outbreaks have happened which are connected to this Beta coronaviruses strains. In Figure 2 structures and genomes SERS-CoV2 is shown. COVID-19 was isolated from a pneumonia patient who worked as the seafood marked of Wuhan, it was found that one stain of SAS-CoV-2 size was 29.9 kb (Wu et al; 2020) the whole genome of Wuhan-Hu-1 coronavirus i.e. WHCV. MARS-CoV and SARS-CoV both have RNA genome of 30.1 kb and 27.9 kb respectively (de Wit et al; 2020). Earlier it is shown that the CoV genome is variable ranging from 6-11 of ORFs i.e. open reading frame (Song et al; 2020). The virus RNA's two-third is mainly presented in the 1st ORF i.e. ORF1 a/b which decodes into two pp1a, pp1ab and polyproteins and encodes into non-structural proteins total 16 (NSP), the rest ORFs are encodes into structural proteins and accessory. The virus genome remaining part encodes into 4 necessary structural proteins like small envelop protein (E), nucleocapsid protein (N), spike glycoprotein (S) and small matrix protein (M) (Cui et al; 2019) and other various kinds of proteins which interact with the host innate immune response. Wu et al. currently executed deep meta-transcriptomic WHCV sequencing that consist of total 16 expected NSP. WHCV showed some phylogenetic and genomic resemblance to SARS-CoV, mainly in receptor-binding domain i.e. RBD and S-glycoprotein gene, showed the ability of direct transmission to humans. Comparing with MERS-CoV and SARS-CoV the novel SARS-CoV-2 has similar genomic sequence like that of bat CoVs along with containing few differences. In the protein level no amino acid substitution is present in NSP13, NSP7 matrix, envelop on in the accessory proteins 8b and p6, only change NSP3, NSP2, underpinning subdomain i.e. RBD and spike protein (Wu A et al; 2020).

Figure 2. SARS-CoV-2 genome structure

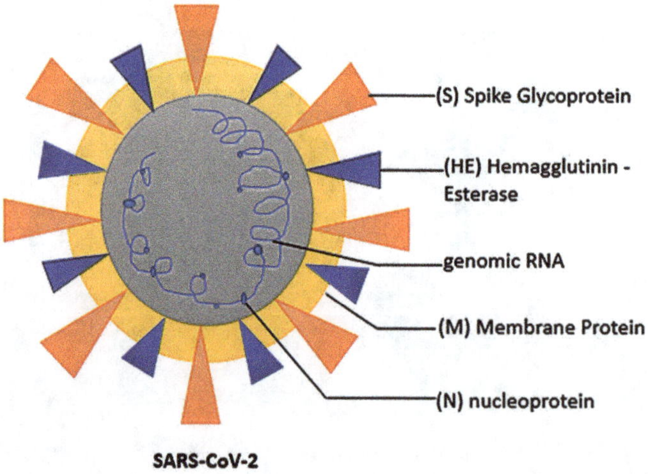

TRANSMISSION OF SARS-CoV-2 (COVID-19)

COVID-19 spreads rapidly (WHO; 5th March; 2020), it is transmitted through droplets and close interaction. Also, the disease is reported to be airborne transfer (Livingston et al; 2020). In the airborne cases very less to no RNA concentration is reported (Zheng et al; 2020). In positive cases, no RNA is identified in serum or urine samples (Dong et al; 2020). Viral RNA can be spotted on fomites as well as plastic (Zumla et al; 2020). On an average, the incubation period is reported to be 3 to 9 days (Guan et al; 2020), within a range between 0 to 24 days (Li et al; 2020). The mean consecutive interval is reported to be 3 to 8 days, which reports to be the end of incubation (Wang et al; 2020). This reports that one can be asymptomatic but infected (Zheng et al; 2020). Before the symptoms are noticed, 44% of transmission is expected to take place already. (Wang et al; 2020). It is risky to come in contact with an infected person as it can affect the life of a non-infected person. Although, the probability getting infected is still not confirm. Burke et al. examined 445 people who came in contact (at least 6 feet from the source for a minimum of 10 min) with 10 COVID-19 positive cases. Only two cases were reported to be positive after the two weeks of testing. Both the patients were household members who were kept isolated from the infected persons. Five cases came in contact with the infected patients but were never reported positive. Even the health workers are reported to be negative (Poutanen et al; 2003). The two other researches are reported to be almost same (Zheng et al; 2020). All positive cases from mainland China estimated that 3.8% are the healthcare workers (1716/44672) (Jin et al; 2020).There are 18% asymptomatic cases (Bosch et al; 2003) (Lee et al; 2003) (Assiri et al; 2013). Most researches prove that disease can get transmitted from asymptomatic patient (Wang et al; 2016) (Huang et al; 2020). Irrespective of lab and CT scan report, they can be infectious as well as asymptomatic (Zumla et al; 2020). Due to the immunity resistance, younger ones are mostly asymptomatic, while the elder are symptomatic (Zheng et al; 2020). It is estimated that 86% of positive cases have no documentation, and among them 55% of cases were infectious (Li et al; 2020). It is mainly due to the contagious time before the arrival of symptoms, the rate of asymptomatic cases that are not documented which is tested by RT-PCR (Agostini et al; 2018). After 10 days, symptoms are visible (Savarino et al; 2003). Although after the disappearance of symptoms, viral shedding continues (Vincent et al; 2005). Viral shedding of COVID-19 RNA continues for 19 days (via feces) or 18 days (by nasopharyngeal swab) (Zheng et al; 2020). Minor and asymptomatic cases incline to shed in 10 days (between 8–15 days) after the symptom determination (Huang et al; 2020), with 90% of cases curing after 10 days and almost all the cases are curing after 15 days (Wu et al; 2020). In case of severely infected patients, primary symptom arises which takes 25 days to shed. In severely infected cases, the viral load is 60% more than in the mild ones (Arabi et al; 2020). Although the probability of severe infected cases is still not discovered.

CLINICAL FEATURES OF COVID-19

SARS-CoV-2 is extremely transmittable in elder humans and peoples having other diseases with low immunity. The average transmittable age is between 47-60 years among these 41.5 to 45.7% were women (Guan et al; 2020). Like it is mentioned everywhere that SARS-CoV-2 patients showed many similar symptoms like dry cough, malaise and fever (Wang et al; 2020). Many patients like children and adults showed mild flu-like symptoms few of them went to critical condition having symptoms like acute respiratory distress symptoms, multi organ failure, death and severe pneumonia (Poutanen et al; 2003). Transmission of the virus through various routes are studied by Zheng et al. (Zheng et al; 2020) by performing swab tests and blood tests. In the basis of various studies and epidemiological study it is found out that the incubation period of the SARS-CoV-2 is 1-14 days mainly 3-7 days. The in the latency stage the virus is transmittable and contagious (Jin et al; 2020). The host-virus interaction stages are as follows a) attachment, b) penetration, c) biosynthesis, d) maturation and e) release. First the virus attaches with the host cell i.e. attachment then the virus genetic material enters the host cell by membrane fusion or endocytosis i.e. penetration. As soon as the genetic material of the virus i.e. the RNA enters the host cell it further inters the nucleus of the cell and instructs the cell to replicate many virus copies this stage is known as biosynthesis i.e. mRNA is utilized for making of the viral protein. After that maturation of the new viruses occurs in the cell and finally gets released from the host cell by destroying it. The cycle is then repeated when ultimately the high viral load is reached. At this point the virus antibodies are detected in the blood. SARS-CoV-2 contains four structural proteins (Bosch et al; 2007), which are as follows a) envelop (E), b) Membrane (M), c) nucleocapsid (N) and d) Spike (S). The most common symptoms as reported from many patients are dry cough and fever, gastrointestinal and upper respiratory symptoms are very rare symptoms for the critical cases which shows that the symptoms are non-specific and depends on person to person i.e. viral tropism is different when compared with MERS-CoV (Lee et al; 2020), influenza and SARS-CoV. Prof. Nan-Shan Zhong along with his team members performed 1099 confirmed lab cases sampling. They found out that the percentage of symptoms found mostly among 1099 cases were fever having percentage 88.7 which is the most common and vomiting having percentage 5.0 less common among the other symptoms. The other symptoms are a) cough 67.8% b) sputum production 33.4%, c) fatigue 38.1%, d) headache 13.6%, e) sore throat

13.9% (Guan et al; 2019) and shortness of breath 18.6%. Elderly and underlying disorders patients like cardiovascular disease, chronic pulmonary disease, hypertension and diabetes showed various severe symptoms like multi-organ failure, acute respiratory distress syndrome, coagulation dysfunction, septic shock, metabolic acidosis difficult of correct and death (Huang et al; 2020).

DIAGNOSIS OF COVID-19

COVID-19 detection is done by various process like clinical manifestation, epidemiological history and few auxiliary examinations like CT scan, detection of nucleic acid, blood culture, immune identification technology (point-of-care Testing of POCT of the IgM and IgG and ELISA (Enzyme linked immune sorbent assay). The symptoms of COVID-19 are atypical which includes fever, cough, respiratory symptoms, dyspnea as well as viral pneumonia. For this reason, auxiliary detection is mandatory the detection of COVID-19, like the epidemiological history.

Nucleic Acid Identification Process

The most common nucleic acid identification technologies for SARS-COV-2 are high-throughput sequencing and real-time quantitative polymerase chain reaction (RT-qPCR), which is shown in Figure 3. The high-throughput sequencing technology and the virus blood culture are the most commanding method of identification of SARS-CoV-2 (Xu et al; 2020). Because of high cost and dependency of equipment the uses of high-throughput sequencing technology is the clinic is less. Because of these reasons RT-qPCR is most effective, straightforward and most common procedure for the pathogenic virus detection in blood from respiratory secretion (Lim et al; 2020). Soon after the COVID-19 spread in China various countries started using RT-qPCR for testing in the clinic. The use of probes in the ORF1ab and N gene and specific primers in the SARS-CoV-2 region detection was done by using RT-qPCR. Lab-confirmed infection was defined in the patient when both the targets comes out positive. Two different portions of the virus genome i.e. N and ORF1b was described by two 1-step assays of RT-qPCR i.e. TaqMan-based fluorescence signal was reported by Chu. et al. (Chu et al; 2004). The negative ones are confirmed by negative control of the samples and the positive ones are confirmed by the SARS-CoV-2 samples collected i.e. respiratory specimen from the infected person by using this process. From one of the study there is reported that saliva can be used for detection of SARS-CoV-2 about 91.2% (11/12) positive rate in the individuals by running RT-qPCR i.e. non-probes SYBR based fluorescence signal, test on the saliva of the infected persons this provides a noninvasive diagnosis of SARS-CoV-2. Thus saliva proves to be a promising specimen for detecting, infection control and monitoring of individuals infected with SARS-CoV-2 (Tian et al; 2020). High specificity and sensitivity was shown by RT-qPCR for MARS-CoV-2 as well as SARS-CoV-2 (Letko et al; 2020). Five individuals showed negative RT-qPCR but showed CT result on chest positive and after repeated swap testing by RT-qPCR the individuals were tested positive for SARS-CoV-2 (Wenham et al; 2020). SARS-CoV-2 sensitivity of detection is within a range of 50 to 80% which mainly depends various factors like testing protocol type, clinical specimen number etc (Walls et al; 2020). So, the improvement of the RT-qPCR for

SARS-CoV-2 infection needs to be done. Other disadvantages of the RT-qPCR are long time for results, burdensome nucleic acid detection, biological safety hazard brought by operation of patient samples and retention.

Figure 3. RT-PCR testing for COVID-19

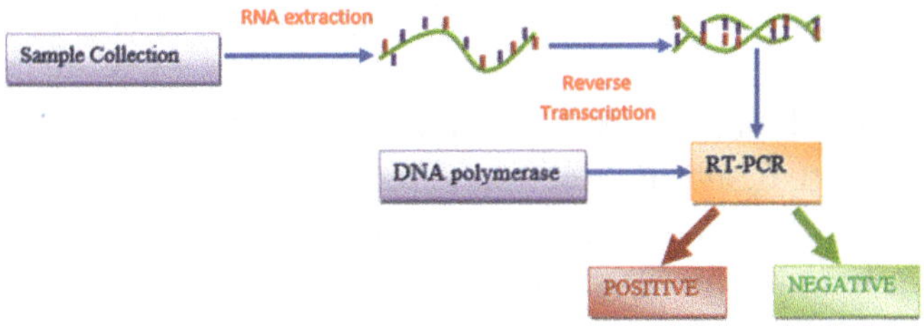

Ct Scans and Various Other Analytical Methods

Because of unavailability of COVID-19 antibody detection kit RT-qPCR is the main diagnosis method for the identification of SERS-CoV-2 but ignoring the false negative rate can be dangerous for both the patient as well as to the others because of high infection rate so to overcome the minimal false negative some clinic started using CT scans along with RT-qPCR because of it high sensitivity. Individuals whose RT-qPCR comes out negative should go through CT scan which minimizes the false negative chance. High resolution CT scan in short HRCT should be done on the individuals on the chest of early diagnosis of the COVID-19 infection (Huang et al; 2020). Various studies have studies deeply the CT scan results of the chest of the infected individuals (Lim et al; 2020). Classical CT images of the infected individual chest showed consolidative pulmonary opacities and bilateral pulmonary parenchymal ground-glass, few times with a peripheral lung distribution and a rounded morphology. Peripheral predominance in the Lung as also been seen individuals of MERS-CoV and SARS-CoV infections in the lungs and the results if the CT showed appearance of ground-glass opacities like the one in SARS-CoV-2 infection in the lungs (Tian et al; 2020). Because of the earlier findings of these things in lungs for the case of both SARS-CoV and MERS-CoV, CT scan found its place in the auxiliary diagnosis method of SARS-COV-2 highly in the high COVID-19 infection areas. Inspire having various advantages of the CT scan, drawbacks are also there for this diagnosis method they are they cannot distinguish the pneumonia in the lungs are from the COVID-19 or from any other infections and CT image abnormal hysteresis. As stated the drawbacks of the two detection method of the COVID-19 infection labs should immediately use some antigen antibody detection kit which detects specific virus antigen of antibody in the sample collected as the sensitivity of these diagnosis method is very high so the chances of false-negative are very rare. Presently ELISA kits for SARS-CoV-2 and POCT of IgM/IgG is made and is tested by various companies and showed much higher rate of detection compared to the other detection methods unfortunately still there is no published article and product available in the market. The SARS-CoV N-based IgG ELISA sensitivity is much higher near about 94.7% than that of S-Based ELISA os SAR-CoV which is nearly 58.9% (Lim et al; 2020), still the IgG/IgM SARS-CoV-2 sensitivity needs to be studied. So, inventing other specific and sensitive auxiliary process of COVID-19 detection is urgently needed.

TREATMENT OF COVID-19

There is no specific antiviral drug available for SARS-CoV-2 presently just like MERS-CoV and SERS-CoV infection (Zheng et al; 2020). The current treatment includes conservative fluid management, oxygen therapy, uses of wide range of antibiotics for killing the secondary bacterial infections related to the viral infection (Tian et al; 2020). On the based on the research done on the genomic organization of SARS-CoV-2 and research on molecular mechanisms of coronavirus infection (Huang et al; 2020) there are various possible targets of therapeutics for existing drug repurposing or inventing an effective mediation against the COVID-19.

Identify the Virally Targeted Inhibitors

An antiviral drug popularly known as Remdesivir which targets the RNA polymerase and inhibits the viral production of RNA, because of this this drug showed to be effective against huge range of viruses having RNA which includes MERS and SERS-CoVs cultured in culture cell and in mice and also in models of nonhuman primates (Jin et al; 2020). The administration of the antiviral drug remdesivir intravenously was done first by the Washington Department of Health which was found to be highly effective for SARS-CoV-2 inhibition in vitro (Zheng et al; 2020). So, other various nucleoside analogues like galidesivir, favipiravir and ribavirin (Zheng et al; 2020) can also be applicable clinically against the SARS-CoV-2 infected individuals. Non-structural proteins like papain-like protease (PLP) and Chymotrypsin-like (3C-like protease, 3CLpro) inhibits the replication of the coronavirus and also inhibits the innate host immune response (Xu et al; 2020). Because of these 3CLpro inhibitors like flavonoids and cinanserin as well as PLP inhibitors like diarylheptanoids, are also good choices for the treatment of COVID-19 infected individuals. ACE2 arbitrates SARS-CoV-2 entrance in the host cell as a functional receptor of SARS-CoV-2. So by stopping the binding of ACE2 with the S protein is a helpful approach for stopping the COVID-19 infection (Xu et al; 2020).

Antibody and Plasma Therapy

Just like in the cases of MERS-CoV and SERS-CoV trials the recovered individuals of from the COVID-19 started donating plasma as reported in various studies. Initially, it acquired good results both in the case of severe and acute SARS-CoV-2 individuals. This method the generation of recombinant human monoclonal antibody (mAb)is honestly not the final solution to fight against the novel virus. The development for the potential candidate therapeutics of the COVID-19 infection, can be done by binding receptor-binding domain (RBD) of SARS-CoV-2 with CR3022, a SARS coronavirus-specific human monoclonal antibody (Zheng et al; 2020). Other neutralization of monoclonal antibodies SARS-CoV like CR3014, m396 can be a different treatment method of COVID-19 patients (Xu et al; 2020). Vaccines against the SARS-CoV-2 which should be effective are needed for viral shedding, transmission and for reducing disease severity for stopping the outbreak. Various strategies of vaccination against MERS and SERS-CoV are tested in various animals, like subunit vaccine, protein vaccine, recombinant DNA, viral vectors, live-attenuated virus etc (Zhang et al; 2020). Studies are in development but for a vaccine to develop the time needed for it to pass all tests takes many months to many years. Presently there can be many targets for COVID-19 but still more lab and clinical studies needs to be done. Chinese scientists working with WHO for launching up to 80 trials for clinical testing for probable treatment for SARS-CoV-2. A homoeopathic medicine Arsenic Album 30 taken 1 time for 3 days and repeated after one month have be suggested by many homoeopathic doctors for preventive as well as curative against the novel virus. Many traditional Chinese medicines showed to be effective as a supportive treatment for the virus. Many drugs like stem cell and were HIV drugs showed in the clinical trials.

FUTURE WORK

Till date, no antivirus vaccine or others specific treatment for COVID-19 is not available. So, it has become a world emergency situation where there is need of antivirus vaccine or any other treatment for COVID-19 disease. The current status to prevent the COVID-19, is to build a strong immunization within the individuals; basically it comes with maintaining the biological clock, good healthy food, drink and cleanliness. Presently the future technologies processes like modern drug research and development, IOT (Internet of things), AI (Artificial Intelligent) has an imminent characteristics in the improvement of epidemiological research and analysis. With the joined applications and effort of a efficient methodology, Covid-19 will endure much lesser than the largeness of the world and the forthcoming capability of human beings to face this type of epidemic. The main issues of this epidemic are to reduce spread of this virus and to make the antivirus vaccine.

CONCLUSION

SARS-CoV-2 is main responsible for the pandemic of COVID-19. It is imagined to be belong from bat Coronavirus and is also one of the seven human transmissible disease. The first human case of corona virus was noticed at Wuhan, China, December of 2019. Those who have corona test positive are diagnosed as COVID-19 patients. The present COVID-19 disease is obviously a worldwide problem of public health concern. There have been quick progresses in what we identify about the corona virus pathogen, clinical features of disease and also identify the causes of infection. To develop the disease regulatory system for future, it is essential to create complete public health laws and guidelines, and make a disease control system in line with the countrywide conditions, so as to it can perform when it will required and active role in any upcoming infectious disease epidemic.

ACKNOWLEDGMENT

The authors acknowledge the Centre for Healthcare Science and Technology, Heaton Hall, IIEST-Shibpur, India.

REFERENCES

Huang, C., Wang, Y., Li, X., Ren, L., Zhao, J., Hu, Y., Zhang, L., Fan, G., Xu, J., Gu, X., Cheng, Z., Yu, T., Xia, J., Wei, Y., Wu, W., Xie, X., Yin, W., Li, H., Liu, M., ... Cao, B. (2020). Clinical features of patients infected with 2019 novel coronavirus in Wuhan, China. *Lancet*, *395*(10223), 497–506. doi:10.1016/S0140-6736(20)30183-5 PMID:31986264

Zhou, P., Yang, X. L., Wang, X. G., Hu, B., Zhang, L., Zhang, W., Si, H.-R., Zhu, Y., Li, B., Huang, C.-L., Chen, H.-D., Chen, J., Luo, Y., Guo, H., Jiang, R.-D., Liu, M.-Q., Chen, Y., Shen, X.-R., Wang, X., ... Shi, Z.-L. (2020). A pneumonia outbreak associated with a new coronavirus of probable bat origin. *Nature*, *588*(7836), E6. Advance online publication. doi:10.103841586-020-2951-z PMID:32015507

Lu, R., Zhao, X., Li, J., Niu, P., Yang, B., Wu, H., Wang, W., Song, H., Huang, B., Zhu, N., Bi, Y., Ma, X., Zhan, F., Wang, L., Hu, T., Zhou, H., Hu, Z., Zhou, W., Zhao, L., ... Tan, W. (2020). Genomic characterisation and epidemiology of 2019 novel coronavirus: Implications for virus origins and receptor binding. *Lancet*, *395*(10224), 565–574. doi:10.1016/S0140-6736(20)30251-8 PMID:32007145

Riou, J., & Althaus, C. L. (2020). Pattern of early human-to-human transmission of Wuhan 2019 novel coronavirus (2019-nCoV), December 2019 to January 2020. *Eurosurveillance*, *25*(4), 2000058. doi:10.2807/1560-7917.ES.2020.25.4.2000058 PMID:32019669

WHO. (2020). *Coronavirus disease (COVID-2019) situation reports*. https:// www.who.int/emergencies/diseases/novel-coronavirus-2019/situationreports

Giovanetti, M., Benvenuto, D., Angeletti, S., & Ciccozzi, M. (2020). The first two cases of 2019-nCoV in Italy: Where they come from? *Journal of Medical Virology*, *1–4*(5), 518–521. Advance online publication. doi:10.1002/jmv.25699 PMID:32022275

Paraskevis, D., Kostaki, E. G., Magiorkinis, G., Panayiotakopoulos, G., Sourvinos, G., & Tsiodras, S. (2020). Full-genome evolutionary analysis of the novel corona virus (2019-nCoV) rejects the hypothesis of emergence as a result of a recent recombination event. *Infection, Genetics and Evolution*, *79*, 104212. doi:10.1016/j.meegid.2020.104212 PMID:32004758

Hampton, T. (2005). Bats may be SARS reservoir. *Journal of the American Medical Association*, *294*(18), 2291. doi:10.1001/jama.294.18.2291 PMID:16278351

Banerjee, A., Kulcsar, K., Misra, V., Frieman, M., & Mossman, K. (2019). Bats and coronaviruses. *Viruses*, *11*(1), E41. doi:10.3390/v11010041 PMID:30634396

Li, W., Shi, Z., Yu, M., Ren, W., Smith, C., & Epstein, J. H. (2005). Bats are natural reservoirs of SARS-like coronaviruses. *Science, 310*(5748), 676–679. doi:10.1126cience.1118391 PMID:16195424

Wu, F., Zhao, S., Yu, B., Chen, Y. M., Wang, W., Song, Z. G., Hu, Y., Tao, Z.-W., Tian, J.-H., Pei, Y.-Y., Yuan, M.-L., Zhang, Y.-L., Dai, F.-H., Liu, Y., Wang, Q.-M., Zheng, J.-J., Xu, L., Holmes, E. C., & Zhang, Y.-Z. (2020). A new coronavirus associated with human respiratory disease in China. *Nature, 579*(7798), 265–269. Advance online publication. doi:10.103841586-020-2008-3 PMID:32015508

Onder, G., Rezza, G., & Brusaferro, S. (2020). Case-fatality rate and characteristics of patients dying in relation to COVID-19 in Italy. *Journal of the American Medical Association*. Advance online publication. doi:10.1001/jama.2020.4683 PMID:32203977

Livingston, E., & Bucher, K. (2020). *Coronavirus disease 2019 (COVID-19) in Italy*. Journal., doi:10.1001/jama.2020.4344

Zheng, M., Gao, Y., Wang, G., Song, G., Liu, S., Sun, D., Xu, Y., & Tian, Z. (2020). Functional exhaustion of antiviral lymphocytes in COVID-19 patients. *Cellular & Molecular Immunology, 17*(5), 533–535. Advance online publication. doi:10.103841423-020-0402-2 PMID:32203188

Dong, Y., Mo, X., Hu, Y., Qi, X., Jiang, F., Jiang, Z., & Tong, S. (2020). *Epidemiological characteristics of 2143 Pediatric patients with 2019 coronavirus disease in China*. Journal., doi:10.1542/peds.2020-0702

Zumla, A., Chan, J., Azhar, E., Hui, D., & Yuen, K. (2016). Coronaviruses - drug discovery and therapeutic options. *Nature Reviews. Drug Discovery, 15*(5), 327–347. doi:10.1038/nrd.2015.37 PMID:26868298

de Wit, E., van Doremalen, N., Falzarano, D., & Munster, V. J. (2016). SARS and MERS: Recent insights into emerging coronaviruses. *Nature Reviews. Microbiology, 14*(8), 523–534. doi:10.1038/nrmicro.2016.81 PMID:27344959

Song, Z., Xu, Y., Bao, L., Zhang, L., Yu, P., Qu, Y., Zhu, H., Zhao, W., Han, Y., & Qin, C. (2019). From SARS to MERS, thrusting coronaviruses into the spotlight. *Viruses, 11*(1), E59. doi:10.3390/v11010059 PMID:30646565

Cui, J., Li, F., & Shi, Z. L. (2019). Origin and evolution of pathogenic coronaviruses. *Nature Reviews. Microbiology, 17*(3), 181–192. doi:10.103841579-018-0118-9 PMID:30531947

Guan, W. J., Ni, Z. Y., Hu, Y., Liang, W. H., Ou, C. Q., He, J. X., Liu, L., Shan, H., Lei, C., Hui, D. S. C., Du, B., Li, L., Zeng, G., Yuen, K.-Y., Chen, R., Tang, C., Wang, T., Chen, P., Xiang, J., ... Zhong, N. (2020). Clinical characteristics of coronavirus disease 2019 in China. *The New England Journal of Medicine, 382*(18), 1708–1720. Advance online publication. doi:10.1056/NEJMoa2002032 PMID:32109013

Wang, D., Hu, B., Hu, C., Zhu, F., Liu, X., & Zhang, J. (n.d.). Clinical characteristics of 138 hospitalized patients with 2019 novel coronavirus-infected pneumonia in Wuhan, China. Academic Press.

Wang, D., Hu, B., Hu, C., Zhu, F., Liu, X., Zhang, J., Wang, B., Xiang, H., Cheng, Z., Xiong, Y., Zhao, Y., Li, Y., Wang, X., & Peng, Z. (2020). Clinical Characteristics of 138 Hospitalized Patients With 2019 Novel Coronavirus–Infected Pneumonia in Wuhan, China. *Journal of the American Medical Association*, *323*(11), 1061. Advance online publication. doi:10.1001/jama.2020.1585

Poutanen, S. M., Low, D. E., Henry, B., Finkelstein, S., Rose, D., Green, K., Tellier, R., Draker, R., Adachi, D., Ayers, M., Chan, A. K., Skowronski, D. M., Salit, I., Simor, A. E., Slutsky, A. S., Doyle, P. W., Krajden, M., Petric, M., Brunham, R. C., & McGeer, A. J. (2003). Identification of severe acute respiratory syndrome in Canada. *The New England Journal of Medicine*, *348*(20), 1995–2005. doi:10.1056/NEJMoa030634 PMID:12671061

Jin, Y. H., Cai, L., Cheng, Z. S., Cheng, H., Deng, T., Fan, Y. P., Fang, C., Huang, D., Huang, L.-Q., Huang, Q., Han, Y., Hu, B., Hu, F., Li, B.-H., Li, Y.-R., Liang, K., Lin, L.-K., Luo, L.-S., Ma, J., ... Wang, X.-H. (2020). A rapid advice guideline for the diagnosis and treatment of 2019 novel coronavirus (2019-nCoV) infected pneumonia (standard version). *Military Medical Research*, *7*(1), 4. doi:10.118640779-020-0233-6 PMID:32029004

Bosch, B. J., van der Zee, R., de Haan, C. A., & Rottier, P. J. (2003). The coronavirus spike protein is a class I virus fusion protein: Structural and functional characterization of the fusion core complex. *Journal*, *77*(16), 8801–8811. doi:10.1128/JVI.77.16.8801-8811.2003 PMID:12885899

Lee, N., Hui, D., Wu, A., Chan, P., Cameron, P., Joynt, G. M., Ahuja, A., Yung, M. Y., Leung, C. B., To, K. F., Lui, S. F., Szeto, C. C., Chung, S., & Sung, J. J. Y. (2003). A major outbreak of severe acute respiratory syndrome in Hong Kong. *The New England Journal of Medicine*, *348*(20), 1986–1994. doi:10.1056/NEJMoa030685 PMID:12682352

Assiri, A., Al-Tawfiq, J. A., Al-Rabeeah, A. A., Al-Rabiah, F. A., Al-Hajjar, S., Al-Barrak, A., Flemban, H., Al-Nassir, W. N., Balkhy, H. H., Al-Hakeem, R. F., Makhdoom, H. Q., Zumla, A. I., & Memish, Z. A. (2013). Epidemiological, demographic, and clinical characteristics of 47 cases of Middle East respiratory syndrome coronavirus disease from Saudi Arabia: A descriptive study. *The Lancet. Infectious Diseases*, *13*(9), 752–761. doi:10.1016/S1473-3099(13)70204-4 PMID:23891402

Agostini, M. L., Andres, E. L., Sims, A. C., Graham, R. L., Sheahan, T. P., Lu, X., Smith, E. C., Case, J. B., Feng, J. Y., Jordan, R., Ray, A. S., Cihlar, T., Siegel, D., Mackman, R. L., Clarke, M. O., Baric, R. S., & Denison, M. R. (2018). Coronavirus susceptibility to the antiviral remdesivir (gs-5734) is mediated by the viral polymerase and the proofreading exoribonuclease. *mBio*, *9*(2), e00221–e18. doi:10.1128/mBio.00221-18 PMID:29511076

Savarino, A., Boelaert, J. R., Cassone, A., Majori, G., & Cauda, R. (2003). Effects of chloroquine on viral infections: An old drug against today's diseases? *The Lancet. Infectious Diseases*, *3*(11), 722–727. doi:10.1016/S1473-3099(03)00806-5 PMID:14592603

Vincent, M. J., Bergeron, E., Benjannet, S., Erickson, B. R., Rollin, P. E., Ksiazek, T. G., Seidah, N. G., & Nichol, S. T. (2005). Chloroquine is a potent inhibitor of SARS coronavirus infection and spread. *Virology Journal*, *2*(1), 69. doi:10.1186/1743-422X-2-69 PMID:16115318

Arabi, Y. M., Asiri, A. Y., Assiri, A. M., Aziz Jokhdar, H. A., Alothman, A., Balkhy, H. H., AlJohani, S., Al Harbi, S., Kojan, S., Al Jeraisy, M., Deeb, A. M., Memish, Z. A., Ghazal, S., Al Faraj, S., Al-Hameed, F., AlSaedi, A., Mandourah, Y., Al Mekhlafi, G. A., Sherbeeni, N. M., ... Hussein, M. A. (2020). Treatment of Middle East respiratory syndrome with a combination of lopinavir/ritonavir and interferon-β1b (MIRACLE trial): Statistical analysis plan for a recursive two-stage group sequential randomized controlled trial. *Trials*, *21*(1), 8. doi:10.118613063-019-3846-x PMID:31900204

Xu, Z., Shi, L., Wang, Y., Zhang, J., Huang, L., Zhang, C., Liu, S., Zhao, P., Liu, H., Zhu, L., Tai, Y., Bai, C., Gao, T., Song, J., Xia, P., Dong, J., Zhao, J., & Wang, F. S. (2020). Pathological findings of COVID-19 associated with acute respiratory distress syndrome. *Journal*, *8*(4), 420–422. doi:10.1016/S2213-2600(20)30076-X PMID:32085846

Lim, J., Jeon, S., Shin, H. Y., Kim, M. J., Seong, Y. M., & Lee, W. J. (2020). Case of the index patient who caused tertiary transmission of COVID-19 infection in Korea: The application of lopinavir/ritonavir for the treatment of COVID-19 infected pneumonia monitored by quantitative RT-PCR. *Journal of Korean Medical Science*, *35*(6), e79. doi:10.3346/jkms.2020.35.e79 PMID:32056407

Chu, C. M., Cheng, V. C., Hung, I. F., Wong, M. M., Chan, K. H., & Chan, K. S. (2004). Role of lopinavir/ritonavir in the treatment of SARS: Initial virological and clinical findings. *Thorax*, *59*(3), 252–256. doi:10.1136/thorax.2003.012658 PMID:14985565

Tian, S., Hu, W., Niu, L., Liu, H., Xu, H., & Xiao, S. Y. (2020). *Pulmonary pathology of Early-phase 2019 Novel Coronavirus (COVID-19) pneumonia in two patients with lung cancer*. doi:10.1016/j.jtho.2020.02.010

Letko, M., Marzi, A., & Munster, V. (2020). Functional assessment of cell entry and receptor usage for SARS-CoV-2 and other lineage B betacoronaviruses. *Journal*, *5*(4), 562–569. doi:10.103841564-020-0688-y PMID:32094589

Wenham, C., Smith, J., & Morgan, R. (2020). Gender and C-W Group, COVID-19: The gendered impacts of the outbreak. *Journal*, *395*, 846–848. PMID:32151325

Walls, A. C., Park, Y. J., Tortorici, M. A., Wall, A., McGuire, A. T., & Veesler, D. (2020). *Structure, function, and antigenicity of the SARS-CoV-2 spike glycoprotein*. doi:10.1016/j.cell.2020.02.058

Zhang, W., Du, R. H., Li, B., Zheng, X. S., Yang, X. L., Hu, B., Wang, Y.-Y., Xiao, G.-F., Yan, B., Shi, Z.-L., & Zhou, P. (2020). Molecular and serological investigation of 2019-nCoV infected patients: Implication of multiple shedding routes. *Emerging Microbes & Infections*, *9*(1), 386–389. doi:10.1080/22221751.2020.1729071 PMID:32065057

KEY TERMS AND DEFINITIONS

COVID-19: The pandemic situation due to spreading SARS-CoV-2, a pandemic occurs in 2019 and still continue.

Epidemiology: A scientific study process where a data driven systematically to find out the risk factor and causes of healthcare-oriented conditions and facts in definite inhabitants.

SARS-CoV-2: A virus which effects human bodies and extremely transmittable also pathogenic viral infection which first spread from the seafood market of Wuhan, China from 12th Dec 2019; now spreads worldwide.

Treatment: A process where a patient is given medical facilities to recover or fight against the disease or illness.

WHO: World Health Organization is a statutory organization of the United Nations that observes the main health related issues worldwide.

APPENDIX

Additional Information

COVID-19 is a rapidly infectious disease caused by SARS-CoV-2 (Scaused by severe acute respiratory syndrome coronavirus 2), which arisen in Dec, 2019 Wuhan, China. This virus basically originated from the family of Coronaviridae in order of Nidovirales. Corona signifies crown-like spikes which is basically situated the outer surface of the layer; so it was known as a CORONAVIRUS. This types of viruses are microscopic in size in between 65–125 nm in dia. and enclose a single-stranded RNA as a nucleic material, the length is basically in between 26 to 32kbs. There are many organizations are working for developing the corona vaccines, for example Inovio Pharmaceuticals, Moderna Therapeutics, Vir Biotechnology, Novavax, Stermirna Therapeutics, Johnson & Johnson, etc.

Chapter 3
Mental Health and Psychosocial Support for Persons in Quarantine and Isolation Facilities During the COVID-19 Pandemic in Namibia:
A Multi-Sectoral Response

Rachel J. Freeman
University of Namibia, Namibia

Simon George Taukeni
University of Namibia, Namibia

Eveline Kalomo
Wichita State University, USA

ABSTRACT

In this chapter, the authors describe the essential need of mental health and psychosocial support for people accommodated in mandatory quarantine and isolation facilities during the outbreak of COVID-19 pandemic in Namibia through a multi-sectoral response. Namibia recorded its first two index cases on 13 March 2020 when a married couple arrived in the Windhoek district in Namibia from Madrid, Spain on 11 March 2020. Namibia has since March 2020 provided supervised quarantine services to 12,128 persons in facilities around the country. The Ministry of Health and Social Services provides mental health and psychosocial support services, which were critical in the short and long-term response to COVID-19 pandemic. Public health measures were developed in line with WHO guidelines to contain the virus. These measures include the need of setting up quarantine and isolation facilities. Recommendations for future research in strengthening mental health and psychosocial support services and coping strategies are provided in the chapter.

DOI: 10.4018/978-1-7998-4414-3.ch003

INTRODUCTION

In the light of the worldwide outbreak of the COVID-19 pandemic, His Excellency, Dr. Hage Geingob, President of the Republic of Namibia demonstrated strong leadership in declaring a State of Emergency in terms of Sub-Article (5) of Article (26) of the Namibian Constitution of 1990. In the Namibian Government's containment efforts to curb the transmission and spread of COVID-19, special measures under the State of Emergency have been put in place through phase Lockdown measures. One of the measures under the State of Emergency was the Stage 1 Lockdown of 21 days (from 27 March – 17 April 2020), which was applicable to the Khomas- and Erongo regions, inclusive of the Okahandja and Rehoboth Municipality areas. This lockdown was extended with fourteen (14) days from 18 April until 04 May 2020. The 3rd Stage of Lockdown was effective from the 1st of June 2020 until 29 June 2020. The 4th Stage of Lockdown has been effective from 29th June until 17th September 2020, which will also terminates the six months of State of Emergency declared. With reference to the afore-mentioned, further directives were given by the President of the Republic of Namibia to provide mandatory quarantine and isolation facilities for returning Namibian citizens and permanent residents for a period of fourteen (14) days of supervised quarantine. Furthermore, directives were issued by the President of the Republic of Namibia to provide alternative accommodation to persons without shelter for a period of at least three (3) months, effective from April to June 2020.

In response to the afore-mentioned Lockdown measures, the Government of the Republic of Namibia activated a National Health Emergency Coordination Committee on COVID-19 under the leadership of the Ministry of Health and Social Services. In addition, an Incident Management System was established to strengthen the operationalization of the National Public Health Emergency Operation Center (NPHEOC), which become the central hub from where all COVID-19 responders operated. In prioritizing the health of all Namibians amid COVID-19, a multi-sectoral response team was established, which comprised of government sectors, development partners, higher education institutions, private sector, faith-based organizations and civil society organizations. All these multi-sectoral partners collaborated efforts in the development of a Multi-Sectoral National Response Plan for COVID-19 in Namibia.

In accordance with the WHO Guidelines (2020), informed by the country context, a customized Multi-Sectoral National Response Plan for COVID-19 in Namibia comprised of nine technical pillars namely:

1. Country Coordination, Planning and Monitoring
2. Risk Communication and Community Engagement
3. Surveillance & Contact Tracing
4. Points of Entry
5. Laboratory Coordination
6. Case Management
7. Infection Prevention and Control
8. Operations and Logistics
9. Mental Health and Psychosocial Support

This chapter only focuses on the provision of mental health and psychosocial support services under Pillar 9 on the Multi-Sectoral National Response Plan for COVID-19. The core functions of this pillar include providing psychosocial support and counselling services to all people in mandatory quarantine and isolation facilities, arrange temporary shelter for persons and children on the streets without shelter as well as, to mobilize corporate sponsorships and church donations such as food, shelter, water, sanitation and other basic necessities (WHO Namibia, 2020). The chapter provides solutions and recommendations as well as future research directions.

BACKGROUND

This section provides broad definitions and discussions on the mental health and psychosocial support for persons in mandatory quarantine and isolation facilities. Mental health and psychosocial support for persons undergoing stress and anxiety are highly recommended to help instil sense of resilience and better coping mechanisms among those affected by the COVID-19 pandemic. As part of national response and preparedness, Namibia has made available facilities to accommodate persons who tested positive to COVID-19 and for persons who were in direct contact with those tested positive. A quarantine facility is a designated place for persons who had direct contact with any infected persons or who travelled to countries with widespread ongoing transmission or who had symptoms including fever and cough (WHO, 2020). When the town of Walvis Bay in Namibia became epicenter of COVID-19, many people who tested positive were informed to self-quarantine and isolation due to adequate mandatory quarantine facilities and the public responded with mixed feelings. Centron and Landworth (2005) assert that quarantine maybe applied at the individual or group level or at home or a designated facility. On the other hand, isolation facility is a designated place that is situated in hospital setting under the supervision of medical professionals. Thus, isolation involves the separation of persons infected with COVID-19 pandemic from others for the purpose of protecting non-infected persons (Suppawittaya, Yiemphat & Yasri, 2020). Mental health and psychosocial support endure that people should be empowered to care for themselves, their families and communities to instil self-confidence and build resilience. This, in turn will encourage positive recovery and strengthen their ability to deal with challenges in the future (MHSS, 2020).

MENTAL HEALTH AND PSYCHOSOCIAL SUPPORT FOR PEOPLE IN MANDATORY QUARANTINE AND ISOLATION FACILITIES

According to Freeman (2020) in response to prioritize the mental health and psychosocial needs of Namibians, there was an urgent need to lobby and advocate the Incident Manager of COVID-19 Response Team and WHO for the establishment and inclusion of the Mental Health and Psychosocial Support Pillar. Pillar 9 based on Namibia's need and demand for such services. The tasks of Pillar 9 included providing psychosocial support and counseling services to the following respective groups, namely persons in quarantine, persons in isolation, their families, as well as to vulnerable individuals, including persons without shelter in the community.

Pillar 9 comprises of multi-sectoral stakeholders (social workers from MHSS, Higher Education (UNAM), Namibian Defence Force (NDF), Ministry of Gender Equality, Poverty Eradication and Welfare (MGEPEW); UN Agencies in Namibia (e.g. IOM, WHO, UNICEF, etc.); Namibian Police Services (NAMPOL), City of Windhoek Police; Nurses, Psychologists (State & Private Sector), Psychiatrists, Occupational Therapists, Community Counsellors; Community leaders (e.g. regional & local counsellors); Home Based Care Volunteers; Community Healthcare workers; Social Welfare Committees; COVID-19 patients & Families; Persons without shelter; Non-Governmental Organisations; Community Based Organizations; Faith Based Organizations).

The Ministry of Health and Social Services (2020) in response to citizens' needs for psychosocial support and counseling services under the auspices of Pillar 9 provided public health education, psychosocial support and counseling services to people under quarantine, for patients diagnosed with COVID-19 and their families. Pillar No.9 ensured the provision of psychosocial support and counseling services to persons in quarantine facilities, patients in hospital isolation, including vulnerable populations and healthcare workers by social workers and psychologists. Facilities that satisfy the minimum standard as prescribed under the national guidelines were identified and reserved for the purpose of quarantine and isolation. All persons identified through contact tracing were place under supervised quarantine for a period of 14 days. Furthermore, to mandatory quarantine and isolation additional containment measures such as, stay at home, physical distancing and restricted movement directives adversely affect social and mental wellbeing of healthy individuals by inhibiting social interaction, social connectedness and engagement in healthy lifestyles. Other measures in place include the provision of 24 hour access to COVID-19 public health information, tele-counselling services and psychological care via hotline numbers 0800 100 100. A total number of 513 people without shelter were housed at two sites in Windhoek. Provision of food, accommodation and internet connectivity were provided by the Ministry of Health and Social Services to people in quarantine. Leaflets on gender-based violence, alcohol and drug abuse, suicide prevention and prevention of elder abuse during COVID-19 were developed with input by multi-sectoral stakeholders (MHSS 2020).

The key objectives of the MHPSS Pillar are to:

- Enhance the social functioning of people in distress in order for them to deal with their needs and problems in an effort to cope with their stressful situation.
- Instill hope, strengthen the capacity of people to become resilient and to improve their quality of life.
- Advocate for the needs, plights and rights of the poor and the vulnerable.
- Link people in need with the necessary services, resources and opportunities.
- Provide comprehensive and holistic care services to the poor and the vulnerable through a multi-disciplinary team approach.
- Empower caregivers and significant others to provide efficient and effective care and support to the infected and affected by the life-threatening disease such as, COVID-19 and other challenges.

COVID-19 has multiplied by forced quarantine to combat the spread of the disease applied by nationwide lockdowns, which have the potential to produce acute panic, anxiety, obsessive behaviors, paranoia and depression as well as post-traumatic stress disorder (PTSD) in the long run (Dubey et al, 2020). It was also revealed in a study by Dubey et al (2020) that during lockdown, outbursts of racism, stigmatization and xenophobia against particular communities were being widely reported. In Namibia, for example, outburst xenophobia remarks were expressed on social media towards Chinese nationals as well as, towards the first two index COVID-19 cases, who travelled from Spain. Effects such as, posttraumatic stress disorder have been reported as symptoms of which have been positively associated with the duration of quarantine (Hawryluck, Gold, Robinson, Pogorski, Galea, & Styra, 2004). People who are in isolation facilities are likely to suffer from anxiety due to uncertainty about their health status and develop obsessive-compulsive symptoms such as repeated temperature checks and sterilization (Li, Yang, Liu, Zhao, Zhang, Zhang et al, 2020).

The multi-sectoral MHPSS pillar developed the following documents in strengthening the provision of Mental Health and Psychosocial Support:

- Guideline on Psychosocial Support, Counselling and Mental Health on COVID-19.
- Directives on Psychosocial Support, Counselling and Mental Health for persons without shelter, alcohol and drug related centres, residential care for older persons, and services for mental health facilities (Part of Directives No. 107, issued on 21 April 2020).
- Terms of Reference (TOR) for Mental Health and Psychosocial Support in response to COVID-19.
- Draft Guide on Services to Persons in Quarantine in Response to COVID-19.
- Draft Guide on Services to Bereaved Families affected by COVID-19.
- Draft Guide on Pre- and Post-Testing for COVID-19.

MENTAL HEALTH AND PSYCHOSOCIAL SUPPORT FOR PERSONS WITHOUT SHELTER

Persons without shelter may be at higher risk of contracting COVID-19 or developing complications due to COVID-19, as they may not be able to access and use mainstream and basic services. Their circumstances may affect their ability to follow public health advice, such as being able to effectively isolate/self-isolate from others and perform proper hand and personal hygiene. The different multi-sectoral key stakeholders identified approximately 900 people in the Windhoek area in need of shelter. Various material and social needs were identified in order to render mental health and psychosocial services. Persons without shelter were classified in the following categories:

- Persons without shelter (persons living in the street).
- Persons living in backyards (stay in backyard temporarily because of lack of permanent shelter).
- Persons living in riverbeds.
- Persons occupying land unauthorized (e.g. in Kleine Kuppe, Dumpsite) who refused to be resettled, but are in need of basic services to meet their needs (e.g. food, water, sanitation, etc.)

- A rapid assessment on persons without shelter was conducted and approximately 900 persons in need of shelter were identified.
- Social workers conducted individual need assessments of which a comprehensive report will be compiled in order to determine the needs of persons without shelter. The need assessment covers reintegration, repatriation, rehabilitation, skills auditing, skills training, employment creation as well as current and future needs.
- A total number of 420 persons without shelter are housed at Katutura Multi-Purpose Youth Centre under the supervision and support by 5 Social Workers, 1 Part time Occupational Therapist and 21 Volunteers. A total number of 113 persons without shelter are housed at Khomasdal Soccer Stadium under the supervision and support by 4 Social Workers, 1 part time Occupational Therapist and 8 Volunteers. Mobile Teams serve a number of 132 persons without shelter at the Dumpsite, Kleine Kuppe, Truckport, etc.) which include 1 Social Worker, 3 Police Officers from the City of Windhoek.
- A mobile Nursing Team consisting of 4 nurses and 1 social worker attended to the physical and mental health of the persons without shelter.
- Food, water, as well as, psychosocial support and public health education are provided to the above-mentioned groups on a daily basis. Temporarily accommodation is provided in tents (with mattresses and blankets sponsored by the social corporate responsibility Community Engagement project of UNAM, called UNAM *Cares*). Meals were prepared daily and served by the Uni-Social Church and the Namibia Council of Churches, Church Task Force prepared with assistance by the residents and the volunteers. Sunday lunches were provided for Katutura by the Seventh Day Adventist Church.
- Previously during Stage 1 Lockdown, all necessities to fulfil the needs of persons without shelter were donations, with some raw food from Office of the Prime Minister's (OPM) National Disaster Management Programme. Although, most food is procured via the OPM Disaster Management Programme, some donations are solicited from local businesses and individuals. It is stored and distributed from a central store.
- Several multi-sectoral stakeholders' meetings in regards to persons without shelter were conducted with the office of the Khomas Regional Governor, the CEO of the City of Windhoek and Disaster Management Team from OPM, Khomas Regional Commander Office and others.

Reintegration

- A family of 11 at Klein Kuppe and Okuryangava vendors were relocated to their own house in Otjomuise. However, some returned to find a new place to live.
- Six persons without shelter were successfully re-integrated with their families. Two from Khomasdal stadium, one went to Windhoek and one to Gobabis, Omaheke region. Two males and one female left for Rundu, to work in the construction business. Seven persons from Katutura Youth Centre; two males went to Gobabis, Omaheke region, while the others went to Oniipa, Oshikoto region. Two females, one went to Okapya Village, Oshana region, while the other one went back to Shandumbala, Khomas region. More recently, one male has been reintegrated with his family in Otjomuise, another male was reem-

ployed by his previous work (with accommodation), and one female has been availed a shack in Freedom Square.

- The mobile team visited Hosea Kutako International Airport, where two (2) women and eleven (11) men were found at this site. A needs assessment was conducted and food was distributed. Some were motivated to be reintegrated with families or joined the sites. Two (2) women were integrated with their families. Seven (7) men went back to their families at Omitara, one (1) went to Blue camp at Hosea Kutako International Airport, while three (3) went to Otjivelo. Very few people are still at the site.

Repatriation

- Thirty one (31) residents from the Commando group were returned to their respective regions of origin, with one male resident returning due to medical reasons.
- Eleven (11) female youth residents went back to Opuwo in the Kunene region.
- Twelve (12) male residents went back to Opuwo, Kunene region.
- Six (6) children went back with their parents or caretakers to Opuwo, Kunene region.
- One (1) child went back to Otjinene in the Omaheke region.
- After a further assessment by the social workers, 39 out of 208 people from the Commando group at Katutura Youth Centre are willing to go back to their homes in Opuwo.

Special Cases (Residents who Need Special Care)

There were five persons in need of special care at Katutura Youth Centre.

- One older person with possible psychiatric issues/dementia- needing full time care
- One man with psychiatric issues, needing full time supervision.
- Two different women with schizophrenia, who is receiving social grant, but is in need some assistance.
- One man with physical disability (foreign national without documents), who are mostly independent.

At Khomasdal Stadium, there were:

- 14-15 people with mental illness (some supervision needed for hygiene and medical, basic needs).
- Two people with physical disabilities (both are mostly independent).
- Three patients are suffering from tuberculosis and need assistance/ supervision most of the times: one mostly remains in the tent, one has is occasionally unwell and needs medical assistance, and one was hospitalized.

Older Persons

- Three persons older than 60 years are residing at Katutura Youth Centre.
- There was also an older couple, who were found without shelter and were placed at Senior Park (Old Age Facility) in Pionierspark, Windhoek.

Foreign Nationals

There are three residents with foreign citizenship at the shelters. Two of them at Katutura Youth Centre, and one at Khomasdal stadium. Two are Zimbabwean nationals and one claimed to be Kenyan National. Additionally, there is one foreigner still living on the street.

Case 1: Zimbabwean National

Presently, this client has no valid permit to stay in Namibia, nor documents indicating his original entry permit in the country. He has been in Namibia for 10 years. The Zimbabwe's Embassy is aware of his stay in the country. They are equally aware that he is willing to return to his country.

Case 2: Zimbabwean National

This client has also no valid permit to stay in Namibia. His passport was seized by Home Affairs, however, he was issued with a Temporary Travel Document by the Zimbabwean Embassy, expiring in September 2020 preceding the country lockdown due to coronavirus.

Case 3: Kenyan National

This client states that he is a Kenyan. According to him, he entered the Namibian territory from South Africa where he was residing as a temporary asylum seeker. The client has a copy of an expired Asylum Seeker Temporary Permit issued by South Africa. He has no valid permit to stay in Namibia, nor document indicating his entry permit. The client stated that his immigration related documents were all stolen the day he entered the country, but he does not have a Police Declaration confirming the incident.

Case 4: Chinese National

The Chinese National was found at an old house owned by a fellow Chinese, who is currently residing in Kavango. The house has no water, no electricity and he had no food. According to the client he was married to a Namibian national, however he reports he cannot remember her name.

Network and Coordination

- Various needs were identified by the social workers and vulnerable people were linked to the constituency counselors for food supplies.

- Identify and co-opt other stakeholders to serve on the Regional Task Force COVID-19 as per President's Directives.

Capacity Building

At both the Katutura Youth Centre and Khomasdal Stadium, individual social work and Occupational Therapy Assessments and some interventions continue to be made. Different churches continue to occasionally come to give other spiritual encouragement. Red Cross provides residents with public health education training on COVID-19, and have trained 3 residents from each of the sites to continue with the same at some remuneration in generating an income to address some of the psychosocial needs of some of the persons without shelter.

At Katutura, there is four psychosocial groups, which addresses different topics, including lifestyle change, effective parenting skills, tobacco cessation, and substance abuse. Vocationally, there are 5 people making tyre plant pots, and some women have been learning domestic skills in order to be employed as such. Three times a week, the 'African Unicorn' Organization come to run group activities with the children. Additionally, there are occasional once-off events made, such as for African Childrens' Day, 'No Tobacco' Day, and International Day Against Drug Abuse and Illicit Trafficking.

At Khomasdal, there are 2-3 psychosocial groups on substance use held each week due to the many clients with this issue. Additionally, there are 3 other psychosocial groups weekly for 'Healthy Relationships', Entrepreneurship skills, and general life skills. Vocationally, groups held have been to make masks (for COVID-19), and firebricks (used instead of wood). Two clients work respectively on leatherwork and wire cars ('draad werk'), but teach others from time to time. Four other residents initiated a vegetable garden and continue in sustaining it. The Fatherhood Foundation, a Faith-Based organization conducted once a week Bible study groups, and movie nights on a Friday as part of edutainment.

Challenges

- Lack of re-integration opportunities (e.g. acceptance by the family members, employment opportunities).
- Lack of resources (human and material support) to meet urgent needs.
- Inadequate variety in food- the meals the clients are mostly eating now after lockdown level one is pap with very simple soup. There is very little fruit and vegetables available to provide nutrients.
- Inadequate toiletries such as, soap and toothpaste are often experienced by residents of the sites, the residents are mostly reliant on donations.
- Need for permanent resettlement land, alternative housing and basic services.
- The current shelters do not provide a conducive environment for rehabilitation due to complexity and group dynamics of the residents. There are also not adequate structures, equipment, and personal protective equipment in place to give vocational training.
- Often client motivation at the shelters for the activities on offer is low. Only some residents take interest, or are inconsistent with their attendance. Reasons can be possibly

because of the high rate of drug and alcohol use, also some have mental illnesses/ other challenges and thus do not have the concentration/ organization of self to participate.

- Many of the clients have skills, but only want to try what they know already or are not motivated at all. It is difficult to obtain materials for everybody's requests.
- It is difficult to offer vocational activities with more safety hazards on the Khomasdal site, such as furniture making and tyre cutting. This is due to residents turning up after having used substances (dangerous, impairs judgment), also not having enough safety equipment- e.g. gloves, boots, etc., residents, who often fight amongst each other, and theft of equipment.
- Security issues are high due to theft and violence, meaning some staff and clients have victimized, and individual and group materials stolen.
- The relaxation of lockdown measure with regards to access to alcohol among some of the residents in the shelters resulted in problems such as physical violence and other behavioral problems.
- Some clients in substance groups, who would like to give up their alcohol and/or substances report that they are struggling to do since most people in the camp also use substances.
- Lack of alcohol and substance abuse rehabilitation centers in the country.
- Individual needs assessment took longer than anticipated due to psychosocial problems experienced by individuals in need of shelter.

SOLUTIONS AND RECOMMENDATIONS

The psychosocial issues such as stigma must be addressed as a matter of urgency. There is a strong need to provide health education and awareness as provided for by WHO in order to address stigma and other psychosocial issues associated with COVID-19.

- Office of the Prime Minister (Disaster Risk Management), Ministry of Urban and Rural Development and Regional Councils to make provision for non-medical basic needs of persons in need of shelter (food, utensils, cleaning material, and blankets). More variety in food is urgently needed.
- Mental Health and Psychosocial Response Team to continue with provision of psychosocial support services to persons in need of shelter, including finalization of individual assessment report, alcohol and drug rehabilitation services.
- Provision of reintegration packages (e.g. acceptance by the family members, employment opportunities).
- Decision on access of alcohol during State of Emergency should be revisited at Presidential level to limit its consumption.
- Some Commando people are willing to be integrated back to the home town but would like higher level government interventions and transport for repatriation, as promised by the Vice President.
- There is a need for permanent resettlement land, alternative housing and basic services to be provided by relevant stakeholders.

- It is highly recommended that persons without shelter should not be placed all together in one place when the 'State of Emergency" is over, as this is not a conducive situation considering the known behavior of some them, such as alcohol and substance use, violence, begging, and other non-conducive behaviors. It would mean that the people cannot rehabilitate so well as there are less members of 'mainstream society' to role model better behaviors to them.
- We recommend placing small groups of people together in different places who are good supports for each other. We also recommend placing people together according to their individual needs assessment.
- People with special needs as mentioned above need to be given priority and action taken now already. This is because the volunteers caring for them have not been trained and their health is at risk, and ethics comes into question. We need to give special attention to accommodation and support needs now already.
- Many of the clients will need long term rehabilitation due to emotional issues from past traumas, mental illnesses and very entrenched substance habits. We recommend that more professionals be employed to deal with these issues (such as social workers, psychologists, occupational therapists)- perhaps as a specialized permanent team, as other countries often have. Until people are able to have their individual rehabilitation needs met and function on a higher level, it will be difficult to involve them in vocational activities in the community successfully.
- Residents need to be provided with a conducive environment for rehabilitation (vocational training, capacity building, skills training).

FUTURE RESEARCH DIRECTIONS

In the future for better dealing with mental health and psychosocial issues of different strata of the society, psychosocial crisis prevention and intervention models should be urgently developed by the government, health care personnel and other stakeholders. Psychosocial preparedness by setting up mental organizations specific for future pandemics is certainly necessary (Dubey et al, 2020). Even though, health education, psychosocial support and post counseling services to people under quarantine, COVID-19 confirmed cases and their families were provided as per provisions of Ministry of Health and Social Services, further research is needed to assess their impacts.

CONCLUSION

The overall picture the authors could draw called for all stakeholders to work together in addressing mental health and psychosocial impact of COVID-19. Toll free helpline numbers for communication national center should be effectively managed by social workers, counselors and psychologists for alleviating psychological distress among the public. Mental health and psychosocial support require further attention to help people in quarantine and isolation facilities tackle their anxiety, stigma and other psychological effects. Services to persons in quarantine and isolation as well we persons without shelter require a multi-sector approach and a long-term strategy. Every sector and organization in the National Response Plan on COVID-19 is a key stakeholder in order to ensure the successful reintegration and recovery of persons in quarantine, without shelter and in isolation. Solutions can be find if we work hard as a multi-sectoral response team to address the highlighted psychosocial and counseling needs. The main aim of mental health and psychosocial support is to improve quality of life and sustaining livelihoods. The provision of psychosocial support and counseling services will address needs and problems that people experience in an effort to empower them in the physical, mental, social, emotional, spiritual, psychological and economic domains.

REFERENCES

Brooks, S. K., Webster, R. K., Smith, L. E., Woodland, L., Wessely, S., Greenberg, N., & Rubin, G. J. (2020). The psychological impact of quarantine and how to reduce it: Rapid review of the evidence. *Lancet, 395*(10227), 912–920. doi:10.1016/S0140-6736(20)30460-8 PMID:32112714

Centron, M., & Landwirth, J. (2005). Public health and ethical considerations in planning for quarantine. *The Yale Journal of Biology and Medicine, 78*(5), 329. PMID:17132339

Dubey, S., Biswas, P., Ghosh, R., Chatterjee, S., Dubey, M. J., Chatterjee, S., Lahiri, D., & Lavie, C. (2020). Psychosocial impact of COVID-19. *Diabetes & Metabolic Syndrome, 14*(5), 779–788. doi:10.1016/j.dsx.2020.05.035 PMID:32526627

Government Gazette of the Republic of Namibia. (2020). *Proclamation No.9. State of Emergency-COVID-19 Regulations*. Namibian Constitution.

Hawryluck, G., & Robinson, P. (2004). SARS control and psychological effects of quarantine, Toronto, Canada. *Emerging Infectious Diseases, 10*(7), 1206–1212. doi:10.3201/eid1007.030703 PMID:15324539

Kluge, H. N. P. (2020). *Statement-physical and mental health key to resilience during COVID-19 pandemic*. Academic Press.

Lai, C. C., Shih, T. P., Ko, W. C., Tang, H. J., & Hsueh, P. R. (2020). Severe acute respiratory syndrome coronavirus 2 (SARS-CoV-2) and coronavirus disease-2019 (COVID-19): The epidemic and the challenges. *International Journal of Antimicrobial Agents*, 55.

Li, Y., Liu, Z., & Zhang, Z. (2020). Progression of mental health services during the COVID-19 outbreak in China. *International Journal of Biological Sciences, 16*, 1732–1738.

Ministry of Health and Social Services. (2020). *Namibia COVID-19 situation report No.46*. Windhoek: Author.

Namibia, W. H. O. (2020). *COVID-19: Namibia WCO Bulletin*. Windhoek: Author.

Rubin, G. J., & Wessely, S. (2020). The psychological effects of quarantining a city. *British Medical Journal*, 368.

Suppawittaya, P., Yiemphat, P., & Yasri, P. (2020). Effects of social distancing, self-quarantine and self-isolation during the COVID-19 pandemic on people's well-being and how to cope with it. *International Journal of Science and HealthCare Research*, *5*(2).

World Health Organization. (2020). *Mental health and psychosocial considerations during the COVID-19 outbreak*. Accessed online: https://www.who. int/docs/default-source/coronaviruse/mental-health-considerations.pdf

KEY TERMS AND DEFINITIONS

Confirmed Case: A person/s who tested positive that is confirmed by one or more of the laboratory methods listed in the case definition.

Contact Tracing: The process of identifying, assessing, and managing people who might have come in contact and been exposed to a virus in order to prevent transmission.

Counseling: A process in which two people meet to explore personal problems and to identify solutions through meaningful discussions and well-informed choices.

COVID-19: An infectious disease caused by coronavirus. It is the acronym for the full name coronavirus of 2019. It means "the coronavirus disease of 2019, which is caused by severe acute respiratory syndrome coronavirus 2" (SARS-CoV-2) (WHO, 2020).

Isolation Facility: The public health practice of separating sick people with a contagious disease from people who are not sick.

Loneliness: An unpleasant emotional response to perceived isolation that causes a person/s to feel empty, alone and unwanted due to lack of connection with other people.

Psychosocial Support: Psychosocial support is a process of facilitating resilience within individual, families, and communities by respecting the independence, dignity and coping mechanisms of individuals and communities. It promotes restoration of social cohesion and infrastructure.

Quarantine Facility: The public health practice of separating and limiting the movement of people who were exposed to a contagious disease to see if they become sick during a given period.

Recovery: A person who was infected with the virus and has survived a virus with no long-term health effects. This simply means that one's immune system has found and destroyed the virus in the body.

Stigma: This involves negative attitudes and beliefs toward someone or group of people based on their health status which lead to prejudice and discrimination. For example, some people who tested positive with Covid-19 were stigmatized and discriminated against as people perceived to spread the virus.

Section 3

Measurements and Interventions

Chapter 4
Towards the Development of IT-Enabled Immunization Monitoring Framework

Suma Dawn
Jaypee Institute of Information Technology, India

Ankur Jain
Jaypee Institute of Information Technology, India

Shivam Agrawal
Jaypee Institute of Information Technology, India

Shresth Pandey
Jaypee Institute of Information Technology, India

ABSTRACT

In this chapter, the authors present a system that uses smart immunization and develops structures to allow collaboration between parents, healthcare workers, and government agencies to cooperate at a grass-roots level to help spread immunization, collect and upload demographics, and allow for its multi-instance analysis. This system will enhance the spread of vaccination and reduce vaccine hesitancy. Information is coagulated and presented as statistical results that are presented in an engaging visualization form. Further, a reminder system has been set up to enable automated email service for parents by reminding them of proper and timely vaccinations. It collates the immunization data to present usable demographics for timely interventions, as may be necessary. The immunization perspective is retrained by easy storage and retrieval and quick remedial measures to contain the spread of vaccine-preventable diseases and reduction in child mortality. Statistical analysis has been done to predict immunization spread among different regions and detect any possible epidemic.

DOI: 10.4018/978-1-7998-4414-3.ch004

INTRODUCTION

Vaccines have proven their mettle in reducing the occurrences of many diseases. This has helped protect children from a multitude of life-threatening diseases. But along with vaccination, its progress monitoring is also of immense importance as many vaccines must be administered over a period of time, having varied doses, and other parameters. The monitoring of immunization records critically reduces the influence of vaccine-preventable diseases.

Improvements in mobile communications and multimedia technologies have fuelled solutions to mobile and smart healthcare solutions such as accessibility, affordability, a reminder system, behavior and statistical analysis. Such systems can assist in ensuring that vaccination targets, set by government healthcare agencies, are achieved. The inability of attaining such pre-set immunization targets can cause the breakdown of healthcare in community. Herd immunity is very important to reduce the risk of an outbreak. It ensures that a large percentage of the community is thoroughly vaccinated. This helps in providing protection for vulnerable individuals who are unable to get vaccinated, such as children such as neonates or immune-compromised individuals. Surveillance of immunization records and their maintenance can aid in asserting and observing the growth of immunization with the community. It can also help in identification of compromised zones and hence help in quick action. This work highlights the coverage of vaccination, impact of immunization performance, its growth rate and convergence of procedures by all healthcare stakeholders.

Immunization coverage in India is not as adequate as it should be for a rapidly developing nation. This has led to many challenges for public health agencies. Complete eradication of vaccination-preventable diseases is still lagging due to a lack of such monitoring. Diligent monitoring of immunization records allows government authorities, healthcare personnel, and general public to take swift corrective and preventive measures in cases of fluctuating vaccination estimates. The timely revelation of an inconsistent vaccination rate, for instance, an unexpected fall in usage of flu vaccines, can prompt the deployment of campaigns for flu vaccination campaigns & such necessary actions.

Addressing such important issues has led to the proposal of a generic system that can handle storage and retrieval of a child's medical case history along with the mandated vaccination records and their schedule. Indian Academy of Paediatrics, 2014, provided numerous updates in the immunization schedule for children aged 0 through 18 years. The various stakeholders of immunization include doctors, healthcare workers, and parents who are considered in this application. Each stakeholder has certain privileges. Such an application can have widespread use by government monitoring agencies. Not only generic mobile phone users but also smart-phone users have increased considerably in the Indian subcontinent. SMS service and timely reminders via emails can be incorporated in this application to make it more user-friendly for parents till the time the child's vaccination coverage is incomplete. Capture and storage of immunization records in a region can help in reducing the dispersal of paper-based record keeping. This, in turn, can help in understanding statistics such as the spread of vaccination, its rate, its impact on society and its acceptance by public. Immediate medical assistance of a needful child or even a particular geographic zone becomes more efficient, hazel free and subjective treatment to child(ren). Analyzing such data helps in healthcare-related research and development activities as well as provides data-driven actions (Kumari et al., 2017).

The United Nations works tirelessly to reduce child mortality rates, improving maternal health and fighting other related diseases. Many of these, especially with respect to children, can be arrested by using proper and timely vaccinations (UNICEF's strategy for health (2016-2030), n.d.), (World Health Organization (WHO), n.d.). Further, there is a large variation in the state-wise monitoring of immunization records (Healthcare in India, n.d.). This is happening in spite of the multiple schemes being run by the central and state governments (Vaccine India, n.d.). All such observations were presented after careful deliberation and study. However, no quick response tool and information analysis are currently in use that can present a computation dashboard for visualization. Hence, a change in focus can be brought about by presenting a system that can encompass many stakeholders and present data analysis as well as appropriate visualization in Immunization and Vaccination Healthcare area.

The purpose of this systematic procedure are to keep a track of children being vaccinated, their progress monitoring in terms of immunization records, providing information about the upcoming vaccine, an associated reminder system (thereby reducing vaccine-hesitancy) (Jarrett et al., 2015), timely action in cases of detection of outbreak of vaccine-preventable diseases, and finally analysis across multiple demographics. Further, some vaccines have certain side-effects that may need more wide study and analysis. Gathering such side-effects immunoinformatics and help in resolving many doubts and beliefs.

The system has the potential to increase the rate of immunization using timely reminders and engaging general public and it also reports the number of immunized people every year. Doctors and related healthcare workers can analyze the vaccination history details along with any previous medical records so as to provide the diagnostically correct vaccination to the child. This immunization system can also help in increasing the number of immunized people in the given geographical region. The updates in a child's vaccination shot detail record can be uploaded to reflect the latest amendments in the system. This immunization system will also help in combating deadly diseases like malaria, tuberculosis, etc., and achieve the aim of universal health coverage. Through immunization, several diseases can be prevented and thus, the aim of the United Nations & Indian Government of sustainable development can be achieved. The analysis can be performed by mining data and utilizing computational methods based on decision making and classification algorithms.

The organization of the paper is as follows: Section 2 presents the related work and current state of art in this domain. The architecture of the proposed system is presented in section 3 and section 4 presents the assessment metrics used. The results of the implementation are discussed in section 5. Section 6 concludes the proposed work.

RELATED WORKS AND LITERATURE

India's urbanization has fuelled a huge lead in her economic development (Kumari et al., 2017). Comprehensive development in social, industrial institutional and infrastructural front will append to the quality of life in her fold of growth (Healthcare in India, n.d.; UNICEF's strategy for health (2016-2030), n.d.; Vaccine India, n.d.; World Health Organization (WHO), n.d.). The development of smart and integrated city is the vision. News of vaccine-preventable diseases still percolates through and cause impediment in the eradication of vaccine-preventable diseases such as polio and measles. Children outside the protection coverage of vaccine suffer adversely not only in terms of health issues but also in socio-economic fronts. Moreover, many parents and guardians still have misconceptions about vaccinations and are vaccine-hesitant (Jarrett et al., 2015), (Lauridsen & Pradhan, 2011).

With proper and timely usage of various IT-enabled technologies and inclusion of ubiquitous computing, data mining, IoT and Wireless sensors, and many others, health systems can be improved. The data can be used for mining various analysis objectives that can succor eradication of vaccine-preventable diseases (Sahu et al., 2010), (Doherty et al., 2016). Vaccine hesitancy and sometimes side-effects of certain vaccines have put a break in the progress of achieving high immunization rates (Tomori, 2011), (Thacker & Shendurnikar, 2004). Hence, it also becomes mandatory to study and analyze such outbreaks and side-effects. Vaccine strategies much emerge from factors such as local healthcare attributes, infrastructure and administration, funding, immunization monitoring, public acceptance, and others (Hardt et al., 2016), (Pan et al., 2016). Collection of vaccination details and related medical case histories are imperative for providing quality and quantity service. Mobile healthcare systems (Wilson et al., 2015) and apps (Chen et al., 2013) though are in existence, their influence has been very constrained.

Hence, a system is required that can collate the aggregated data, provide dashboard-kind analysis for quick visualization so that immunization drives can be more successful.

PROPOSED ARCHITECTURE

Improvement in disease impact and vaccine coverage can happen with timely interventions. The chief objectives of this application include: having viewing rights of a child's vaccination record by doctor or healthcare worker; analysis of the growth rate of a particular vaccination; analysis of the acceptance of the vaccine by community; quick identification of any cases of vaccine-preventable disease and checking its spread; having a reminder system to prompt the Guardian / parent to take measures by undergoing timely vaccination depending on the child's birth date details.

To achieve such a system, a smooth interaction is a must between the various stakeholders. The various persons involved in the system are presented in Figure 1. The activities of healthcare personnel and the interaction diagram are listed in supplementary documents, as figures 4 and 5 respectively.

Due to the enormous increase in the use of mobile phones and internet connection, online access to the application can be done instantaneously. Reminder to parents on the date of upcoming vaccination shots, sent via email and/or SMS push notification can help parents in avoiding any delay in administering vaccine to their children. Presenting the case history to a doctor can help in quick identification of the required vaccination. Government agencies can use statistics to understand the spread of the vaccination, its acceptance, and usefulness to the community.

Figure 1. People involved in the vaccination drive

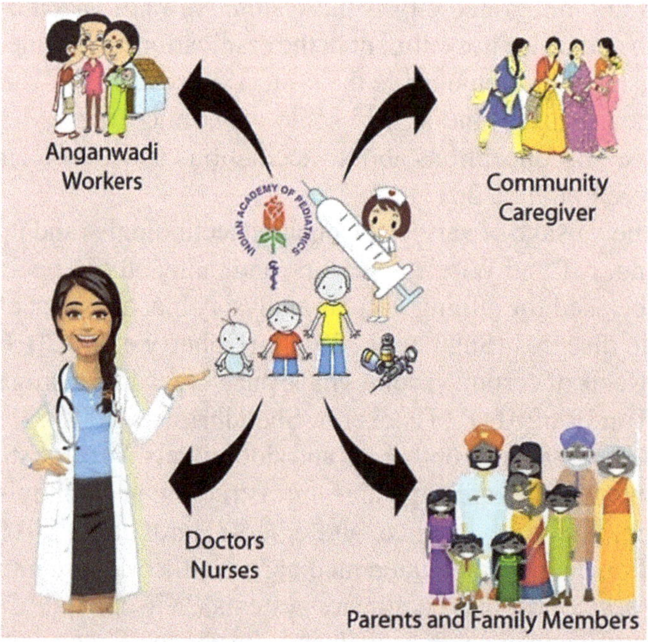

The client-server form of IT architecture has been proposed for this immunization analysis application. For web application design, Django technology shall be used to build applications. Python-based technologies such as Pandas and NumPy will be used to write scripts for back end analysis. A relational database, SQLite3 shall be used for storing and retrieving the data. Using Django-treebeard and Django-import-export, web applications will be integrated into the system. A web-based application has been designed for storage and retrieval of a child's medical record. IT-enabled equipment can help in forming the architecture of this application.

Parents or Guardians of the child can access his/her child's vaccination record and medical history details. The doctor or the healthcare worker can not only view and search the child's complete vaccination and previous medical history records details but also can update the same whenever any updation is performed. The system itself has been tuned, based on the input from the Indian Academy of Paediatrics, to include the timeline for vaccination. Based on this timeline, reminders are sent to the parent / Guardian via SMA and/or email service. The system interaction is shown in Figure 2.

Data visualization solutions have been implemented in this healthcare application based on vaccination drive monitoring and patient profiling to stipulate projection and capacity planning. Contemporary dashboards having an analysis of various data can allow users to access data in a visually appealing and easy-to-use manner. The design of the application also follows certain design principles that allow for intuitive access and navigation.

The various stakeholders of the proposed application include - Doctor / Medical Assistant; Healthcare /Anganwadi Workers; Parents / Guardian of the child; Administrator and Government Personnel. Figure 2 discerns the interaction between the various stakeholders and the modules that are actually involved with the communication platforms and their relations.

Figure 2. System overview of user design and Interaction between the stakeholders of the Vaccination Monitoring Framework

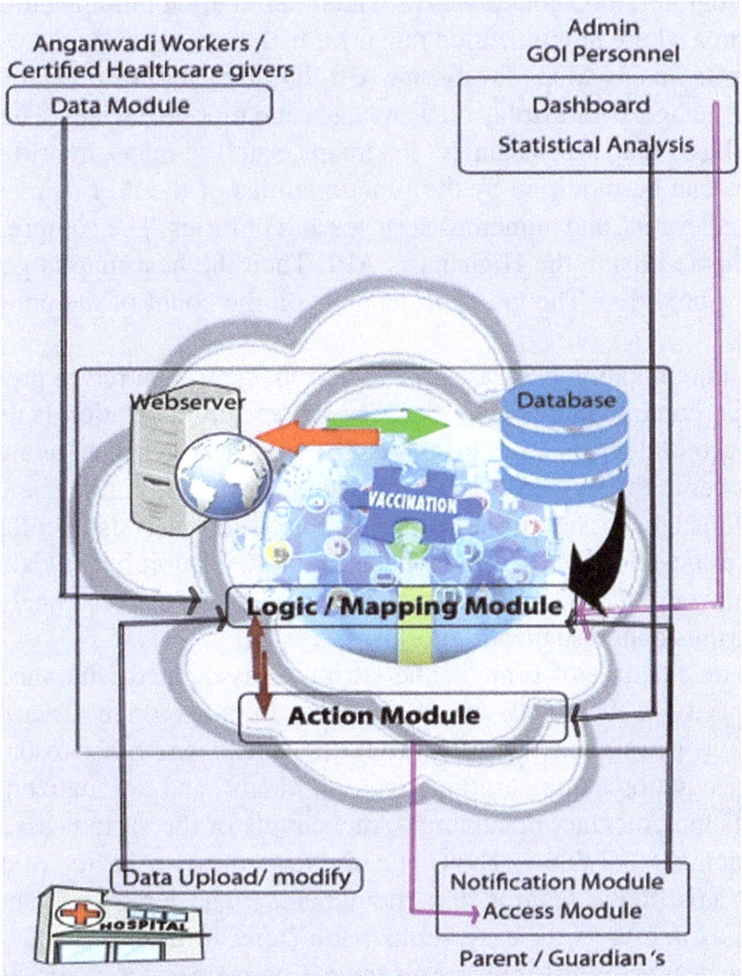

EXPERIMENTAL ASSESSMENT

In this section, the experimental assessment has been depicted. Numerous metrices too are used that can be used to interpret valuable data are also presented herein.

Observational Dataset and Results

India is witnessing the rapid adoption of healthcare analytics. Data emanating from numerous sources such as patient's medical history, surveys, complaint registers, and care assessment records can be used to analyze and provide better service. Collated data can be more useful when presented in a good application system. Such collation has been performed and its homepage is designed.

Further, based on the aggregation of the data, when queries are fired, heat map depiction can be done. The heat map gives us information about the spread of immunization in the world or any geographical region. The color code is provided based upon immunization protection rate. For example, the area where immunization rate is high, that area is assigned with red color. This has been implemented using Maps JavaScript API. It allows for customization of maps as per the content and the imagery for display on web pages and mobile devices. The Maps JavaScript API features four basic map types namely, roadmaps, satellite maps, hybrid maps, and terrain maps. These maps can be modified by the functionalities of the API using layers and styles, various controls and events, and numerous services and libraries. The comprehension functions have been implemented using the Highcharts API. Then the heat map is generated based on the gradient values provided. The gradient depends on the count of the entities chosen based on the query.

As the rate of immunization decreases, the color changes from red to green. With the help of heat map we can come to know about the areas where immunization is needed, so the rate of immunization can be increased in those areas. The data were taken as input from Healthcare personnel, either in *.CSV file or as an individual, row-wise entry. The interconnection is included in Supplementary. The format of the data used for analysis is collated from various datasets such as https://catalog.data.gov/dataset?tags=immunization, https://data.unicef.org/topic/child-health/immunization/. The synthetic data was used to evaluate and analyze the dashboard formation, and various data visualization forms.

Table 1 shows an example of some of the attributes associated with vaccination and their analysis. The disparity in the counts of vaccination can happen due to various reasons such as vaccine hesitancy, people moving away from their areas, and other reasons. These lead to breakage in the vaccination administration. Such problems can be visualized by depictions, as shown in table 2 (supplementary document). An example of the various assessments includes the following depictions in Table 1. The first row shows the distribution of count of boys and girls vaccinated in a particular year for 10 particular areas. The depiction is shown as individual pie charts as well as line plots for easy comparison (refer to table 2 in supplementary document). Further, the year-wise distribution of vaccination records for a particular area pin-code can also be found. A graph depicting number of people immunized v/s year with number of people immunized on y-axis and year on x-axis is also included. The data on y-axis is taken at an interval of 100 units and that of x-axis is at an interval of 1 unit. It reports the number of people immunized every year and the rate of immunization by looking at the trend of the past years, the graph will also help in predicting the number of people who will be immunized in the future. Visualization for spread across area was also demonstrated. The analysis result can also be depicted in terms of values such as Mean, Median, Mode, and others. Such results can be used to understand the acceptance of the immunization drive across areas and understand the spread of vaccine hesitancy. These visualizations can then help in formulating protocols and measures for not only improving the drive acceptance but also act as zones for quick responses in cases of emergencies.

Such analysis can help in understanding not only the vaccine-hesitancy but also the spread of any side-effects of a particular vaccine.

Table 1. Example of attributes associated to analyze side-effects and its spread for a particular vaccine

Health-care Personnel	Child's Govt. Issued ID	Name	Phone No.	Date of Birth	Gender	Area Pincode	Vaccine Effect	Symptoms
1969_36520	835548199222	Keya	9761662657	8-26-2016	Female	201206	5	seizure
1977_98478	612286585615	Vedika	9802061899	9-18-2016	Female	245101	0	
1964_23548	981510566297	Eva	9825345076	10-19-2001	Male	201009	0	
1969_36520	473981446028	Hrishita	9332533787	11-23-2010	Male	245101	5	seizure
1965_36511	450851002445	Navya	9604191370	4-23-2005	Female	245208	4	extreme drowsiness
1972_26450	704265401293	Vihaan	9966709609	10-21-2008	Male	201009	1	mild fever, redness at injection site
1965_36511	276151997629	Pranay	9806428520	11-15-2008	Female	245304	1	mild fever, redness at injection site
1977_10025	579927435477	Sana	9733690958	7-13-2001	Male	245208	0	
1972_26450	284396947796	Pihu	9228048459	2-15-2016	Female	201206	0	
1972_26450	714927902983	Neysa	9568395815	3-21-2003	Male	245101	2	fainting
1964_23548	412076491663	Arnav	9899171958	5-6-2006	Female	245201	0	
1975_13207	274310648397	Aayush	9391477959	12-19-2007	Female	245201	0	
1972_26450	959323526461	Harikiran	9939649303	1-16-2014	Female	201206	2	fainting
1964_23548	456917075521	Darshit	9542193072	11-8-2010	Male	245201	1	mild fever, redness at injection site
1975_13207	205778160211	Dhruv	9099231516	7-28-2001	Male	201009	3	high fever
1972_26450	984071898311	Ranbir	9919425921	1-5-2002	Male	245205	1	mild fever, redness at injection site
1969_36520	703125222217	Shray	9221709046	1-15-2014	Male	201009	1	mild fever, redness at injection site

Regression analysis is a standard tool to establish a relationship between two entities. In this case, we have used it to analyze the effect of vaccine hesitancy between outbreak of an epidemic that could have been controlled by vaccination drives. Poisson regression was calculated area-pincode zone-wise to present the effect of vaccine hesitancy. The study duration was assumed to be a block of 5 years. Except for a few outliers the Poisson regression gave a good prediction mechanism. This is shown the last row of Figure 3.

Figure 3. Prediction of observed data vs. predicted data using Poisson Regression

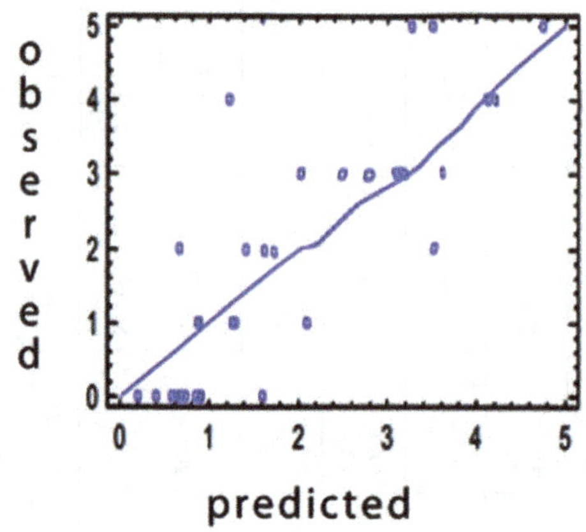

Further, based on the aggregation of the data, when queries are fired, heat map depiction can be done. The heat map in Figure 4 gives us the information about the spread of immunization in the world or any geographical region. The colour code is provided based upon immunization protection rate. For example, the area where immunization rate is high, that area is assigned with red colour. This has been implemented using Maps JavaScript API. It allows for customization of maps as per the content and the imagery for display on web pages and mobile devices. The Maps JavaScript API features four basic map types namely, roadmaps, satellite maps, hybrid maps, and terrain maps. These maps can be modified by the functionalities of the API using layers and styles, various controls and events, and numerous services and libraries. For understanding various other statistics, the visualization of the queries can be easily understood. The comprehension functions have been implemented using the Highcharts API. This API is a charting library that was used in our proposed work. By using this library API in proposed work, renders the interaction to be much uncomplicated between the user and admin with the site. The charts/maps can resize itself according to the screen size of device i.e., they are mobile optimized. The API is basically a scalable vector graphics based API. Its other features include documentation, very advanced responsiveness and accessibility support. Initially a map function is called with respect to the specified longitude and latitude values. Then the heat map is generated based on the gradient values provided. The gradient depends of the count of the entities chosen based on the query.

Figure 4. Graph to display increase in immunization

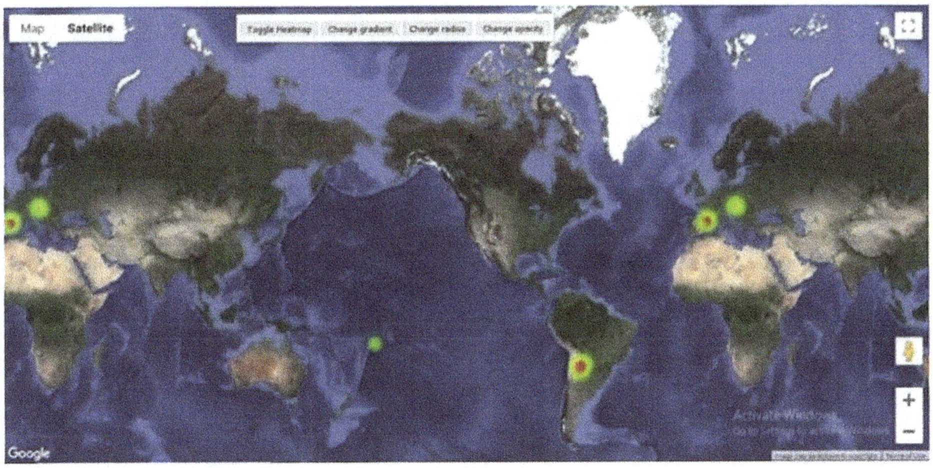

As the rate of immunization decreases, the colour changes from red to green. With the help of heat map we can come to know about the areas where immunization is needed, so the rate of immunization can be increased in those areas. The data taken as input from the Heathcare personnel as either CSV file or as an individual entry. The interconnection is depicted as shown below, in Figure 5.

Figure 5. Relationship between the various entities

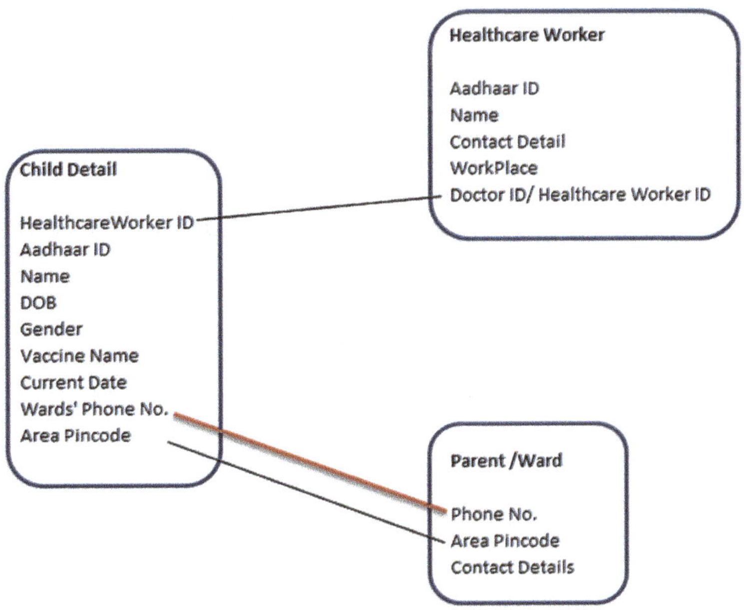

An example of the various assessments includes the following depictions in Figure 6, Figure 7, Figure 8, and Figure 9.

Figure 6. Distribution of Boys and Girls for various areas for a particular year

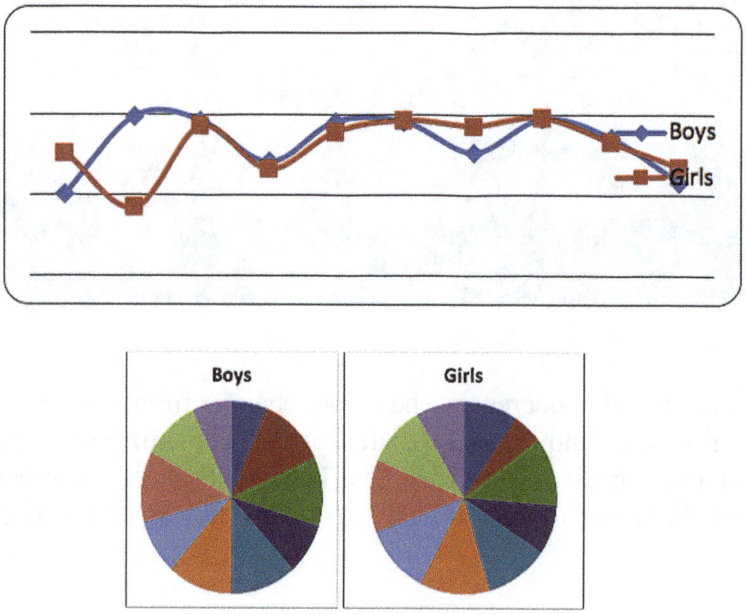

The figure shown above, figure 6, displays the distribution of count of boys and girls vaccinated in a particular year for 10 particular areas. The depiction is shown as individual pie charts as well as line plots for easy comparison. Further, year wise distribution of vaccination records for a particular area pin-code can also be found, as shown in Figure 7.

Figure 7. Year-wise Vaccination of children for an Area given by pincode (eg: 201001)

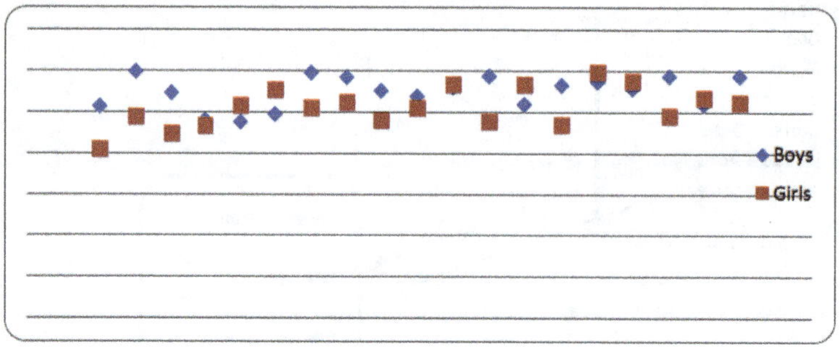

The disparity in the counts of vaccination can happen due to various reasons such has vaccine hesitancy, people moving away from their areas, and other reasons. These lead to breakage in the vaccination administration. Such problems can be visualized by depictions, as shown in Figure 8.

Figure 8. Comparison of children who have been vaccinated as compared to who have not been vaccinated

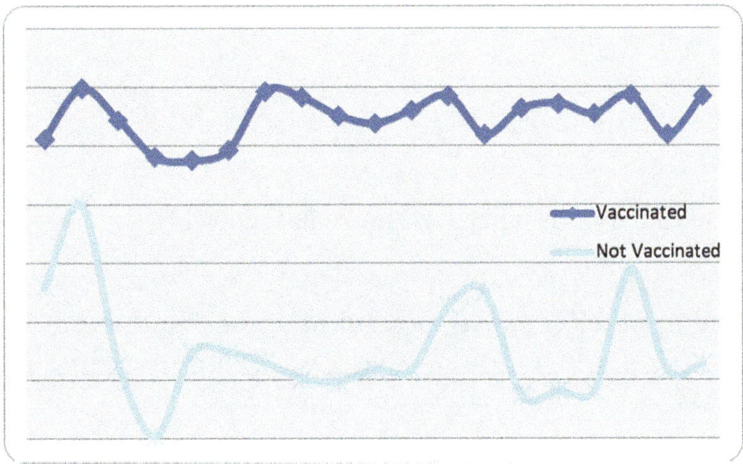

The graph in Figure 9 is of number of people immunized v/s year with number of people immunized on y-axis and year on x-axis. The data on y-axis is taken at an interval of 100 units and that of x-axis is at an interval of 1 unit. It reports the number of people immunized every year and the rate of immunization by looking at the trend of the past years, the graph will also help in predicting the number of people who will be immunized in the future.

Figure 9. Graph to display increase in immunization usage across a duration of almost 6 decades

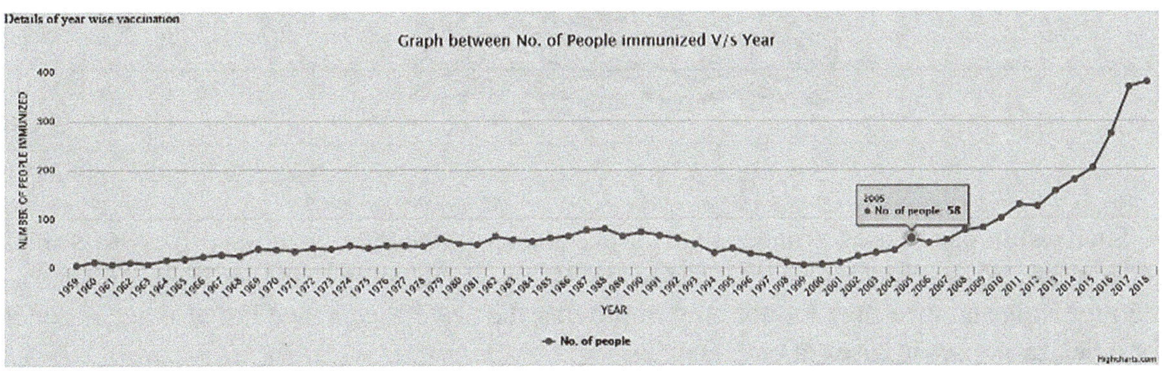

The analysis result can also be depicted in terms of values such as Mean, Median, Mode, and others. One such depiction is shown in Figure 10.

Figure 10. Statistical Analysis Example

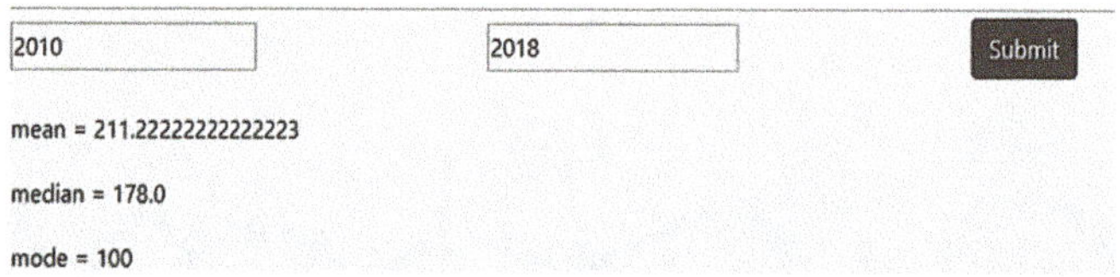

Across area spread can also visualized as shown in Figure 11.

Figure 11. Depiction of the spread of various vaccinations across areas (vertical lines depicting areas)

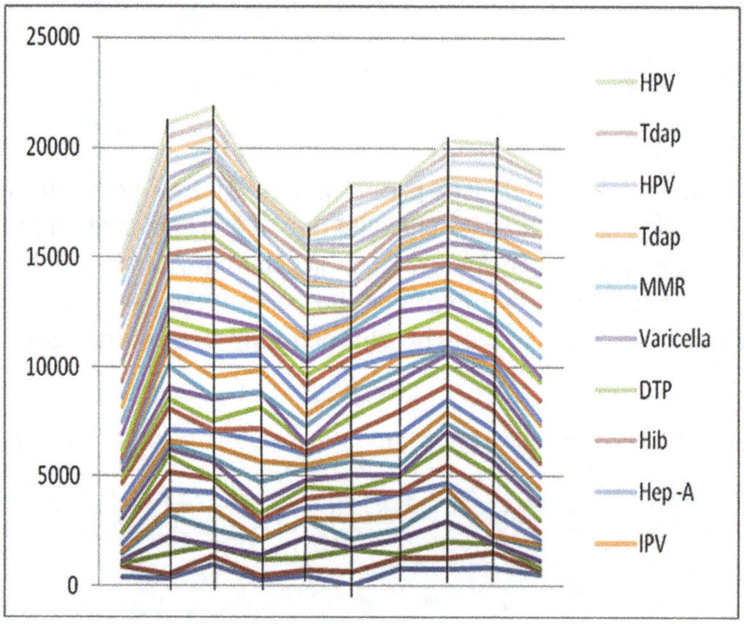

Such results can be used to understand the acceptance of the immunization drive across areas and understand the spread of vaccine hesitancy. These visualizations can then help in formulating protocols and measures for not only improving the drive acceptance but also act as zones for quick responses in cases of emergencies.

CONCLUSION AND FUTURE STUDY

Children are the future of the nation. For India to be strong, our next generation must be healthy too. Digital India has grown on many fronts. Health and wellness is a basic need of any human being. Children, especially newborns and toddlers are prone to high number of infections, many of which can be controlled by proper and timely vaccination. Hence, vaccination drives are so important. This work aims to present with a system that not only helps parents by reminding them of proper and timely vaccinations, as decided by the Immunization Association of India but also collates the immunization data to present usable demographics for timely interventions, as may be necessary. Smart healthcare, including common platform to store and retrieve the immunization records, allows for easy diagnosis and remedy to happen. Such a system can help in retaining the health perspective for kids, easy storage and retrieval, quick remedial measures to contain the spread of vaccine-preventable diseases and reduction in child mortality. In addition, the system is also able to perform statistical analysis on the collected and simulated data to find mean, median, mode, variance and standard deviation to predict immunization spread among different regions and detect any possible epidemic. Measuring the relationship between vaccine-hesitancy and outbreaks due to lack of immunization was also performed by regression analysis. An email-based remembering system too is setup which would send automated (no-reply) emails to parent's registered email ids.

Further, the system also implements building a referral program, so that a user can refer this program to the close relatives and friends. The graph-based relationship depicts the spread of immunization and its importance is also implemented in this work. The whole idea is to integrate network sciences principles to improve vaccination coverage in given social network. For this purpose, an automated email is sent to the referred person to get immunized them immunized and automatically update their medical records in this smart healthcare system.

CONFLICT OF INTEREST

On behalf of all authors, the corresponding author states that there is no conflict of interest.

REFERENCES

Atkinson, K. M., Westeinde, J., Ducharme, R., Wilson, S. E., Deeks, S. L., Crowcroft, N., & Wilson, K. (2016). Can mobile technologies improve on-time vaccination? A study piloting maternal use of ImmunizeCA, a Pan-Canadian immunization app. *Human Vaccines & Immunotherapeutics*, *12*(10), 2654–2661. doi:10.1080/21645515.2016.1194146 PMID:27322109

Chen, H. M., Liou, Y. Z., Chen, S. Y., & Li, J. S. (2013, June). Design of mobile healthcare service with health records format evaluation. In *2013 IEEE International Symposium on Consumer Electronics (ISCE)* (pp. 257-258). IEEE. 10.1109/ISCE.2013.6570215

Doherty, M., Buchy, P., Standaert, B., Giaquinto, C., & Prado-Cohrs, D. (2016). Vaccine impact: Benefits for human health. *Vaccine*, *34*(52), 6707–6714. doi:10.1016/j.vaccine.2016.10.025 PMID:27773475

Hardt, K., Bonanni, P., King, S., Santos, J. I., El-Hodhod, M., Zimet, G. D., & Preiss, S. (2016). Vaccine strategies: Optimising outcomes. *Vaccine*, *34*(52), 6691–6699. doi:10.1016/j.vaccine.2016.10.078 PMID:27887796

Healthcare in India. (n.d.). Available: https://en.wikipedia.org/wiki/Healthcare_in_India

Jarrett, C., Wilson, R., O'Leary, M., Eckersberger, E., & Larson, H. J. (2015). Strategies for addressing vaccine hesitancy–A systematic review. *Vaccine*, *33*(34), 4180–4190. doi:10.1016/j.vaccine.2015.04.040 PMID:25896377

Kumari, S., Haripriya, A., Aruna, A., Vidya, D. S., & Nithy, M. N. (2017). Immunize—Baby steps for smart healthcare: Smart solutions to child vaccination. In *2017 International Conference on Innovations in Green Energy and Healthcare Technologies (IGEHT)* (pp. 1-4). IEEE. 10.1109/IGEHT.2017.8094048

Lauridsen, J., & Pradhan, J. (2011). Socio-economic inequality of immunization coverage in India. *Health Economics Review*, *1*(1), 11. doi:10.1186/2191-1991-1-11 PMID:22828353

Pan, Y., Zhang, M., Chen, Z., Zhou, M., & Zhang, Z. (2016, June). An ARIMA based model for forecasting the patient number of epidemic disease. In *Service Systems and Service Management (ICSSSM), 2016 13th International Conference on* (pp. 1-4). IEEE.

Sahu, D., Pradhan, J., Jayachandran, V., & Khan, N. (2010). Why immunization coverage fails to catch up in India? A community-based analysis. *Child: Care, Health and Development*, *36*(3), 332–339. doi:10.1111/j.1365-2214.2009.01003.x PMID:19735269

Thacker, N., & Shendurnikar, N. (2004). Current status of polio eradication and future prospects. *Indian Journal of Pediatrics*, *71*(3), 241–245. doi:10.1007/BF02724277 PMID:15080411

Tomori, O. (2011). From smallpox eradication to the future of global health: Innovations, application and lessons for future eradication and control initiatives. *Vaccine*, *29*, D145–D148. doi:10.1016/j.vaccine.2011.09.003 PMID:22185830

UNICEF's strategy for health (2016-2030). (n.d.). Available: https://www.unicef.org/health

Vaccine India. (n.d.). Available: https://www.vaccineindia.org/

Wilson, K., Atkinson, K. M., & Westeinde, J. (2015). Apps for immunization: Leveraging mobile devices to place the individual at the center of care. *Human Vaccines & Immunotherapeutics*, *11*(10), 2395–2399. doi:10.1080/21645515.2015.1057362 PMID:26110351

World Health Organization (WHO). (n.d.). Available: http://www.who.int

Yahmed, M A B., Bounenni, M. A., Chelly, Z., & Jlassi, A. (2013, April). A new mobile health application for an ubiquitous information system. In *6th Joint IFIP Wireless and Mobile Networking Conference (WMNC)* (pp. 1-4). IEEE.

Chapter 5
Disease Interactome:
An Assessment Case Study Based on Analysis and Measures to Predict Secondary Diseases

Suma Dawn
Jaypee Institute of Information Technology, India

Nidhi Jain
Jaypee Institute of Information Technology, India

Tulika Gangwar
Jaypee Institute of Information Technology, India

ABSTRACT

The disease interactome is a network of genes that are related to each other through some attributes. These genes, being part of various diseases, show a high correlation among many diseases. Genes being a major part of the interactome thus can be used to determine the relationship between various diseases, their symptoms, clinical similarity, and co-morbidity. Subgraphs and similarity factors such as Jaccardian distance, cosine similarities, and others have been exploited to calculate the relationship between two or more diseases. Many diseases that did not show much resemblance on the basis of gene similarity or symptom similarity were seen to be closely related according to network interactome. The quantitative analysis between disease-disease was also done. Clustering algorithms like hierarchical clustering involving single, complete, and average linkage were applied to get a visual representation in the form of a dendrogram. Thus, disease-disease interactome was created, analyzed for finding related secondary diseases, and their basic nature was understood.

DOI: 10.4018/978-1-7998-4414-3.ch005

INTRODUCTION

A disease network interactome can be explained to be a network of genes interrelated to each other through some attribute, in our case, there are seven attributes namely regulatory, binary, literature, metabolic, kinase, and complexes and signaling. Any kind of relationship between any two genes leads to an addition of edge in the network and thus the increase in the completion of the interactome. Ongoing research is being sought and promoted aggressively, however, due to the incompleteness of the interactome and limited knowledge of disease-gene association prediction mapping of available data is challenging.

The disease-gene network modules of each disease are interrelated to each other in the form of subgraphs and thus have certain distance factor associated to them which can be exploited to calculate the mathematical relationship between two or more diseases. Mathematical conditions to identify the similarity between any two diseases on the basis of network interactome using shortest distance thus can be determined. Measures such as Jaccardian distance, cosine similarities, amongst others, have been used to determine the similarity between disease-gene associations. A prediction can also be made as to which diseases are strongly correlated and thus are likely to happen along with a primary disease. A quantitative comparative study of disease similarity or dissimilarity can thus be achieved along with the classification of similar or dissimilar diseases. Furthermore, the diseases can be clustered into groups using hierarchical clustering and visual representation in the form of plots has also been prepared. The interactome comprising of 13460 genes and 141296 connections have also been plotted.

The disease interactome is a network of genes which are related to each other through some attribute. These genes, being part of various diseases, show a high correlation among the diseases. Thus, the purpose of the project is to understand the gene-gene interactome and find a disease – disease relationship so as to define the quantified relationship between any two pair of diseases and to predict the secondary disease associated to the given primary disease which is much likely to happen together. Thus, the main objectives of the project are to

- Quantify the similarity between the diseases.
- Find distance measures between all diseases and the most similar secondary disease which is much likely to happen along with the primary one.
- Plot a disease-disease interactome.
- Determine distance matrix between diseases on the basis of network separation which can be further used for research work.
- Cluster diseases on the basis of the distance matrix thus received.
- Use the dataset prepared to calculate a distance matrix representing number of mutations required by a gene to convert into another gene.
- Plot a mutation path between these genes.

Based on experimental results, it was found that there is a close relationship between diseases that could be determined using network-based distances and similarity measures. Many diseases that did not show much resemblance on the basis of gene similarity or symptom similarity were seen to be closely related according to network interactome. Thus a prediction could be done as to whether the diseases are interrelated or not and if they are what is the extent to which they are related. Comorbidity could even be predicted and a similarity matrix could thus be calculated. Clustering can also be implemented on the basis of the similarity calculated above.

To quantify the similarity between the diseases, network-based distance measures such as Jaccard distance, Cosine Similarity, and Relative Risk Ratio were applied. A distance matrix was then made for all diseases available in the dataset signifying the similarity between the diseases on the basis of these mentioned methods. The related secondary diseases were determined with the help of similarity matrices. The disease exhibiting minimum distance or maximum similarity can be inferred to be the secondary disease. Further, the distance matrix so calculated is also used to implement hierarchical clustering algorithms like single linkage, complete linkage, and average linkage. The complexity to calculate the network-based similarity between the diseases was reduced from n^4 to n^2 by applying the concept of dynamic programming's memorization method.

LITERATURE SURVEY AND CURRENT STATE OF THE ART

Diseases cause a lot of imbalance in the host body and hence a single disease can be an invitation to other diseases too. In this section, we have summarized some of the related papers and tried to present the current state of the art in this dome of disease-disease interactome and various relationships thereafter.

Authors Menche et al., have proposed that according to the disease module hypothesis the cellular components associated with a disease segregated in the same neighbourhood of the human interactome, the map of biologically relevant molecular interactions (Menche et al., 2015). The paper derives mathematical conditions for the identifiability of disease modules and shows that the network-based location of each disease module determines its pathobiological relationship to other diseases. In (Ghiassian et al., 2015) authors Ghiassian, Mench, and Barabási have discussed that protein network can be viewed as maps by which diseases can be identified with localized perturbation within a certain neighbourhood. In this paper, they propose a method to find the disease module with a particular phenotype. In the paper by authors Caldera, Buphamalai and Jorg (Caldera et al., 2017), there is a map which includes the complex behaviour of interacting molecules. This interactome can be interpreted as a map and human diseases. This paper shows network-based approaches that can help in finding the specific neighbourhood perturbation in a certain disease. Authors Akram and Liao (Akram & Liao, 2017) have shown a method to predict common genes with a disease pair and the identification of common genes associated with diseases can be critical in understanding their pathobiological mechanism. Searching for missing common genes is formulated by minimizing network-based module separation by mapping genes associated with genes on to interactome. The paper by Xim Gulbachce and Yu (Wang et al., 2011) reviews recent, state of the art, network-based methods used for prioritizing disease genes as well as unravelling the molecular basis of human diseases. Yu, et al., (Yu et al., 2016) have discussed a new method to predict the associations between drugs and diseases. The method is based on a module distance, which is originally proposed to calculate distances between modules in the incomplete human interactome. Sharma et al., (Sharma et al., 2013) proposed a network-based analysis of GWAS data to provide novel candidate genes for lipid-lipoprotein traits. Observations built the basis for a large collection of computational approaches to find previously unknown genes associated with certain diseases. In their paper, Das et al (Das et al., 2014) explored mechanisms of human diseases based on certain structurally resolved protein interactome networks. This includes the study of the molecular basis of human disease. Functional interaction patterns in protein-protein interaction networks were discussed by Turunalp and Can (Turanalp & Can, 2008). The goal in this study was not only to discover novel complexes or pathways, which is studied extensively by many researchers but also try to discover recurring functional interaction patterns to understand whether such patterns are reused in different contexts in a PPI network. The importance of an interactome and its study was shown in (Vidal et al., 2011). Although an interactome usually used for protein-protein interactions, they may also refer to metabolic networks or gene-regulatory networks. Drugs interact with different molecular targets to exert their effect. Interactome maintenance is another tedious task as shown by authors Luz Garcia-Alonso et al., in (Garcia Alonso et al., 2014). They have also proposed several hypotheses to explain high mutational load too. Mapping and interpreting protein-protein interaction networks were worked upon by Lage as shown in (Lage, 2014).

Usage of Jaccard coefficient values for finding keyword-based similarity was discussed by Niwattanakul et al., (Niwattanakul et al., 2013). This helped in formulating the similarity measures to facilitate researchers in accessing the required results promptly. Usage of Cosine similarity was discussed by author Usharani (Usharani & Iyakutti, 2013). Relative risk calculations and its usage were shown by Tenny and Bhimji in (Strauss et al., 1991). Nguyen and Lió (Nguyen & Lió, 2009) discussed various similarity measures between gene expression profiles including the Bayesian method. The measure based on implicit semantic similarity was discussed by Turanalp and Can in (Mathur & Dinakarpandian, 2012). To find a similarity between diseases, associations are used to find pairs of similar diseases from a different perspective as shown by Cheng et al., (Cheng et al., 2014). Machine learning methods have been used in identifying disease genes as depicted by Asif et al., in (Asif et al., 2018). In this paper, the classifiers are trained on functional similarities to predict complex disease genes. Zhou and Fu too have used similar methods (Zhou & Fu, 2018) to understand the association between genes and diseases to help in the prevention, diagnosis, and therapy of diseases.

The main objective of collecting genes and categorizing into disease is to group them in clusters on the basis of their similarities and these similarities are found by Euclidean distance and are found by Pearson correlation. To predict function modules, grouping of genes to clusters becomes mandatory. By using this clustering further decision can be made. Protein-Protein Interaction (PPI) network is a network which represents physical interactions between pairs of proteins of an organism. Topological organization of PPI, evolution of PPI and identification and discovery of PPI is done by most researches. Identifying disease genes from a large collection of genomic data is very difficult so the machine learning methods are used. The classifiers are to predict complex disease genes. Functional similarity uses RWR to find the difference between disease and non-disease genes. So the relative risk is greater than 1 that that means that the other disease is more likely to occur if the exposure is possible. PPI consist all genomic biological processes. It is the mapping of most genes in humans and other organisms. For this exercise, OMIN database is used as it provides data for thousands of diseases with their relative risks to other diseases for homosapeins.

Because the interactome is so vast, the genes are viewed as nodes in the interactome and the edges between them represents the relation between them. That relation between nodes can represent any type of relationship i.e. functional or semantic similarity or high degree of relative risk. To understand prevention, therapy and diagnosis of diseases the understanding between the disease and genes is really important. But applying all the experimental methods are definitely too expensive. To compensate some approaches in bioinformatics, provide some candidate gene and disease linkage before applying methods on large scale database

IMPLEMENTATION REQUIREMENTS AND DATASETS

Since the disease genes are not randomly distributed in the network graph they tend to agglomerate in their near vicinity hence form a network subgraph referred to a network module. Mathematical conditions to identify the similarity between any two diseases on the basis of network interactome using shortest distance can thus be determined.

Software Requirements

The implementation has been done in Python 2.7.13

The libraries used are networkx, numpy, optparse, csv, and sys, matplot, pyplot, scikit.

Dataset

The databases are extracted from known sources of NCBI and GenBank. The extracted data are represented in the forms of *.tsv files and *.csv files.

- Database1: interactome.tsv: This file consists of 1,41,296 gene-gene interaction.
- Database2: DataS2_disease_genes: This file consists of 299 diseases with the list of genes associated with them.
- Database3: dict.csv: This file consists of the network-based separation of a disease with itself. (dAA). This file was generated as the output of the code calculatedistancematrixforentiredata.py.
- Database4: distancemattttrrriiixxx.csv: This file consists of the distance matrix between the diseases read from databae2. This file was generated as the output of the code calculatedistancematrixforentiredata.py.
- Database5: main_data.tsv: The file consists of gene ids and their genomic sequences. This file is read by edit.py . The genomic sequences were generated from the OMIM database. The dataset consists of 1100 genes ids with the length of genomic sequences equal to or greater than 30000 genomic sequence length.
- Database6: editdistanceresult.csv: This file consists of the mutation matrix. It was generated as the output of the code edit.py .
- Database7: mutation.tsv: This file consists of pairs of gene ids and the minimum number of mutations between them

Interactome

The interactome as defined above is a graph of genes where genes form the nodes and any relation between two genes is represented by an edge. The relationship between two genes can be regulatory, binary, literature, metabolic, kinase, complexes or signaling. This data is mentioned in the file interactome.tsv and is implemented using the network library in python.

Network-Based Distance Calculations

Each disease constitutes of various genes related to it. These genes are distributed all about the interactome. So, every disease itself forms a network of genes which leads to a distance factor between the genes of a particular disease itself (D_{AA}). For multiple diseases, there would be an intra-network separation between the genes of the disease (dxx) and an inter-network separation between the diseases themselves (D_{AB}). In order to determine how similar two diseases are one has to determine both the intra- as well as inter-network similarity which in the network interactome is given as $S_{AB}= D_{AB}-(D_{AA}+D_{AB})/2$ where Sab signifies the separation between two diseases A and B i.e. network based separation of a disease pair.

Calculation of Intra-Network Distance

In order to calculate distances between the genes of a particular disease, they have to find the shortest distance between all the genes. The mean of the minimum distance of each gene is the shortest closest distance within a disease (D_{AA}).

Calculation of Inter-Network Distance

In order to calculate the internetwork distance i.e. the distance between the genes or protein pair of the two diseases, they have to find the mean of the minimum shortest distance for each gene, belonging to both disease D_A and D_B. The mean of the minimum distance of every gene from every other gene of the other Disease is the distance between the two diseases (D_{AB}).

Calculation of Similarity

S_{AB} compares shortest distances between genes within each disease D_{AA} and D_{BB} to the shortest distance between the A-B disease pair. The set of genes (protein pairs) both genotypes and phenotypes associated to both diseases A and B have d_{AB} =0, therefore, S_{AB} for such disease pairs will be $-(D_{AA} + D_{BB})/2$ which means a negative value. Hence it can be deduced that the smaller the distance-based separation between two genes the similar would the two be. Thus a negative separation value indicates a higher similarity level.

The dataset consists of diseases along with their respective associated genes as different sets. Thus, to implement it two rows of the dataset DataS2_disease_genes are used as the two sets in order to determine the similarity measure.

Jaccard Distance

This similarity measure tells the quantitative similarity between two sets of data. The greater the value of the Jaccard coefficient the more is the similarity between the two sets. It is calculated as

$$J(A,B) = \frac{|A \cap B|}{|A \cup B|}$$

The dataset consists of diseases along with their respective associated genes as different sets. Thus, Jaccardian coefficient tells the similarity measure.

Cosine Similarity

Cosine similarity is a measure of similarity between two non-zero vectors of an inner product space that measures the cosine of the angle between them. The cosine of 0° is 1, and it is less than 1 for any angle in the interval (0,π]radians. Two vectors with the same orientation have a cosine similarity of 1; two vectors oriented at 90° relative to each other have a similarity of 0.

$$Similarity(A,B) = \frac{A.B}{|A|X|B|}$$

The dataset consists of diseases along with their respective associated genes as different sets. Thus, to implement it two rows of the dataset DataS2_disease_genes are used as the two sets in order to determine the similarity measure.

Relative Risk Ratio

Risk ratio (RR) or *relative risk* is the ratio of the probability of an outcome in an exposed group to the probability of an outcome in an unexposed group. Thus, it is the ratio of intersection of two sets to the difference of intersection from their union. It is given as RR = A.B/(A.B – 2* (AUB))

The dataset consists of diseases along with their respective associated genes as different sets. Thus, to implement it two rows of the dataset DataS2_disease_genes are used as the two sets in order to determine the similarity measure. Figure 1 depicts the network similarity measure.

Hierarchical Clustering

1. **Single Linkage:** Single linkage clustering is the type of hierarchical clustering. It is based on a bottom-up manner. It is done by combining two clusters that contain the closest pair of elements. And these elements do not belong to the same cluster. Hierarchical clustering considers every element as a single cluster. The result is often represented by dendrogram. The complexity of a single linkage is O(n^2). Such a dendogram of a single linkage cluster is depicted in Figure 2.

Figure 1. Example of Network Similarity Measures.

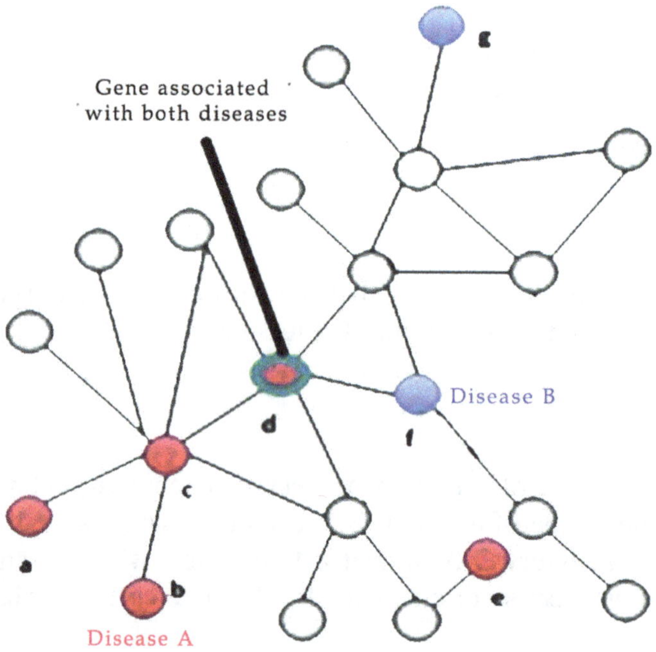

Figure 2. Dendogram of a Single Linkage Cluster.

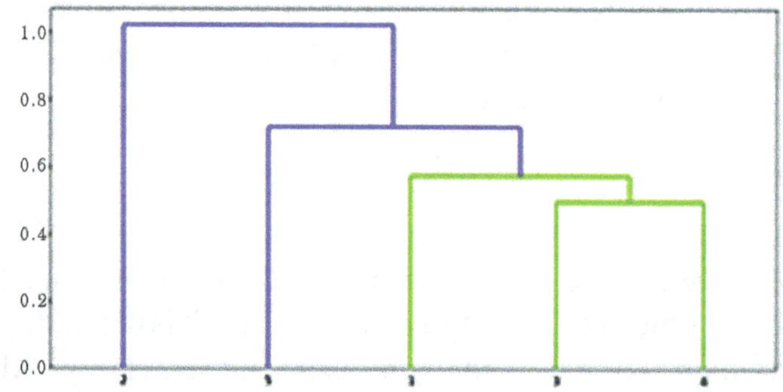

2. **Complete Linkage:** Complete linkage clustering is one of the agglomerative hierarchical clustering. In the beginning, every element is considered as a single cluster. Then it is combined into larger cluster and it is done till all the clusters end up into the same cluster.

This method is also known as farthest neighbour clustering. In genetics, it is defined as the state where two loci are s close that can be never virtually separated. The less is the distance between them, the less are the chances of separation between them. The dendogram depicting complete linkage is shown in figure 3.

Figure 3. Dendogram of a Complete Linkage.

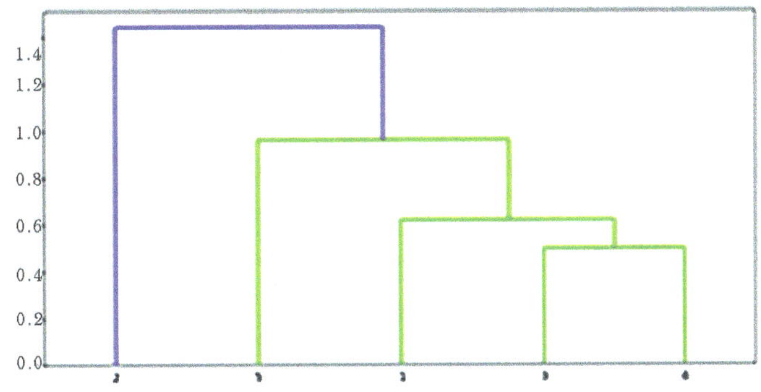

Reading data from DataS2_disease_genes.tsv into a 2D dictionary of was tested using the code written by the name read_data.py to check if the diseases are read in the correct manner in the dictionary and all the genes have been retrieved.

Network-Based Similarity is implemented using the **def read_network (network_file).** This method reads interactome.tsv and creates a network graph. Another method, **def get_pathlengths_for_single_set(G, gene_set)**, calculates the shortest distance between genes of a single disease and returns a 2D matrix of the shortest distance between all genes. The method **def get_pathlengths_for_two_sets(G,given_gene_set1,given_gene_set2)** calculates shortest distances between genes of two diseases and returns a 2D matrix of shortest distance between the genes of two diseases. **def calc_single_set_distance(G, gene_set)** method calculates mean of shortest distance corresponding to each gene of a single disease. For calculation of mean of the shortest distances of each gene pair for both the diseases, **def calc_set_pair_distances(G,given_gene_set1,given_gene_set2)** is used. The method **def calculate_sab(G, final, diseaseA, diseaseB, all_genes_in_network)** calls the above methods and receives values of D_{AB}, D_{AA} and D_{BB} to calculate the value of S_{AB} for each disease pair. **def calculate_distance_matrix(G, final, all_genes_in_network)** method calculates similarity matrix for all the diseases present in the dataset. The method **def calculate_daa_for_all_diseases(G,all_genes_in_network, final)** calculates dAA for all diseases and saves them in a file dict.csv. For plotting of graphs, **def plotmatrix(distance_matrix_disease)** is used. It plots the graph connecting diseases on the basis of the distance matrix calculated.

Various similarity measures are used to quantify the similarity between diseases. Jaccard similarity is calculated using the method **def jaccard_similarity_score(gene_list1,gene_list2)** that takes input of 2 disease details and finds the similarity. For Jaccard distance testing, the pseudo data set was made in order to test the working of Jaccard similarity which was consistent with the expected output. Cosine Similarity is calculated by the function **def get_cosine_similarity(gene_list1,gene_list2)**. Cosine distance testing is performed by using the pseudo data set was made in order to test the working of Cosine similarity which was consistent with the expected output. Relative Risk is defined by the function **def relative_risk(gene_list1, gene_list2)** for a pair of diseases. Relative Risk testing is performed on pseudo data set was made in order to test the working of relative risk which was consistent with the expected output. The dataset used was testing all three methods was done on jaccarddata.tsv

Similarity calculation for any two user-specified genes was tested using module mergetry. py which is a menu driven program for user to enter the diseases of their choices to get the similarity measure. This is depicted in table 1.

Table 1. Similarity values with respect to various parameters

Similarity Parameter	Value
Jacardian measure	0.222222222
Cosine measure	0.0571428571429
Relative Risk measures	O. 2S

Requirement and unit testing have been applied during implementation, to test the robustness of the system so designed. Testing of S_{AB} is also implemented. Two diseases namely PD and MS were stored in two different files and then network similarity was applied to it. The values calculated for D_{AA}, D_{AB}, D_{BB} were then used to check the value of S_{AB} which was consistent with the output received. This was done in the calculation.py module and is shown in Table 2. For calculating the mutation pathway, similarity between two genomic datasets is required which form the basis of the pathway. The algorithm is presented in Algorithm1.

```
Algorithm1: minEditDistance(s1, s2)
Input: s1, s2
Function:
1.         Calculate length of s1, s2
2.         If (length(s1) > length (s2))
Interchange (s1, s2)
3.         Dist = range(length(s1) +1)
4.         Loop (index2, char2 in enumerate(s2))
newDistance= [index2 + 1]
loop (index1, char1 in enumerate(s1))
                         if (char1 =char2)
                                 newDistances.append(distances[index1])
                         else
newDistances.append(1+ min(distances[index1], distances[index1+1], newDistanc-
es[-1]))
5.         Return distances[-1]
```

Table 2. Example of distance measure between two diseases

Disease A: Multiple Sclerosis Disease B: Peroxisomal Disorder
Measurement Parameters: No. of Genes: 69 D_{AA}: 1.85507246377 D_{BB}: 1.05 D_{AB}: 2.73033707865 S_{AB}:1.27780084677

IMPLEMENTATION AND RESULTS

The basic implementation summarizes the process and the modules that are used to depict the resultants are shown in Figure 4 and Figure 5 as module diagram and sequence diagram respectively.

Figure 4. Module Diagram

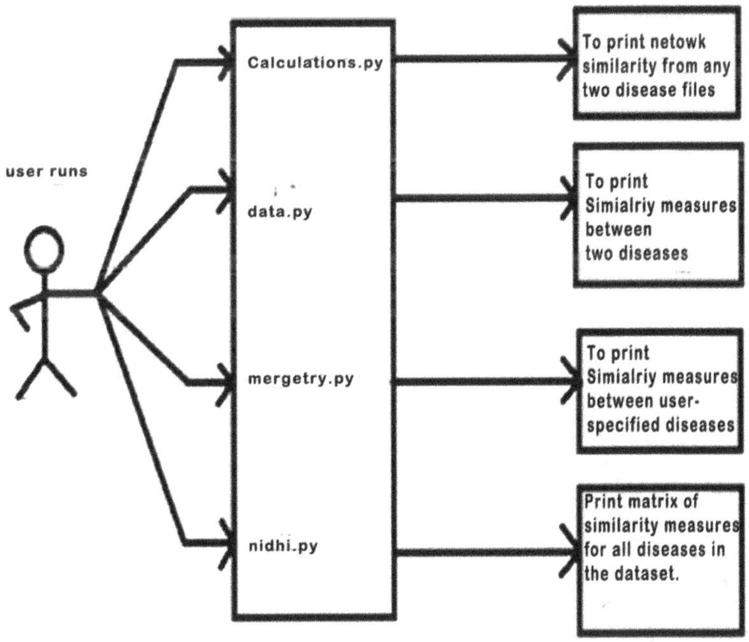

Many a times, there can be cases when there is no path between two pair of genes thus the shortest distance between the two cannot be determined which leads to an exception. Thus to handle these distances between such genes are not considered in the calculation of mean shortest value. The plotting of plotting interactome of the genes was performed. Pseudo data was made to test plotting data with nodes representing genes and edges representing a connection between them. An example of this is depicted in Figure 6.

Figure 5. Sequence Diagram

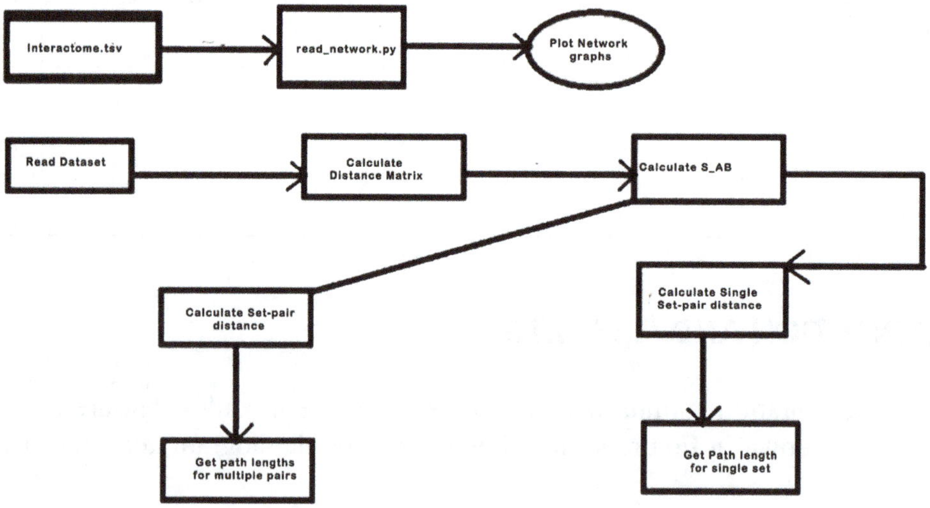

Figure 6. Example of the Graph Plot for Finding the Connection Between the Genes

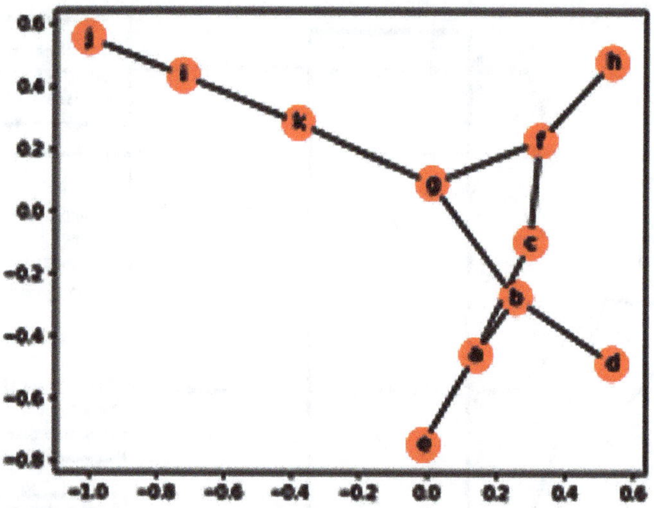

The earlier code implemented to calculate the distance matrix was calculating the distance matrix in time complexity of O(n^4). However, this could be reduced to O(n^2) by memoizing the repeating data to daa dictionary with the help of dynamic programming. The interactome, so obtained, can be plotted in the form of a graph with the help of matplotlib.pyplot and networkx library's method draw_networkx().The resultant of 'distancematrixforentiredata.py' is shown in Figure 7.

Figure 7. Resultant of 'distancematrixforentiredata.py'

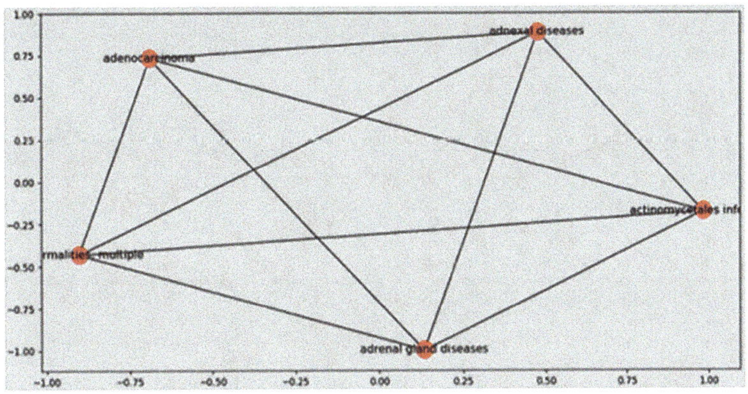

Plotting the Mutation Path

The dataset created consisting of gene ids and genomic sequences that helped in calculating the mutation distance between various genes corresponding to many diseases. The dimension of the mutation matrix thus created was 110 x 110. Each cell in the matrix represents the mutation distance between the gene ids with respect to its row and column. The minimum mutation distance corresponding to each gene id was calculated and this distance was further used to devise the mutation map. The plot of the interactome is shown in figure 8, with the red nodes being the genes and the edges representing a connection between the two diseases. The mutation map consists of nodes representing different gene ids and the edges representing the minimum number of mutations required to convert one gene id to another. A generic mutation path is depicted using figure 9.

Figure 8. Plot of the Interactome with the Red Nodes being the genes and the edges representing a connection between the two diseases

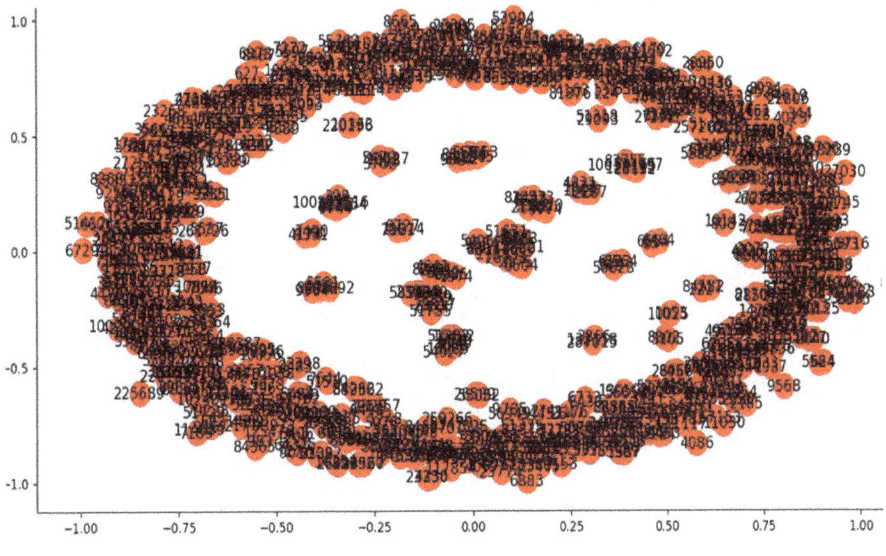

Figure 9. Mutation Path without Notations

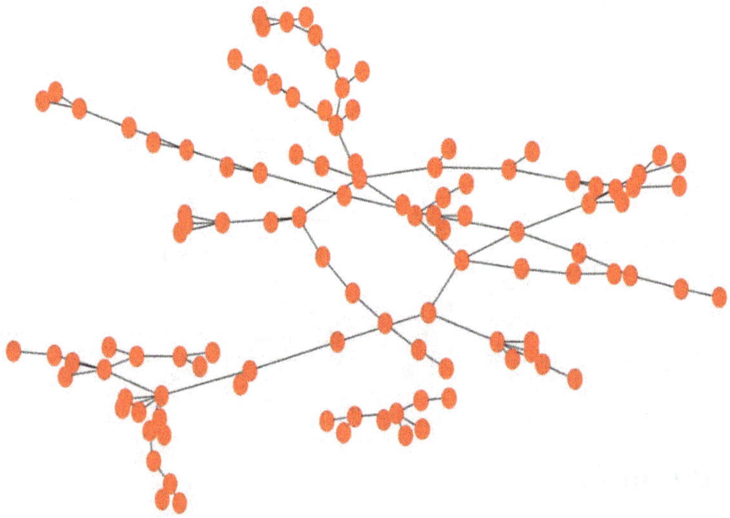

CONCLUSION AND FUTURE RESEARCH DIRECTIONS

Based on experimental results, it was found that there is a close relationship between diseases that could be determined using network-based distances and similarity measures. Many diseases that did not show much resemblance on the basis of gene similarity or symptom similarity were seen to be closely related according to network interactome

Further, a strong relationship can also be achieved quantitatively between multiple diseases using various similarity measures like network similarity based on shortest distance pair, Jaccard similarity, cosine similarity, and relative risk. We can also compare the diseases and analyze them to predict other diseases similar to them. Comorbidity i.e. secondary disease which is most likely to happen along with a primary disease because of strong similarity to it can also be predicted. Moreover, a comparison in the results of various similarity measures can also be done. Thus, it can be concluded from the results received that the closer two diseases are in the interactome the more are its chances to have a strong similarity quantitatively as well as qualitatively.

The genes were analyzed on the basis of their genomic sequences. During the analyses the mutation cost was calculated for each gene pair. The mutation cost for each gene pair was calculates with respect to all the other genes and the gene having minimum mutation cost was selected to be a part of the mutation path.

An application has been implemented that can tell different attributes related to a particular disease like number of genes, its localization in the network graph, quantitative separation between genes in the graph and genes of different diseases, its similarity to different disease on the basis of various algorithms, a comparative study between the results of different similarity measures and prediction of diseases which are highly similar to each other and are thus like to happen together. Further, calculates the similarity between the genes of the above used diseases to predict a mutation path.

FINANCIAL SUPPORT STATEMENT

The authors confirm that the project has not received any funding from any agencies.

COMPLIANCE WITH ANIMAL/HUMAN ETHICS GUIDELINES

The article does not require any human/animal subjects to acquire such approval.

REFERENCES

Akram, P., & Liao, L. (2017). Prediction of missing common genes for disease pairs using network based module separation on incomplete human interactome. *BMC Genomics*, *18*(10), 902. doi:10.118612864-017-4272-7 PMID:29244004

Asif, M., Martiniano, H. F., Vicente, A. M., & Couto, F. M. (2018). Identifying disease genes using machine learning and gene functional similarities, assessed through Gene Ontology. *PLoS One*, *13*(12), e0208626. doi:10.1371/journal.pone.0208626 PMID:30532199

Caldera, M., Buphamalai, P., Müller, F., & Menche, J. (2017). Interactome-based approaches to human disease. *Current Opinion in Systems Biology*, *3*, 88–94. doi:10.1016/j.coisb.2017.04.015

Cheng, L., Li, J., Ju, P., Peng, J., & Wang, Y. (2014). SemFunSim: A new method for measuring disease similarity by integrating semantic and gene functional association. *PLoS One*, *9*(6), e99415. doi:10.1371/journal.pone.0099415 PMID:24932637

Das, J., Fragoza, R., Lee, H. R., Cordero, N. A., Guo, Y., Meyer, M. J., & Yu, H. (2014). Exploring mechanisms of human disease through structurally resolved protein interactome networks. *Molecular BioSystems*, *10*(1), 9–17. doi:10.1039/C3MB70225A PMID:24096645

Garcia Alonso, L., Jiménez Almazán, J., Carbonell Caballero, J., Vela Boza, A., Santoyo López, J., Antiñolo, G., & Dopazo, J. (2014). The role of the interactome in the maintenance of deleterious variability in human populations. *Molecular Systems Biology*, *10*(9), 752. doi:10.15252/msb.20145222 PMID:25261458

Ghiassian, S. D., Menche, J., & Barabási, A. L. (2015). A DIseAse MOdule Detection (DIAMOnD) algorithm derived from a systematic analysis of connectivity patterns of disease proteins in the human interactome. *PLoS Computational Biology*, *11*(4), e1004120. doi:10.1371/journal.pcbi.1004120 PMID:25853560

Lage, K. (2014). Protein–protein interactions and genetic diseases: The interactome. *Biochimica et Biophysica Acta (BBA)-. Molecular Basis of Disease*, *1842*(10), 1971–1980. doi:10.1016/j.bbadis.2014.05.028 PMID:24892209

Mathur, S., & Dinakarpandian, D. (2012). Finding disease similarity based on implicit semantic similarity. *Journal of Biomedical Informatics*, *45*(2), 363–371. doi:10.1016/j.jbi.2011.11.017 PMID:22166490

Menche, J., Sharma, A., Kitsak, M., Ghiassian, S. D., Vidal, M., Loscalzo, J., & Barabási, A. L. (2015). Uncovering disease-disease relationships through the incomplete interactome. *Science*, *347*(6224), 1257601. doi:10.1126cience.1257601 PMID:25700523

Nguyen, V. A., & Lió, P. (2009, December). Measuring similarity between gene expression profiles: A Bayesian approach. *BMC Genomics*, *10*(3), S14. doi:10.1186/1471-2164-10-S3-S14 PMID:19958477

Niwattanakul, S., Singthongchai, J., Naenudorn, E., & Wanapu, S. (2013, March). Using of Jaccard coefficient for keywords similarity. In *Proceedings of the international multiconference of engineers and computer scientists* (*Vol. 1*, No. 6, pp. 380-384). Academic Press.

Sharma, A., Gulbahce, N., Pevzner, S. J., Menche, J., Ladenvall, C., Folkersen, L., & Barabasi, A. L. (2013). Network-based analysis of genome wide association data provides novel candidate genes for lipid and lipoprotein traits. *Molecular & Cellular Proteomics*, *12*(11), 3398–3408. doi:10.1074/mcp.M112.024851 PMID:23882023

Strauss, B. H., Serruys, P. W., de Scheerder, I. K., Tijssen, J. G., Bertrand, M. E., Puel, J., Meier, B., Kaufmann, U., Stauffer, J. C., & Rickards, A. F. (1991). Relative risk analysis of angiographic predictors of restenosis within the coronary Wallstent. *Circulation*, *84*(4), 1636–1643. doi:10.1161/01.CIR.84.4.1636 PMID:1914103

Turanalp, M. E., & Can, T. (2008). Discovering functional interaction patterns in protein-protein interaction networks. *BMC Bioinformatics*, *9*(1), 276. doi:10.1186/1471-2105-9-276 PMID:18547430

Usharani, J., & Iyakutti, K. (2013). A genetic algorithm based on cosine similarity for relevant document retrieval. *International Journal of Engineering Research & Technology (Ahmedabad)*, *2*(2), 1–13.

Vidal, M., Cusick, M. E., & Barabási, A. L. (2011). Interactome networks and human disease. *Cell*, *144*(6), 986–998. doi:10.1016/j.cell.2011.02.016 PMID:21414488

Wang, X., Gulbahce, N., & Yu, H. (2011). Network-based methods for human disease gene prediction. *Briefings in Functional Genomics*, *10*(5), 280–293. doi:10.1093/bfgp/elr024 PMID:21764832

Yu, L., Wang, B., Ma, X., & Gao, L. (2016). The extraction of drug-disease correlations based on module distance in incomplete human interactome. *BMC Systems Biology*, *10*(4), 111. doi:10.118612918-016-0364-2 PMID:28155709

Zhou, J., & Fu, B. Q. (2018). The research on gene-disease association based on text-mining of PubMed. *BMC Bioinformatics*, *19*(1), 37. doi:10.118612859-018-2048-y PMID:29415654

Chapter 6
Therapeutic Decision-Making Process:
An Anthropological Study on a Disaster-Prone Bangladeshi Village

Md. Musfikur Rahman
International Centre for Diarrhoeal Disease Research, Bangladesh

Md. Nasir Uddin
https://orcid.org/0000-0001-7422-5761
Prime Minister's Office, Bangladesh

ABSTRACT

Therapeutic decision making is crucial to address any health problems. Household livelihood assets had significant impact on therapeutic decision making in the study village. The researchers administered participant observation, in-depth interview, and FGD for data collection by using purposive sampling during November 2010 to June 2011. Among 250 households, the number of ill persons were 316, of which 297 received treatments from popular, folk, and professional sectors while the rest did not seek any options. The decision makers were varied for newborn, children, adolescent, adult, and aged people, and it depended on the cyclical issues of an illness episode.

INTRODUCTION

Decision-making is nothing but the cognitive course resulting in the assortment of a belief or a process of act among a number of possible options. Each decision-making course constructs a final choice that may or may not term as rapid action. It is the lessons of selecting and choosing different options based on the assessments and preferences of the decision maker. In the village Char Majhira illnesses were not only a therapeutic matter, but also a communal subject that was of concern to family members. As the family structure regulates decision making within

DOI: 10.4018/978-1-7998-4414-3.ch006

the household, it has important effects upon health care options. When the villagers recognized themselves as ill, they were acting a number of things. They were doing nothing. They were attempting to tackle the illness by themselves or with the family. They were talking to friends and relatives about what they should do. They have taken care from a number of different sources, including but not limited to physicians. Indeed, the study carried out in *Char* Majhira indicates that generally 90 to 92% of all illness episodes were never seen by a physician. Many of these illness episodes were treated within the family during the study period. The major alternative to the physician was self/family care, traditional or folk healers in the village. The researchers have found the following practices in the village as a decision-making process in relation to newborns, children, adolescents, adults and aged people.

The objective of the study was to discuss the therapeutic decision-making process of a disaster-prone village that is to investigate how socio-economic, geographic and other factors contribute to the health hazards of this disadvantage people. To achieve the objective of the study, the researchers talked about most common severe illness of the village, the number of ill people of the village and the healing decision making process of the village.

BACKGROUND OF THE STUDY

The research has adopted a framework for analysis and action to explore and improve access to health care in char people, in Bangladesh, namely *The Health Access Livelihood Framework.* The framework links social science and public health research with broader development approaches to improve health system development. Access becomes an issue once illness is recognized and treatment seeking is initiated. Five dimensions of access influence the course of the health-seeking process: Availability, Accessibility, Affordability, Adequacy, and Acceptability. What degree of access is reached along the five dimensions depends on the interplay between (a) the health care services and the broader policies, institutions, organizations, and processes (PIOP) that govern the services, and (b) the livelihood assets people can mobilize and combine in particular vulnerability contexts. Hence, access improves as health care services become better aligned with clients' needs and resources. Sick persons and caregivers seek help not only in health facilities or private practice, but also in drug shops and pharmacies as well as from healers representing a wide array of medical traditions. Access to these health care service providers is governed by cultural norms, policies, laws and regulations, which themselves are influenced by broader trends in society, global health policy, research, and development as a whole.

Whether people actually recognize an illness and seek treatment in drug shops or through other health care services depends to a large extent on their access to livelihood assets of the household, the community, and the wider society. These livelihood assets comprise human capital (local knowledge, education, skills), social capital (social networks and affiliations), natural capital (land, water, and livestock), physical capital (infrastructure, equipment, and means of transport) and financial capital (cash and credit). The availability of these assets is influenced by forces over which people have little control, for instance economy, politics or technology, climatic variability or shocks like floods, river erosion, draughts, armed conflicts or epidemics. Such factors may be referred to as their vulnerability context.

Figure 1. The Health Access Livelihood Framework.

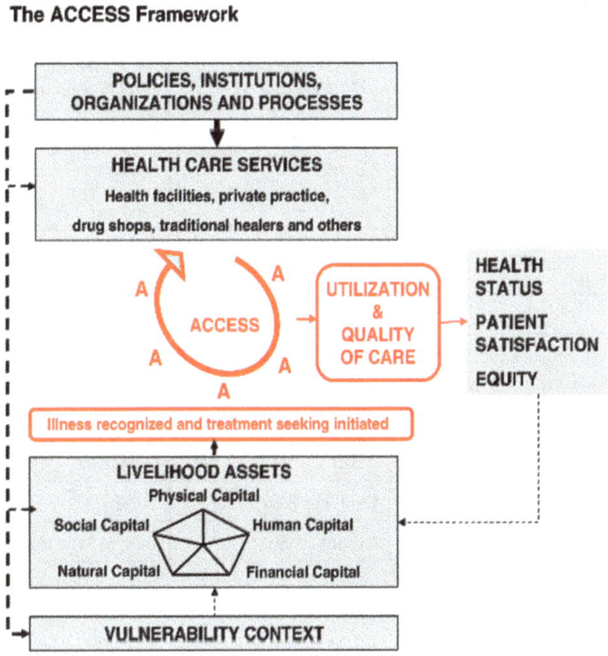

It was developed in the frame of the ACCESS Programme, which focuses on understanding and improving access to prompt and effective malaria treatment and care in rural Tanzania as an empirical case study (Brigit Obrist et al., 2007).

The qualitative research had conducted by using the both emic and etic approaches. The researchers administered participant observation, in-depth interview and FGD for data collection by using purposive sampling of 250 households during November 2010 to June 2011. The head and aged people of the households were considered as the key respondents. As a head and aged member of the family, they have adequate knowledge as well as vast experience regarding health problems. Char Majhira under Sariakandi Upazilla of Bogura district in Bangladesh had selected as the study area. Because, this village is frequently affected by the natural disaster like river erosion, flood in every year and it is a remote village of this Uapzilla.

FINDINGS

Most Common Illness of the Study Village

The study people had identified the following most common illness of their village based on severity ranking. The illnesses mentioned in here were reported symptoms or names of illnesses mentioned by the respondents themselves. The name of an illness mentioned was not validated by a physician. However, when labeling the Bengali terms or symptoms described by the participants by a medical name, a physician was consulted.

Table 1. Most common illness of the study village

Most Severe Illness					
Severity Ranking	**Newborn (1-6 Months)**	**Children (4-8 Years)**	**Adolescents (9-16 Years)**	**Adult (17-55 Years)**	**Aged (56+)**
1	Convulsion	Malnutrition	Malnutrition	Ulcer	Stroke
2	Pneumonia	Rickets	Gastric	Asthma	Paralysis
3	Jaundice	Pneumonia	Malaria	Diabetes	Asthma
4	Measles	Diarrhea	Typhoid	High Blood Pressure	Arthritis
5	Breathing Difficulty	Measles	Diarrhea	Arthritis	Memory Loss
6	Loose Motion	Breast Feeding Child Diarrhea	Tonsil Infection	Ear Infection	Ear Infection
7	Fever	Fever	Skin Illness	Gastric	Lower Back Pain
8	Skin Illness	Cold	Fever	Weakness	Toothache
9	Excessive Crying	Mouth ulcer	Growing Pain	Headache	Hearing Difficulty
10	Cold	Fungal Infection	Conjunctivitis	Fungal Infection	Blurry Vision

Source: Primary Data (2010-11)

Number of Ill People During the Study Period

Among 250 households, 219 had at least an illness person during the study period and rest did not have any problems. The numbers of ill persons were 316 of which 297 received treatments from different options while the rest did not seek any options. As to the table two among the ill persons 194 were females and 122 were males. The researchers have found that, among 316 sick persons adolescent people were in great number 123, among them males were 44 and females were 79, newborns were 27, among them males were 15 and females were 12, children were 49, among them males were 27 and females were 22, adult were 89, among them males were 26 and females were 63 and the elderly people were 28, among them males were10 and females were 18.Total numbers of ill persons of landless households were 153, among them males were 56 and females were 97. It is indicating that, the conditions of females were severe in the village and household's assets have a great impact on illness in this village.

Decision Makers for Newborns, Children and Adolescents Illness

The villagers explained that it was usually the mother only or the parents together who first noticed that there is something wrong with the family members especially for newborn, children and adolescents. In some family's other members, especially the grandmothers were also the ones to scrutinize first illness in the family members.

According to the native culture, older people are honored by all generations, particularly the younger, for their knowledge and expertise in life including how to construct decisions regarding the handling of illness. The Grandfather/Mother (*Dada/Dadi*) is the person who should be kept informed about all family related matters, including the health status of newborn, children and adolescents. The villagers said that the most important reason for contacting *Dada/Dadi* was to show them respect. They also attained in the decision-making process in terms of helping, either sharing experience or others. Still, just about every two-family said that they always contacted the *Dada/Dadi*when any one was ill.

Correspondingly, the majority of the parents said that they would begin treating the ailing members of the family with the medicines they themselves study were the most appropriate. Some of them discussed with other relatives, mainly uncle, brother, sister, father in law, mother in low and neighbors. The data on illness cases that mothers considered to be more serious is shown in the figure 2. On the other hand, uncle, brother, sister, father in law, mother in law and neighbors are the relatives with whom the mother communicated. Discussion in this circum-

Table 2. Number of households based ill persons during the study period

Landless			Small Peasant			Medium Peasant			Rich Peasant		
Newborn (1-6 moths)	Male	5	Newborn (1-6 moths)	Male	4	Newborn (1-6 moths)	Male	3	Newborn (1-6 moths)	Male	3
	Female	5		Female	3		Female	3		Female	1
Children (4-8 years)	Male	13	Children (4-8 years)	Male	8	Children (4-8 years)	Male	5	Children (4-8 years)	Male	1
	Female	9		Female	9		Female	3		Female	1
Adolescent (9-16 years)	Male	23	Adolescent (9-16 years)	Male	11	Adolescent (9-16 years)	Male	9	Adolescent (9-16 years)	Male	1
	Female	54		Female	17		Female	7		Female	1
Adult (17-55 years)	Male	11	Adult (17-55 years)	Male	9	Adult (17-55 years)	Male	6	Adult (17-55 years)	Male	0
	Female	23		Female	27		Female	11		Female	2
Aged 56+	Male	4	Aged 56+	Male	2	Aged 56+	Male	3	Aged 56+	Male	1
	Female	6		Female	7		Female	4		Female	1

Source: Primary Data (2010-11)

Figure 2. Person who was very much alert to the illness of newborn, children and adolescent

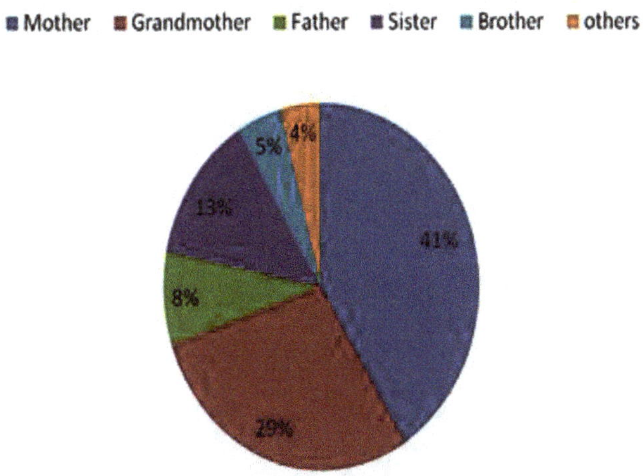

stance marks informal consultation rather than strict advice seeking. It also constitutes a verbal acknowledgement that the family member is ill.

Decision Makers for Adult Illness

In case of adult illness, the decision makers were varied based on the gender in the study village. For 26 adult male patients, 87% of the decisions were taken by patients' elder brothers, 10% by society leaders and the rest were taken by patient's fathers. The researcher observed that, wisdom and experience was the key determinants to select a decision maker among the villagers. On the other hand, consultation with the community leaders who possessed social dignity was another aspect of a decision maker in the village regarding adult illness.

Figure 3. Decision makers for adult (male) illness

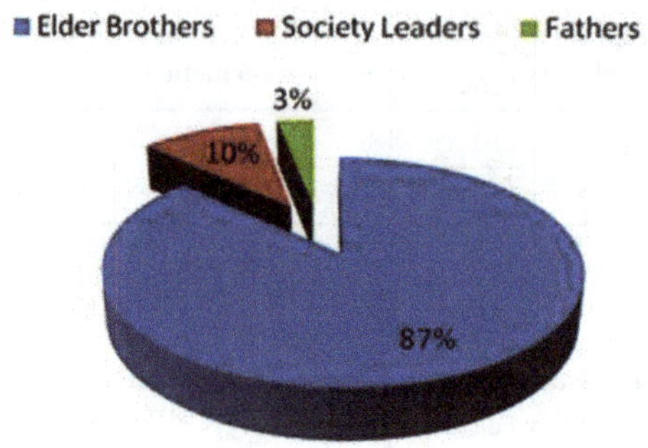

On the other hand, in case of adult 63 females, most of the decisions were taken by the mother in law as to the villagers. Husband has limited scope to take a decision in this case, because, most of the villagers believed that, they had specail knowledge on female illness.

Figure 4. Decision makers for adult (female) illness

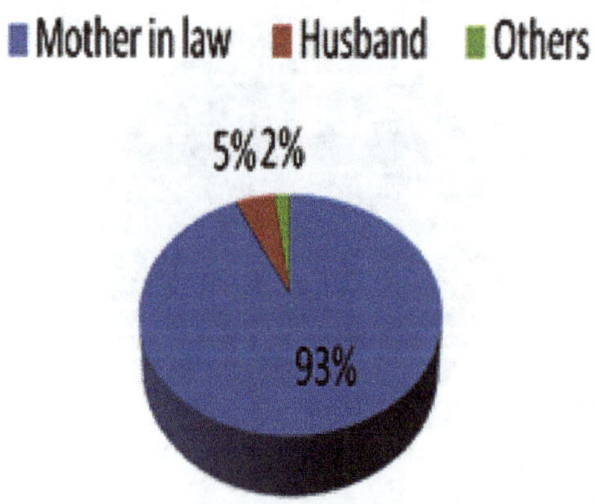

Decision Makers for Aged Illness

In the study village, most of the decisions regarding the elderly illness were taken by elder son. On the other hand, most aged people of the respective decent were playing an important role to take a decision in this regard who have distinctive knowledge regarding the illness.

Figure 5. Decision makers for aged illness

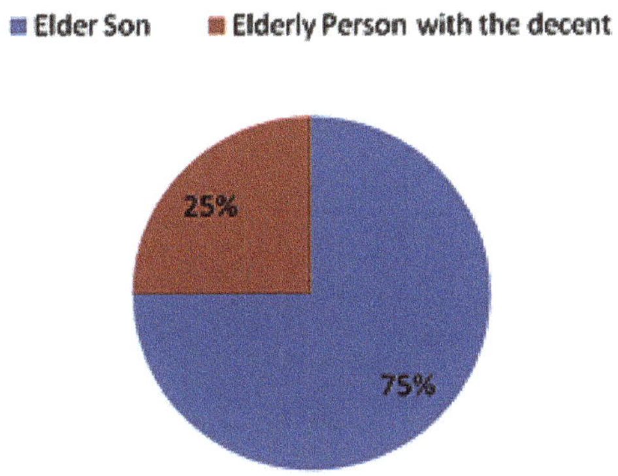

DECISION MAKING PHASE

Time of taking decisions in relation to the illness of study people was not so simple. The researchers have observed that it depended on the cyclical issues of an illness episode.

Expressing as Well as Dissemination of Illness Message to Family/ Community

It was the first step of taking decision for any illness, treatment of the study population as to the villagers. When the patients were expressing their view to the family members as well as other people of the community, then they were treated as illness, persons in case of adolescent, adult as well as aged people. Defining oneself as being ill usually follows a number of subjective experiences, including (Helman, 1994) as to the villagers:

1. Perceived changes in the bodily appearance, such as loss of weight, changes in skin color or hair falling out.
2. Changes in regular bodily functions, such as urinary frequency, heavy menstrual periods, irregular heartbeats.
3. Unusual bodily emissions, such as blood in the urine, sputum or stools.
4. Changes in function of limbs, such as paralysis, clumsiness or tremor.

Figure 6. Cyclical issues of an illness episode

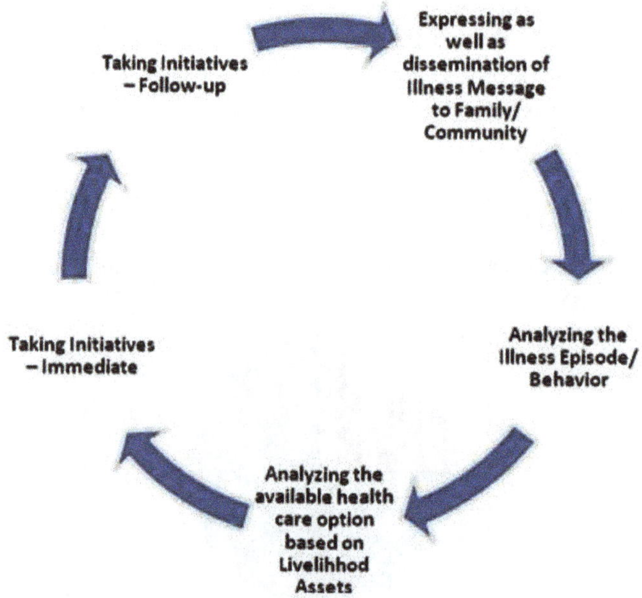

5. Changes in five major senses, such as deafness, blindness, lack of smell, numbness, or loss of taste sensation.
6. Unpleasant physical symptoms, such as pain, headache, abdominal discomfort, fever of shivering.
7. Excessive or unusual states, such as anxiety, depressions, nightmare or exaggerated fears.
8. Behavioral changes in relation to others, such as marital or work disharmony.

ANALYZING THE ILLNESS EPISODE/ BEHAVIOR

After expressing or defining the illness, it was the second steps to analyze the illness episode/ behavior as to the villagers. The researcher observed that it was the notion about an episode of sickness and their treatments that were embodied by all those engaged in the therapeutic process. It was to examine the sorts of questions that the villagers were asked themselves, when they perceived themselves as being ill (Helman, 1994) and how they weave the answers to these questions into the story or narrative of their ill-health. These questions were as to the table no 3.

ANALYZING THE AVAILABLE HEALTH CARE OPTION BASED ON LIVELIHOOD ASSETS

The researchers have observed that, based on the livelihood assets, the villagers were chosen available health care options like the popular sector, the folk sector, the professional sector. We can discuss it to follow the below points.

- Physical capital
- Social capital
- Human capital
- Natural capital and
- Financial capital of the villagers

Physical Capital

The physical capital of this village was relatively so poor compared to other areas of the country. The main crops were paddy, jute, wheat, potato, brinjal, patal, onion, garlic, arum, mustard and chilli. Extinct and nearly extinct crops Indigo (extinct); Til, (sesame), Tisi (linseed), Arhar, black gram, Kawan (Italian millet), yam, etc. Main fruits were Mango, jackfruit, guava, banana, papaya. There were 36 fishery families lived in the *char*s. The communication roads consist of mud roads 15 km and waterways 35 nautical Miles from Upazila headquarters. Materials used in building dwellings included corrugated tin, polythene, straw, leaves, and brick. The leaves were most normally used for structure of roofs (47%), followed by tin (14%), straw (36%), brick (1%), and polythene (2%). About 76% of the households had family members who were members of an NGO (Non-Governmental Organization). 46% of the households had at least one person selling manual labour to make their living. 87% of the households did not have any fixed place of defecation. Of those who had a fixed latrine, 22% had a ring, slab or a cemented latrine, and the remaining households had a fixed place without any protection against faucal contamination. River as a source of drinking water was almost universal with 99% of households reported use of river water for drinking. Twenty three percent of the households were using the latrine. Eight percent of the households had a radio, 4% had a mobile phone at home.

Physical capital has great impact on the issue of distance and thus physical access to health care services. From this village the Union Health and Family Welfare Center (UHFWC) and Upazila Health complex was at 15 km distance, located outside of the village, the 3 pharmacies was at 1.5 km distance and *kobiraj* was nearby at 1 km distance as to the villagers.

In case of insignificant problems village people tend to go to the medicine shops first, and when the illness doesn't get cured and the trouble becomes bigger, they decide to go to Satellite Clinic of NGO's of the *char* because there are more medicines, equipment and qualified doctors available in the clinic. They prefer the Satellite Clinic of NGO's and go by foot, van, votvoti or boat. They rarely visit the Union Health and Family Welfare Center (UHFWC) and Upazila Health complex because the services they got from Satellite Clinic of NGO's was practically the same as in and the distance was thus not worth the care supply. Villagers were reluctant to go to the union clinic as it was too far. When people have to go outer of the *char* for serious illness they depend on foot, van, votvoti or boat. The sand which always creates problems for the villagers need as the transports were so slow. One definite case that has been commonly emphasized was the fact that transport of pregnant women was extremely problematic.

Table 3. Illness episode questions

Questions	Clarification
What has happened?	This includes organizing the symptoms and signs and giving it a name or identity.
Why has it happened?	This explains the etiology or causes of the conditions.
Why has it happened to them?	This tries to relate the illness to aspects of the patients, such as behavior, diet, body-build, personality or heredity.
Why now?	This concerns the timing of the illness and its mode of onset, sudden or slow.
What would happen to them if nothing were done about it?	This considers its likely course, outcome, prognosis and dangers.
What are its likely effects on other people (family, friends, employers, and workmates) if nothing were done about it?	This includes loss of income or employment or a strain on the family as well as social relationships.
What should they do about it – or to whom should they turn for further help?	It includes strategies for treating the conditions, including self-medication, consultation with friends or family or going to take therapeutic options available in the society.

Source: Primary Data (2010-11)

Social Capital

*Char*Majhira consists of 3 *paras, Uttar* (north)*para, Moddhy* (central) *para* and *Dokkhin*(South) *para.* The 44% inhabitants who didn't occupy any cultivable land were landless, 35.2% were small peasant who have 0.01-1.00-acre cultivable land, 19.6% were medium who have 2.51 – 7.50-acre cultivable land and 1.2% was rich who has cultivable land 7.50 acre and/or above.

About 76% of the households had family members who were members of an NGO's (Non-Governmental Organization). 46% of the households had at least one member selling manual labor to make their living. There are one secondary school (private), and one madrasa in the *char.* Among the study people who had been to school, 76% attended secular schools, and 24% attended religious schools.

Gender biases as well as social stratification had adverse impact on the *char* life. The researcher noticed the difference in class. Most people were poor on the *char*, but as a member of the union, the counselor was evidently an especially respected man and richer than the common *char* dwellers. In an in-depth- interview with him, he said that he did not go to the Satellite Clinic of NGO's as well as Union Health and Family Welfare Center (UHFWC) and Upazila Health complex as they don't have any experienced and qualified doctors.

It is worth mentioning that his social status, connected with his economic situation. As to his affordability he went directly to the private hospitals outside the *char* in Bogura. The researcher could derive from the research that the increasing mobility on the *char* was exceptionally difficult.

Higher education is difficult for *char* dwellers to access and only 3 students who were graduated don't come back to the *char* and stay in the Bogura town.

Gender inequality on the *char* was so high. Seven percent of the households in the area were female-headed, and 93% were male-headed. 97% of main earners were male. In general, women almost never own land. It is always their husbands that own the land. Men mostly work in agriculture or fishing in the river. As to the respondent's female paramedics, visiting the *char,* but she was coming from outside the *char* as a part of Satellite Clinic of NGO's. On the *char* the researcher noticed among the women, 76% were housewives, 12% students, the rest were unemployed.

In the use of health care, the researcher noticed much dissimilarity. The researchers noticed one difference when talking about the *kobiraj.* Men clearly have a great deal of respect to the *kobiraj* and are very happy about his services, while women seem to be more serious and went less easily. Because, women were reluctant to consult with male *kobiraj.* The landless, small peasant, medium households were received treatment from popular as well as folk sectors. The figure 7 will show the choice of treatment of the villagers based on household assets.

Figure 7. Choice of treatment

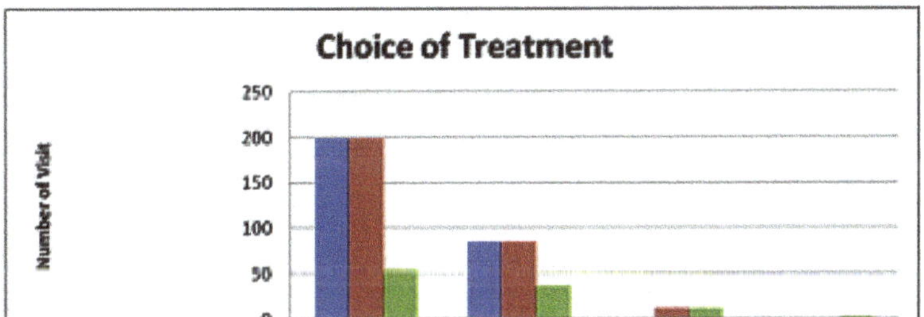

	Landless	Small Peasant	Medium Peasant	Rich
Popular Sectors	199	85		
Both Popular & Folk Sectors	199	85	11	
Professional Sectors	54	37	11	2

If we look at the figure 7, we will find that, 199 landless illness people out of 297 were visited both the popular and folk sectors for their illness sated in the chapter 4. Among the 199 landless illness people 54 were gone to the professional sectors for treatment. 37 patients of small peasant households were gone to the professional sectors while 85 of the same households were consulted with both the popular as well as folk sectors for the treatment. 11 illness, persons from medium households were visited all sectors one after another respectively. But it is worth mentioning that 2 persons from rich households were consulted only professional sectors outside the village.

Human Capital

Human capital represents the skills, knowledge, ability to labor and good health that together enable people to pursue different livelihood strategies and achieve their livelihood objectives. At a household level human capital is a factor of the amount and quality of labor available; this varies according to household size, skill levels, leadership potential, health status, etc. (DFID,

1997). In the study village, most of the people were living hand to mouth. They were not educated. They used to mainly depend on agricultural labor which was not technology based. It has great impact of their choice of treatment already stated in the figure 7 in this section.

Natural Capital

It is not supportable for the livelihood of these people. The area was highly prone to river erosion and floods. It has also the great impact of their choice of treatment already stated in the figure 7 in this section.

Financial Capital

As the researchers have already stated under the social capital issues that, The 44% inhabitants who didn't occupy any cultivable land were landless, 35.2% were small peasant who have 0.01-1.00 acre cultivable land, 19.6% were medium who have 2.51 – 7.50 acre cultivable land and 1.2% was rich who has cultivable land 7.50 acre and/or above. About 76% of the households had family members who were parts of an NGO's (Non-Governmental Organization). 46% of the households had at least one person selling daily labor to make their living. The vulnerable financial situations claimed that the cost of health services constitutes a serious threshold. Particularly treatment outside of the *char* was very costly. Services on the *char* tend to believe the financial capacity of the locals, because a land less villager needs medical assistance, usually he only needs to pay for the medicine. It is indicated that the available popular and folk health services regularly propose treatment free of charge. Mr. Golam Rasul the health assistant, who works at health program of World Vision (NGO), claims that he also lets the landless villagers use his motorcycle charging the cost of fuel as well as fee 275 taka. However, in case of severe illness, villagers indisputably prefer expensive professional sectors outside the *char* like Bogura Sahhid Ziaur Rahman Medical College and Hospital and to the *char*'s own Satellite Clinic of NGO's. It comes into the view that no matter how the landless villagers were, they thought about it worth their while to spend such a huge cost when a life-threatening illness hits their family. The landless need for selling advance in labor, to emergency crops to be able to pay for the sort of cure, others go into debt from NGOs. Five women of medium households even went as far as Bogura to get rid of sexually transmitted infection (STI). Their family has forced to sell their land in order to pay for the expenses about 8700takas as to them. Because of the serious cost of proper medical care in hospitals outside the *char*, villagers tend to reschedule their visit to a qualified doctor. To save money, the villagers tried with the self-treatment first. They usually tend to wait three days or whole weeks until they go to a hospital in Bogura. If some one falls into the position, whether they go to hospital in Bogura or not, it was led him or her die in the meantime. So, the financial capitals represent a life-threatening margin for the disadvantage well as vulnerable people who are living in the village.

TAKING INITIATIVES– IMMEDIATE AS WELL AS FOLLOW UP

The researchers observed that, the villagers were taken immediate as well as follow-up initiatives by considering the above issues. It was an intrinsic cognitive as well as belief system which has great impact on thc cyclical process of an illness episode in the village.

UTILIZATION AND QUALITY OF CARE

The researchers observed that the perception of a facility's worth is even more significant than its accessibility. That's why the researcher deeply examined the locals' first choice and satisfaction. It is transparent from the research that the quality of care is indeed an extremely significant deciding factor in the choices of health care.

There were two chief aspects that seem to characterize why people on the *char* choose a certain type of health care options. Such as

THE EXPLICIT EXERCISE AND INTEREST OF THE HEALTH CARE

Certain health care option specializes in specific problems. Based on the problem and the severity of the illness villagers were chosen the health care options for using. The popular sectors were used by the villagers for the illness stated in the table 4.

Table 4. List of illness treated in the popular sector

Age Group	Illness
Children/Newborn	Diarrhea, Measles, Fungal Infection
Adolescent	Malnutrition, Diarrhea, Skin Diseases
Adult	Asthma, Diabetes, High Blood Pressure, Fungal Infection
Aged	Stroke, Paralysis, Asthma, Toothache, Blurry Vision

Source: Primary Data (2010-11)

On the other hand, the villagers were going to the medicine shops for minor problems like headaches, fever and diarrhea, to the *kobiraj/ Fokir/ Hujur*(folk healers) for cold, fever, skin diseases, loose motion, diarrhea, paralysis, arthritis, lower back pain, etc, and they seldom leave the *char* and gone to Bogura to take medication from hospital for major problems that needs definite cost and qualified doctors.

The medicine shops of the village were close to get help. Villagers collected medicine straight from there.The villagers, and then more particularly the women, have generally great faith in the Satellite Clinic of NGO's. The villagers who have afforded to go to Bogura or Union Health and Family Welfare Center (UHFWC) and Upazila Health complex outside the *char* with a qualified doctor, they have definitely done so. In case of failure in this case they believed that "*Allah is always with them*".

This is decisive from the research that they have an individual fondness for Satellite Clinic of NGO's with qualified doctors. If health care options offering the same services are available and closer to their home, the villagers tend to go there.

PATIENT SATISFACTION

Another aspect was the extent of satisfaction of villagers about the different types of health-care available in the village. The regular shortage of medicine as well as no qualified doctor represents deters villagers from making use of that type of health service. Normally villagers were happy when they got the help and efforts and they were dissatisfied about the particular health care when it didn't work. The researchers could clearly notify this fact from the Satellite Clinic of NGO's in the village. The villagers were satisfied with the services of this clinic when they received medicine as well as advice. But, as satellite clinics were held weekly in a particular location via boats/van with regular intervals (fortnightly or monthly depending on need and funding) with the frequent shortage of medicine, the villagers did not always receive the medicines they needed, which influenced their level of satisfaction to a great extent. The researchers asked the villagers to give marks on the respective health care options available in the village out of 10. They marked them as below.

Figure 8. Marked by villagers to the health care options in the village out of ten

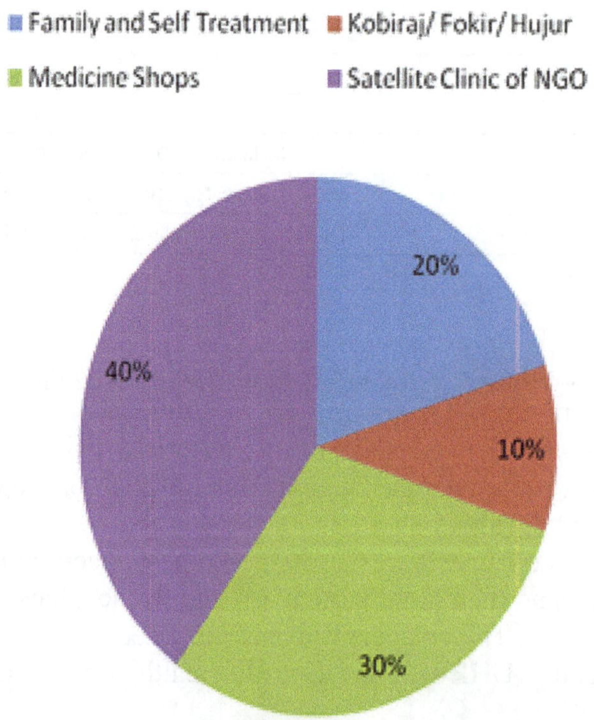

The villagers have given 4 marks to the Satellite Clinic of NGO's, 3 to the medicine shops, 2 to the family as well as self-medication and 1 to the folk sectors like *kobiraj/ Fokir/ Hujur* (folk healers).

CONCLUSION

Explaining the practice of decision making based on above issues or categorization of statements of the villagers may not be sufficient, particularly because health care seeking affect by multifaceted interactions among many individual, household, community, and variables of the supply side. The researchers have analyzed the data through an iterative course that was always revising, and re-examining the themes.

The detail conversations and probing with the respondents pointed out that the cyclical process of an illness episode affect the final decision-making process on health seeking discussed in the above. Seeking treatment for illness is unconfirmed on illness and therefore, detection of the presence of illness is the first appreciation of the decision-making process. Sex, age, suffering, bodily weakness, and signs and symptoms of illness verify the health status of individuals, as well as indicating the extent of harshness of the illness.

When the patients and his family members become assured that the illness was becoming harsher the requirement for medical care was constructed. The necessity of medical care did not essentially decode into taking actual steps for seeking health care options. The gap between the requirement for care and medical care seeking were associated with the cost of obtaining health care services, recognized advantage of the care, affordability of the health care options, willingness to criticize anything to face the healthcare requirement amongst others. When health status appreciation, arises the villagers begin looking for information on availability of health care options. The ring of messages acquired from previous knowledge, knowledge of family members and friends, religious, social and cultural beliefs, customs and attitudes can be termed as indigenous knowledge. Based on this knowledge and other knowledge about therapeutic activities, family members as well as patients build and assess available healthcare options in the village.The substitutes are examined on the basis of assets, needs connected with the employment of the alternative supports and the resources the household had. This examination lets the villagers make a decision where to get the medical care services from, when to ask for care, what to ingest, and what to use and not use. The decision-making process has described in figure 6.

The researchers have analyzed the strategy of the decision-making process of villagers. From the in-depth interviews with the respondents, it has been clear that the participants judged the decision-making process at every phase was as a mutual understanding process of family as well as community members. It is translucent, however, that the cyclical process of an illness episode defined at every phase express an allowable action of decision making founded on the cultural values, norms, customs, experiences, ideas, opinions priorities, and choices of patients, their families and community in the village.

ACKNOWLEDGMENT

The researchers are very much grateful to the study people who have participated in the research as a source of primary information. On the other hand, they are also owed to the researchers who have played a significant role to produce a scientific result from the entire project.

REFERENCES

Department of Agriculture Extension. S. U. (2011). Village Profile 2010, Sariakandi Upazila. Dhaka: Ministry of Agriculture, The People's Republic of Bangladesh.

DFID. (1997). *Sustainable Livelihood Guidance Sheets'*. Retrieved from http:// www.eldis.org/ vfile/upload/1/docume nt/0901/section2.pdf

Helman, C. G. (1994). Culture, health and illness: An introduction for health professionals (3rd ed.). Butterworth Heinemann.

Obrist, B., Iteba, N., Lengeler, C., Makemba, A., Mshana, C., Nathan, R., ... Schulze, A. (2007). Access to health care in contexts of livelihood insecurity: A framework for analysis and action. *PLoS Medicine*, *4*(10), e308. doi:10.1371/journal.pmed.0040308 PMID:17958467

KEY TERMS AND DEFINITIONS

Health Access Livelihood Framework: The framework links social science and public health research with broader development approaches to improve health system development. Access becomes an issue once illness is recognized and treatment seeking is initiated. Five dimensions of access influence the course of the health-seeking process: Availability, Accessibility, Affordability, Adequacy, and Acceptability.

Illness Episode: It is nothing but the illness stories of patients.

Popular, Folk, and Professional Sectors: These are available health care options that the community people frequently used in response to their multiple health hazards. Popular sector deals with the experiences of aged family members to treat illness. Folk sectors deal with the community healers in response to diagnose multiple illness in the community where professional sectors mainly touches the modern medical facilities.

Therapeutic Decision Making: It is a comprehensive process in which people usually make decision to response any physical, psychological, and social illness.

ENDNOTES

1 Primary Data (2010-11).
2 Primary Data (2010-11).
3 Primary Data (2010-11).
4 Primary Data (2010-11).

Chapter 7
Universal Newborn Hearing Screening Programme in Malaysia and Nigeria:
A Comparative Analysis

Iyanda Ismail Abdussalaam
https://orcid.org/0000-0003-1463-2116
University of Fujairah, UAE

Ameen Abdullateef
University of Ilorin, Nigeria

Nurudeen Opeyemi Wahab
https://orcid.org/0000-0003-3688-7507
Olabisi Onabanjo University, Nigeria

ABSTRACT

The developing countries of the world are still lagging in the implementation of the universal newborn hearing screening (UNHS). In other to eradicate unnecessary earshot impairments via suitable rehabilitation processes, there is need for more studies. Thus, this chapter is channeled to bridge this gap. This study used secondary data by comprehensively reviewing the published researches and other relevant and related works and found that UNHS practices in Malaysia and Nigeria have both differences and similarities. The two countries use AABR and OAE as their protocol, and the newborn hearing screening is not binding on the caregivers in both countries. However, their approaches differ in the area of finance, follow-up intervals, and the years of introduction among others. Nevertheless, there are some challenges impeding the effective implementation of the programme which includes include lack of awareness, death of personnel, inadequate diagnostic centers, among others. Given these findings, this chapter could be said to have practical implications for the stakeholders.

DOI: 10.4018/978-1-7998-4414-3.ch007

INTRODUCTION: UNIVERSAL NEWBORN HEARING SCREENING AS A CONGENITAL DEAFNESS

Universal Newborn Hearing Screening (UNHS) programme is an imperative apparatus for initial treatment and diagnosis of hearing impairment. It is an approach that assists in recognising the inherited deafness and earshot damage in new babies before leaving the hospital (Ahmad et al., 2011). Universal Newborn cognitive impairment is perhaps the most frequently diagnosed sensory birth defect and this happens in every 1000 live births with an approximate incidence of 4 to 6 in developing nations (Olusanya et. al., 2007). This implies that UNHS performs a key role in efforts to minimize and/or avoid hearing impairments linked with deficiencies in the social, emotional, language and cognitive development of newborns, despite the presence of risk factors (Kemp, et. al, 2015). Because of the critical number of births occurring outside of medical clinics, vaccination centers have been suggested as an avenue for community based universal hearing screening programmme in order to enhance medical clinic based programmes in developing nations (Olusanya, 2008; Swanepoel, et. al., 2006). In the evolving health model, a whole group of health practitioners and staff are expected to offer patients with the best possible care. Since, in the emerging context of health, integration of treatment around the spectrum is important (Ismail, et. al., 2018).

UNHS has been adopted by virtually all the countries of the world. Meanwhile, the programme is conceded as an indispensable element of communal health upkeep in early infantile in majority of the developed countries in contrast to the developing nations which have low acceptance of the UNHS programme. The numbers of kids universal with earshot injury is cumulative, and these kids face a number of impediments and afflictions, given that spoken linguistic is the biggest medium of communication and social relations. In acknowledgement of the rising and major problem of hearing injury universally, the World Health Assembly (WHA), which comprised health ministers of the United States member states and which is liable for shaping the programmes of the World Health Organisation (WHO), met in 1995 and approved a decision on the reduction and stoppage of key sources of unnecessary hearing damage and on timely discovery in kids, children and babies within the context of primary health care. But it is disheartening that while newborn earshot screening of entire newborns has become a practice of municipal health care system in advanced states, the needs of infants with lifelong hearing impairment have not yet been addressed in developing countries (Olusanya, 2007).

In light of the benefits of UNHS programme and given the nature of the problem being faced by the developing countries, UNHS programme is expected to be significant in these countries, there is a need for the stakeholders' i.e., government, caregivers and parents to do the needful. Therefore, this chapter aims at comparing current UNHS practices in Malaysia and Nigeria with a view to making useful recommendations as regards the steps that could ensure effective implementation of UNHS programme.

BACKGROUND: THE COMPREHENSIVE VIEW OF UNIVERSAL NEWBORN HEARING SCREENING

The reports of the World Health Organisation (WHO) estimate that the total numbers of persons with hearing problems in the world has increased from one hundred and twenty (120) million in 1995 to 278 million in 2005 (Olusanya, Wirz & Luxon, 2008). At global level, about 6 per 1000 Newborns annually experience permanent earshot injury at natal period and at least ninety percent (90%) of them are in emerging states (Olusanya, 2008). For infants, as well, the outright numbers are increasing as the global populace develops. An expected 34 million youngsters right now have incapacitating hearing loss, the vast majority of them are living in Asia Pacific, South Asia, and SubSaharan Africa (WHO, 2018a, 2018b, 2018c; Wilson et al., 2017; Vos et al., 2016). To address this situation, UNHS was initiated to discover early cause of hear impairment in neonates and make necessary interventions and precautions. The origin of newborn hearing screening (NHS) could be traced to the Babbidge Report (1965) in the U.S.A. Babbidge Report (1965) proposed the improvement and employment of the collectively applied techniques for easy classification and assessment of hearing damage (JCIH, 1995). The major milestone in the implementation of UNHS was the establishment of a Joint Committee on Infant Hearing (JCIH) in 1969. Various recommendations have since been made by the committee to improve on the methods and the modalities to tackling issues relating to UNHS.

Also, in 1970, the JCIH delineated the major risk factor responsible for earshot injury and proposed the following: description of inherited infantile hearing deficiency, inborn prenatal infections such as rubella and other non-bacteria fetal infections (e.g., cytomegalovirus, and herpes, chronic facial irregularities, natal heaviness fewer than one thousand and five hundred (1500) grams and a billionaire level larger than twenty). In 1982, microbial meningitis and terrible suffocation were included. Between 1982 and 1994, JCIH added additional risk indicator. All these were the yardsticks used by JCIH for identifying and observing newborns with the alleged earshot damage (JCIH 1982, 1994). The year 2000 JCIH's statement involved the laws and strategies for timely hearing impairment diagnosis and intervention programmes. It was this statement that recommended universal screening before hospital discharge. It endorsed screening before discharge of hospital, follow-up, and identification of babies that require supplementary care and rehabilitation (Muse et al., 2013).

Moreover, the screening to detect hearing loss has two stages. The first stage is called Transient Evoked Otoacoustic Emissions (TEOAE) while the second method is Automated Auditory Brainstorm Response (AABR) (Olusanya & Somefun, 2009). In TEOAE, newborn's ear is tested with incidences between 2000 and 4000 HZ. The effect is signified by a bend that merely displays whether optoacoustic radiation appear or not. If the aural photoemission appears, it implies that earshot of baby does not display deafness higher to thirty to forty (30-40) db. At the second stage, AABR test is used to detect auditory neuropathy. To carry out AABR test, a caregiver would place sensor, which is linked to a processor, on the infant's scalp. The sensor assesses the infants' brainwave activity in reaction to slight choking echoes that are conveyed via slight ear piece. Both TEOAE and AABR take between 5-10 minutes, and each stage is perfectly painless.

Finally, UNHS can both be hospital and community-based. The hospital-based UNHS is adopted for early detection of hearing loss before the newborn is discharged from the hospital. However, community-based UNHS is used as a follow-up to hospital-based UNHS and also to fulfil the needs of the infants who are born outside the hospital. The community-based UNHS is relevant especially in the developing countries where home deliveries are prevalent.

BRIEF ACCOUNT OF UNHS PROGRAM IN THE SELECTED COUNTRIES

Malaysia

Malaysia started implementation of UNHS programmes in 2003 (Ahmed et al., 2011). This as at then was only initiated in the non-public hospital in Malaysia. Then, the programme was implemented in the public hospitals in 2009 (Abdul Majid et al., 2017). Although the Malaysian Government attempted to start the programme earlier than 2003, the implementation could not begin until 2003 and 2009 for non-public and public hospitals respectively. This was due to some challenges being faced by the ministry of health.

In 2005, available statistics in Malaysia "showed that 7.2% of children less than 10-year-old suffered hearing loss which was equivalent to 285,000 children (Noor, 2013). As at 2009, two private hospitals and two teaching hospitals started implementing the UNHS programme. The hospitals are: Summary Medical Centre (SMC), Pusat Perubatan University Kebangsaan Malaysia (PPUKM), Hospital University Sains Malaysia (HUSM) and Sime Darby Medical Centre (SDMC). The hospitals employed both OAE and AABR as the methods of conducting the screening. The country's Ministry of the Health had made some efforts to expand the implementation of UNHS programme, and additional hospitals such as Kuala Lumpur Hospital, Sultanah Bahiyah Hospital in Alor setar, Putarajaya Hospital and all the universities' teaching hospitals have adopted UNHS (Noor, 2013).

At present in Malaysia and according to Malaysian Health Director General Datuk Dr. Noor Hisham Abdullah, UNHS programme is regarded an increasingly best strategy for early detection of hearing loss. With the implementation of the UNHS, it has been held that hearing loss among infants can be identified by the age of 3 months while the intervention can be introduced at the age of six months. Yet, there are many challenges and obstacles obstructing the effective implementation of UNHS programme in Malaysia. These challenges include inadequate equipment, shortage of personnel, and lack of awareness as regards the importance of UNHS programme among the parents, hospital workers and the general public.

Nigeria

One cannot specifically tell the specific date in which Nigeria actually started implementing the UNHS programme, but Nigeria was not unaware of the prevalence of hearing loss in the country. For instance, a study was conducted in 1995 among school-age children in the regular schools. This study showed that about 14% of the sampled children suffer from hearing loss. The 2002 national survey also showed that there is an excessive occurrence of earshot injuries in the country. The two studies signified that infant earshot discovery and interference strategy for Nigeria were initiated in the year 2004 (WHO 2009). Thus, it can be stated that UNHS programme started in 2004 in Nigeria.

Nevertheless, the actual implementation of the programme started in the year 2005, when a native non- governmental association (Hearing International Nigeria) in alliance with the central and State of Lagos Health Ministries introduced a trial newborn earshot screening programme between April-May 2005. Given this, it can be inferred that the current level of UNHS programme in Nigeria is not encouraging as the number of hospitals implementing the programme is not increasing. The duo of professor Abayomi and Professor Julius Ademokoya expressed their sadness that while there is an emphasis on UNHS programme implementation in the developed world, it is not the case in Africa, particularly Nigeria (Ogundipe, Obinna & Oawale, 2016). Furthermore, Professor Julius Ademokoya, the president of Speech Pathologist and Audiologist in Nigeria (SPAAN) observed that many newborns in Africa continue to suffer undetected and unmanaged hearing and speech disorder. He also revealed that lack of diagnostic and rehabilitative equipment, inadequate manpower and training facilities among others are the problems militating against the implementation of UNHS in Nigeria (Ogundipe, Obinna & Olawale, 2016).

Table 1. Comparing UNHS Practices in Malaysia and Nigeria

Criteria	Malaysia	Nigeria
Prevalence (per two life birth)	Total number of screening -58,000 for 2013-2014, 78 out of 58,000 detected with hearing loss.	Total number of screening – 12,000 infants (approximately 7 per 1000 live births were found to have hearing impairment).
Year Introduced	2003 in non-public hospitals and 2009 in public hospitals.	Intervention policy-2004. Actual implementation in hospitals-2005.
Encouragement for coverage per personnel (HP)	Not legally mandated	Not legally mandated
Protocol applied	AABR in HKL Putrajaya hospital; OAE in Bukit Matarjam hospital, miri hospital.	AABR and TEOAE in health centres in Lagos and state-owned hospitals.
Finance	Non-public hospitals – caregivers bears the cost; public hospitals – free screening and diagnosis.	Local non-governmental organisations bear the cost
Government Support	Screening and diagnosis	None
Mean age of Diagnosis	3.6	2.0
Follow-up Interval	Within 42 days	Between 3-4 months

Source: The authors

DISCUSSION

From the table, it can be inferred that to a certain extent both Malaysia and Nigeria differ in their approach towards implementation of the UNHS programme. For example, the programme was introduced in Malaysia in 2003 and 2009 in the country's non-public and public hospitals respectively, but the implementation of the programme actually started in Nigeria in the year

2005. Another area of difference between the two countries is that the cost of the hearing screening programme is borne by caregivers in the Malaysian non-public hospitals while the screening and diagnosis are free of charge in the Malaysian public hospitals. But the cost is shouldered by the local non-governmental organizations in Nigeria. In fact, the programme in Nigeria is free up to the provision of hearing aids through funding support from the local non-governmental organizations. In addition, while the Malaysia government provide support in the area of screening and diagnosis, there is no support from Nigeria government.

Furthermore, the personnel involved in the screening exercise in Malaysia are nurses/audiologists/technicians, but in Nigeria, the screening are done by the audiologists, and the trained community health workers who are given few weeks of training to embark on the screening exercise.

More so, the mean age of diagnosis is 3.6 in Malaysia while that of Nigeria is 2.0. The follow-up intervals in Malaysian is within 42 days while that of Nigeria ranges between 3-4 months. There are some areas of similarities in the approach of the two countries. For instances, both Malaysia and Nigeria use AABR and TEOAE as their protocol. Also, the UNHS programme is not legally binding on anybody in both Malaysia and Nigeria i.e., it is not compulsory.

SOLUTIONS AND RECOMMENDATIONS

The challenges and many other issues of UNHS must be addressed and some of the ways by which these issues can be overcome includes the follow-up system in order to minimize default rates (Olusanya, Wirz & Luxon, 2008). There should also be a wide range of awareness and campaign to sensitize the public regarding the value of UNHS and its impacts. In addition, more screening centers should be established to meet the needs of the newborns. More dedicated and qualified personnel should be recruited and trained and retrained. These recommendations are held to be effective in addressing the issues and challenges confronting UNHS programme implementation. We are therefore confident that this chapter will be useful to the stakeholders and there will be an improvement in the existing level of UNHS programme implementation in Malaysia and Nigeria.

FUTURE RESEARCH DIRECTIONS

- More study should be carried out in other countries in other to have a comprehensive knowledge about universal newborn hearing screening programmes.
- The populace should be educate about the causes of congenital hearing loss and how to prevent it.

CONCLUSION

The chapter concludes that UNHS practices in Malaysia and Nigeria are feasible and viable. From this report, one can deduce that UNHS practices in the two countries have some commonalities and differences. The implementation of the programme in the selected countries is hampered by low public awareness, resource constraints and lack or inadequate government support and donor support. However, the fact still remains that the challenges may be daunting, yet not insurmountable (May et al., 2007).

FUNDING

This research received no specific grant from any funding agency in the public, commercial, or not-for-profit sectors.

REFERENCES

Abdul-Majid, A., Zakaria, M., Abdullah, N. A. C., Hamzah, S., & Mukari, S. S. (2017). Current development, issues and challenges of universal newborn hearing screening program in Malaysia. *International Educational Scientific Journal*, *3*(4), 1–27.

Ahmad, A., Mohamad, I., Mansor, S., Daud, M. K., & Sidek, D. (2011). Outcome of a newborn hearing screening program in a tertiary hospital in Malaysia: The first five years. *Annals of Saudi Medicine*, *31*(1), 24–28. doi:10.4103/0256-4947.75774 PMID:21245595

Babbidge Jr, H. D. (1965). *Education of the deaf.* A report to the secretary of health, education, and welfare by his advisory committee on the education of the deaf.

Ismail, A. I., Abdul Majid, A., Zakariab, M. N., Abdullah, N. A. C., Hamzah, S., & Mukarid, S. Z. (2018). Factors predicting health practitioners' awareness of UNHS program in Malaysian non-public hospitals. *International Journal of Pediatric Otorhinolaryngology*, *109*, 78–84. doi:10.1016/j.ijporl.2018.03.030 PMID:29728190

Joint Committee on Infant Hearing. (1982). Joint Committee on Infant Hearing 1982 Position Statement. *Ear and Hearing*, *4*, 3–4. PMID:6832505

Joint Committee on Infant Hearing. (1994). Joint Committee on Infant Hearing Year 1994 position statement: Principles and guidelines for early hearing detection and intervention programs. *Pediatrics*, *95*, 152–156.

Joint Committee on Infant Hearing. (1995). Joint committee on infant hearing 1994 position statement. *Pediatrics*, *95*(1), 152–156. PMID:7770297

Kemp, A. A. T., Delecrode, C. R., da Silva, G. C., Martins, F., Frizzo, A. C. F., & Cardoso, A. C. V. (2015). Neonatal hearing screening in a low-risk maternity in São Paulo state. *Revista Brasileira de Otorrinolaringologia (English Ed.)*, *81*(5), 505–513. doi:10.1016/j.bjorl.2015.07.010 PMID:26277836

May, C., Finch, T., Mair, F., Ballini, L., Dowrick, C., Eccleset, M., & … . (2007). Understanding the implementation of complex interventions in health care: The normalization process model. *BMC Health Services Research*, *7*(1), 148. doi:10.1186/1472-6963-7-148 PMID:17880693

Muse, C., Harrison, J., Yoshinaga-Itano, C., Grimes, A., Brookhouser, P. E., Epstein, S., Buchman, C., Mehl, A., Vohr, B., Moeller, M. P., Martin, P., Benedict, B. S., Scoggins, B., Crace, J., King, M., Sette, A., & Martin, B. (2013). Joint Committee on Infant Hearing of the American Academy of Pediatrics. Supplement to the JCIH 2007 position statement: Principles and guidelines for early intervention after confirmation that a child is deaf or hard of hearing. *Pediatrics*, *131*(4), e1324–e1349. doi:10.1542/peds.2013-0008 PMID:23530178

Noor, H. A. (2013). Implementation of Universal Newborn Hearing Screening programme to be expanded. *The Malaysian Borneo Post*. Retrieved on the July 18, 2018 from http://www.theborneopost.com/2013/05/17/implementation-of-universal-newborn-hearing-screening-programme-to-be-expanded/

Ogundipe, S., Obinna, C., & Olawale, G. (2016). With advancing age, ear infections are inevitable. *The Nigerian Vanguard*. Retrieved on the April 23, 2018 from https://www.vanguardngr.com/2016/06/with-advancing-age-ear-infections-are-inevitable-professor-julius-ademokoya/

Okhakhu, A. L., Ibekwe, T. S., Sadoh, A. S., & Ogisi, F. O. (2010). Neonatal hearing screening in Benin City. *International Journal of Pediatric Otorhinolaryngology*, *74*(11), 1323–1326. doi:10.1016/j.ijporl.2010.08.017 PMID:20863576

Olusanya, B. O. (2007). Addressing the global neglect of childhood hearing impairment in developing countries. *PLoS Medicine*, *4*(4), 74. doi:10.1371/journal.pmed.0040074 PMID:17407384

Olusanya, B. O. (2009). Newborns at risk of sensorineural hearing loss in low-income countries. *Archives of Disease in Childhood*, *94*(3), 227–230. doi:10.1136/adc.2008.144550 PMID:18786955

Olusanya, B. O., Luxon, L. M., & Wirz, S. L. (2005a). Screening for early childhood hearing loss in Nigeria. *Journal of Medical Screening*, *12*(3), 115–118. doi:10.1258/0969141054855274 PMID:16156940

Olusanya, B. O., Luxon, L. M., & Wirz, S. L. (2005b). Childhood deafness poses problems in developing countries. *BMJ (Clinical Research Ed.)*, *330*(7489), 480. doi:10.1136/bmj.330.7489.480-c PMID:15731158

Olusanya, B. O., & Newton, V. E. (2007). Global burden of childhood hearing impairment and disease control priority project for developing countries. *Lancet*, *369*(9569), 1314–1317. doi:10.1016/S0140-6736(07)60602-3 PMID:17434407

Olusanya, B. O., & Somefun, A. O. (2009). Sensorineural hearing loss in infants with neonatal jaundice in Lagos: A community-based study. *Annals of Tropical Paediatrics*, *29*(2), 119–128. doi:10.1179/146532809X440734 PMID:19460265

Olusanya, B. O., Wirz, S. L., & Luxon, L. M. (2008). Community-based infant hearing screening for early detection of permanent hearing loss in Lagos, Nigeria: A cross-sectional study. *Bulletin of the World Health Organization*, *86*(12), 956–963. doi:10.2471/BLT.07.050005 PMID:19142296

Swanepoel, D. W., Hugo, R., & Louw, B. (2006). Infant hearing screening at immunization clinics in South Africa. *International Journal of Pediatric Otorhinolaryngology*, *70*(7), 1241–1249. doi:10.1016/j.ijporl.2006.01.002 PMID:16483673

Vos, T., Allen, C., Arora, M., Barber, R. M., Bhutta, Z. A., & Brown, A. (2016). Global, regional, and national incidence, prevalence, and years lived with disability for 310 diseases and injuries, 1990-2015: A systematic analysis for the Global Burden of Disease Study 2015. *The Lancet, 388*(10053), 1545–1602. (16)31678-6 doi:10.1016/S0140-6736

Wilson, B. S., Tucci, D. L., Merson, M. H., & O'Donoghue, G. M. (2017). Global hearing health care: New findings and perspectives. *The Lancet, 390*(10111), 2503–2015. (17)31073-5 doi:10.1016/S0140-6736

World Health Organisation. (2009). *Newborn and infants hearing screening: current issues and guiding principles for action.* Retrieved on the May 14, 2018 from https://www.who.int/blindness/publications/Newborn_and_Infant_Hearing_Screening_Report.pdf

World Health Organization. (2018a). *Addressing the rising prevalence of hearing loss.* http://apps.who.int/iris/bitstream/handle/10665/260336/9789241550260-eng.pdf?sequence=1&ua=1

World Health Organization. (2018b). *Deafness and hearing loss—Key facts.* https://www.who.int/mediacentre/factsheets/fs300/en/

World Health Organization. (2018c). *Prevention of blindness and deafness—Estimates: Global estimates on prevalence of hearing loss* [Embedded powerpoint presentation]. https://www.who.int/pbd/deafness/estimates/en/

ADDITIONAL READING

Clemens, C. J., Davis, S. A., & Bailey, A. R. (2000). The false-positive in universal newborn hearing screening. *Pediatrics*, *106*(1), 1–5. doi:10.1542/peds.106.1.e7 PMID:10878176

de Kock, T., Swanepoel, D. W., & Hall, J. W. III. (2016). Newborn hearing screening at a community-based obstetric unit: Screening and diagnostic outcomes. *International Journal of Pediatric Otorhinolaryngology*, *84*, 124–131. doi:10.1016/j.ijporl.2016.02.031 PMID:27063767

Johnson, J. L., White, K. R., Widen, J. E., Gravel, J. S., & James, M. (2005). Multicenter evaluation of how many infants with permanent hearing impairment pass a two-stage otoacoustic emissions/automated auditory brainstem response newborn hearing screening protocol. *Pediatrics, 116*(3), 663–672. doi:10.1542/peds.2004-1688 PMID:16140706

Kumar, S. (2001). WHO tackles hearing disabilities in developing world. *Lancet, 358*(9277), 219. doi:10.1016/S0140-6736(01)05460-5 PMID:11476854

Laguyo, D. (2013). *Hearing intervention critical before 6 months of age.* Retrieved from:http:// www.upm.edu.ph/sites/default/files/CMVILLAMOR%20press%20release%20on%20hearing%20screening%20and%20intervention.pdf

Marquez, E. (2015). *Newborn Hearing Screening.* Retrieved from https:// prezi.com/brzpwo2omx4q/newborn-hearing-screening/

McPherson, B., & Brouillette, R. (2004). A fair hearing for all: Providing appropriate amplification in developing countries. *Communication Disorders Quarterly, 25*(4), 219–223. doi:10.1177/15257401040250040601

Piza, M. R. de T. (2014). Overview of newborn hearing screening programs in Brazilian maternity hospitals. *Revista Brasileira de Otorrinolaringologia (English Ed.), 80*(5), 369–370. doi:10.1016/j.bjorl.2014.07.003 PMID:25303808

KEY TERMS AND DEFINITIONS

Automated Auditory Brainstem Response (AABR): This is a test of how well the brain and the hearing nerve react to the sound.

Caregivers: This is a salaried or un-paid family member of an individual who supports them with everyday life activities.

Congenital Hearing Loss: This is loss of hearing at birth or hearing loss that can occur subsequently but is attributable to hereditary factors or other conditions that have affected the fetus while in the womb.

Infection: This is the penetration of the body by infectious micro-organisms or parasites.

Meningitis: This is an infection of the brain and spinal cord membranes, commonly triggered by disease.

Otoacoustic Emission (OAE): This is sound that is produced from inside the inner ear.

Transient-Evoked Otoacoustic Emissions (TEOAE): This is are Sounds that are produced by the outer hair cells of the cochlea in reaction to a temporary click.

Universal Newborn Hearing Screening (UNHS): This is an approach that assists in recognising the inherited deafness and earshot damage in new babies before leaving the hospital.

World Health Assembly: This is a platform in which the World Health Organization is regulated by its 190 countries and territories and also the highest health policy setting body in the world.

World Health Organization: The specialist body United Nations that is accountable for global public health.

Chapter 8
In Vitro and in Vivo Models for Pathogenic Neisseria gonorrhoeae Infections

Karthikeyan Ramalingam
https://orcid.org/0000-0002-9334-427X
B. S. Abdur Rahman Crescent Institute of Science and Technology, India

Sucharithra Ganesh
B. S. Abdur Rahman Crescent Institute of Science and Technology, India

ABSTRACT

The prevalence of gonorrhea has not discontinued in several countries and still remains as one of the top sexually transmitted diseases (STD) and it's caused by Neisseria gonorrhoeae. This bacterium gains entry into the human host via receptors, and by the usage of several virulence factors, it manages to spread through the cells and leads to severe complications. The study of these bacteria in various in vitro and in vivo models have paved the way for gaining insights on various aspects of bacterial infection, such as the study of pathogenesis of the organism in the host. It also drove the development of more appropriate drugs for the treatment of the gonorrhea illness caused by this 'superbug'. This chapter focuses on providing a concise overview on the general aspects of N. gonorrhoeaeas an update and the in vitro and in vivo models used for understanding this bacterium over the years. Despite gonorrhea not being a rare STD, it is still a big challenge for researchers, healthcare professionals, and communicators with public awareness to communicate effectively with the general community.

INTRODUCTION

Sexually transmitted diseases (STDs) are infections caused by pathogens that are transmitted from one person to another via any type of sexual contact. There are several STDs caused by different pathogens such as virus, bacteria and parasites (Lunzen and Altfeld, 2014). One of the major burdens faced by the world today is the sexually transmitted infection (STI) caused by

DOI: 10.4018/978-1-7998-4414-3.ch008

a species of the genus Neisseria (Trevisan, 1885), *Neisseria gonorrhoeae*, the pathogen which causes the human disease called gonorrhea. This bacterium is known to affect an average of 60-65 million people worldwide every year (Woods, 2005).The disease caused by the bacterium, gonorrhea, is the second most reported sexually transmitted disease in the USA and, reference to its existence can be traced back as far as to "biblical times" (Lev. 15:1-15:19).The causative agent *N. gonorrhoeae* of the disease gonorrhea was discovered by a German physician, Albert Ludwig Sigesmund Neisser, in 1879 (Ligon, 2005). *N. gonorrhoeae*, a gram-negative bacterium, is an obligate human pathogen which often causes infection at the mucosal sites of the urogenital tracts causing STI. Gonorrhea can affect almost anyone who is sexually active; younger women who are less than 25 years of age, older women with many sexual partners, and homosexuals are very susceptible. *Neisseria* infection is both symptomatic and asymptomatic with most women depicting the latter form of the disease. The disease may manifest just a few days or weeks' post-infection leading to several complications (Detels et al. 2011).

Gonorrhea may be posing high susceptibility to HIV (Human Immunodeficiency Virus) and *Chlamydia trachomatis*(which causes the STI chlamydia). It has been studied that infection by *N. Gonorrhoeae*may be posing a high risk for also transmitting HIV (Monty Montano et al, 2007). *N. gonorrhoea* had been initially treated with penicillin and then with other antibiotics such as cephalosporins, fluoroquinolones and tetracyclines, which significantly reduced the incidence of the disease; yet the crisis of antibiotic resistance made the treatment and cure ineffectual leading to the high prevalence of the disease. This antibiotic resistance ability of the bacteria had made the CDC (Communicable Disease Center) CDC categorize them as '*superbugs*' (Unemo et al., 2016).

The basis of gonococcal infection (i.e. from gonococcus, the pus-producing bacterium (*N. gonorrhoeae*) that causes gonorrhea in humans depends on the adherence of the bacterium to the epithelia and anti-adherent agents have been tried and tested as a treatment. One study showed the efficacy of the lactobacillus, a microbiota that produces lactic acid, against the adherence of gonococcus. *N. gonorrhoeae* bacterium is highly capable of immune evasion due to its ability to alter the antigenic determinants (Edwards and Apicella, 2004), i.e. to escape the immune response.

It has been studied that gonococcal lipo-oligosaccharide and peptidoglycan induces proin-flammatory cytokines and chemokines which further initiate a cascade of events. Phagocytic cells are employed at the site, and these initiate immune responses elicited by the body. This produces reactive oxygen and nitrogen species thereby causing cytotoxic effects to the cells (Rahal et al., 2014). But, the strong antioxidant system of the bacteria comprising of catalase, superoxide dismutase, ABC type Mn transporter and cytochrome c peroxidase, enables them to defend and survive in such environments (Speers-Roesch and Ballantyne, 2005). Symptomatic infections are characterized by flooding of numerous polymorphonuclear neutrophils (PMNs), the most numerous granulocytes (white blood cell), and the gonococcus is found intracellular to it (Johnson and Criss, 2011) i.e., infected individuals contain large numbers of PMNs with ingested gonococci (Simons et al., 2005).

There is a strong requirement of appropriate data for the interpretation of the disease related studies which will enable the development of disease selective and sensitive drugs. The use of various relevant animal models, organ and cell line models for the research and developmental studies of *Neisserial* infections has provided significant information for the interpretation and extrapolation of the data, through the years. These models provided valuable toolsf or various molecular mechanism studies and, drug discovery and development studies.

CLINICAL MANIFESTATION

The clinical manifestations of the disease in men include yellow to green discharge from penis, pain in the testicles and epididymis and burning sensation during urination (Brown et al., 2016).In females, similar pain and burning while urination is experienced as well as excessive discharge from vagina and, also, bleeding may take place (Supriya et al., 2001). If left untreated in females, it will lead to pelvic inflammatory disease (PID). Furthermore, affected mothers can transmit this infection to their infant's eyes causing *Opthalmia neonatorum* (ON) or neonatal conjunctivitis, which can cause blindness (Matejcek and Goldman, 2013). Both men and women may suffer sterility and women may come across ectopic pregnancy (Ghanem, 2016).

Patients infected may suffer from: proctitis (inflammation of the rectal lining) (Patton et al., 2014), vulvovaginitis (inflammation of the vulva and vagina), urethritis (inflammation of the urethra) (Barlow and Phillips, 1978), prostatitis (swelling and inflammation of the prostate gland), orchitis (inflammation of the testicles), ovaritis (inflammation of an ovary) and occasionally, endocarditis (infection or inflammation of the endocardial surface of the heart), meningitis (inflammation of the membranes (meninges) surrounding your brain and spinal cord), conjunctivitis or 'pink eye' (inflammation or infection of the transparent membrane (conjunctiva) that lines the eyelid and covers the white part of the eyeball) (Mak et al., 2001), pharyngitis or 'sore throat' (inflammation of the back of the throat or pharynx), salpingitis (infection and inflammation in the Fallopian tubes),dermatitis-arthritis(a form of disseminated gonococcal infection that causes skin lesions and affects multiple tendons, more commonly the fingers, wrists, toes, and ankles)can be detected in spread infections (via blood) (Ghanem, 2016).

EPIDEMIOLOGY OF INFECTION

Gonorrhea was estimated to affect87.7 million people worldwide annually, in the year 2005(Newman et al., 2015). The incidence of the disease increased to 106 million cases per year, as reported in 2015 (Newman et al., 2015). These data were provided by the World Health Organization(WHO). In 2013, there is an estimation of 200 million new cases of Chlamydia and Gonorrhoeae a year (CDC, 2007; Workowski and Bolan, 2015).The European center for disease prevention and control (ECDC) conducted a survey in 28 European countries from 2010 to 2014, and the numbers of cases of gonorrhea were estimated to be 32766, 39817, 47631, 53136 and 66413, respectively. Based on the available data, a gradual increase in the rate of infection over the years is clear (ECDC, 2016). In the Unites States, the disease incidence was estimated to be of 301,174 cases in 2009 (Satterwhite et al., 2013), 309341 cases in 2010 (CDC, 2010), 333004 cases in 2013 (Gregory et al., 2015) and 350062 cases in 2014 (CDC, 2015). Gonorrhea was seen in slightly higher rates in females than in males (Xiong et al., 2016). In India, a survey conducted at a Sexually Transmitted Disease (STD) center with a group of 358 patients that presented co-infections with gonorrhea concluded that the disease affects almost all age groups (Gurung et al., 2010). From 2003 to 2006, the percentage of men infected was far higher than that of infected women; 9.3-12.1%, respectively (Shim, 2011). In the year 2007, the percentage of men infected decreased to about 6.4% (Gesink Law, 2008).But, in the year 2008, there was an increase of about 12.4% and they also reported that about 14.4% of people had co-infections with STIs (Bala et al., 2011).

Back in 1999, the numbers of new cases were found to be 1.56 million in North America, 1.11 million in Western Europe, 27.2 million in South and Southeast Asia, 7.27 million in Latin America and the Caribbean(Smith et al., 2013). In Africa, the incidence of *Neisseria gonorrhoeae* was estimated to be of 17.5 million cases in 2005 and 21.1 million cases in 2008 (Chesson et al., 2017, showing a clear increase of new cases.

PATHOGENESIS AND VIRULENCE

Pathogens are those micro-organisms that are able to cause a disease and thereby elicit an immune response in the body (Klimpel, 1996). This ability to cause disease is termed pathogenicity. *Neisseria gonorrhoeae* is a capnophilic (thrive in the presence of high concentrations of carbon dioxide), virulent obligate human pathogen, i.e. that require a host to complete their life cycle (Balloux and van Dorp, 2017; Quillin and Seifert, 2018).The virulence of a pathogen can be defined as the disease inducing capacity or the degree of pathogenicity (Peterson, 1996). Virulence factors denote the properties of the microorganism that enables its establishment in the host and causes infection and enhances the pathogenicity. The virulence factors of bacterium generally include endotoxins and exotoxins, the protein molecules that aid in attachment, entry, and interaction with host proteins thereby, causing interference with host metabolism, through hydrolytic enzymes (Hung and Christodoulides,2013). *N. gonorrhoea* requires the interaction with human mucosa cells for not only pathogenesis but is also essential for their life cycle to progress (Fig.1).

This gram-negative bacterium, like others, possess lipopolysaccharide (LPS) endotoxins and does not produce any exotoxin (Tzeng et al 2002). The Neisserial LPS is referred to as lipooligosaccharide (LOS) attributing to its structural differences (Rouphael and Stephens,2012). During the course of growth, the outer membrane releases fragments containing LOS called '*blebs*', which are involved in the pathogenesis. The bacterium enters the epithelium by 'parasite mediated endocytosis' (Quillin and Seifert, 2018).

Immune evasion and antiphagocytosis are often confused in the literature. With immune evasion the bacterium hides itself from the immune system. But with antiphagocytosis the bacterium remains actively extracellular, in spite of recognition by the immune system. The bacterium release effector proteins into the host cell cytoplasm or secrete toxins which penetrate through the host cell membrane targeting host cell proteins. This originates direct or indirect impairment of the cytoskeleton assembly that leads to the inability of the host cell to manipulate their membrane to engulf the recognized bacterium (Scheenstra, 2010).

Figure 1. Schematic overview of Neisseria gonorrhoeae virulence factors and pathogenesis mechanisms

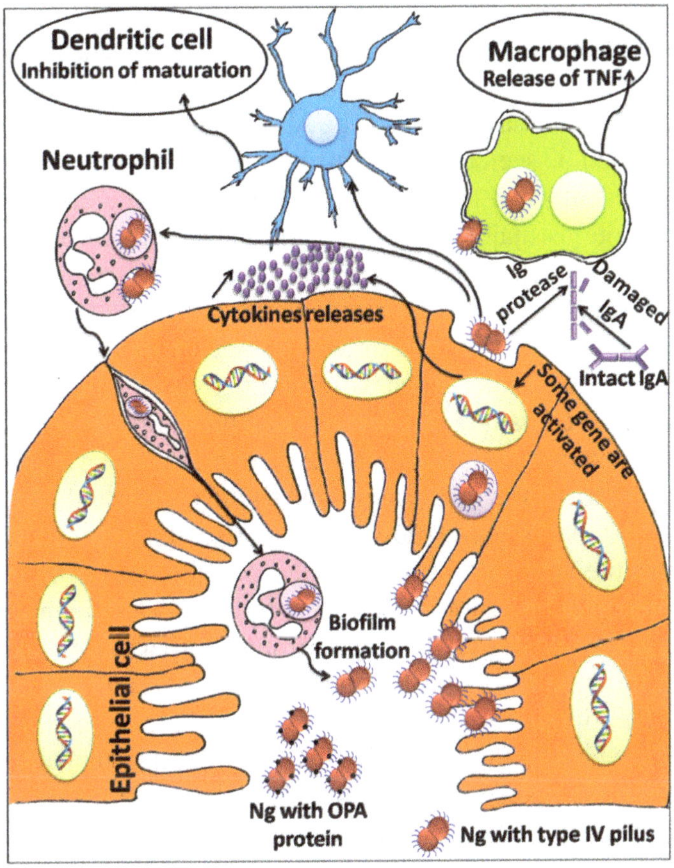

Table 1. Virulence factors from N. gonnorrheae bacterium

Virulence Factor	Function	References
Capsule	Anti-phagocytosis for the entry	Spinosa, et al., (2007)
Porin B	Invasion of bacterium	Ayala et al., (2002)
Opa (Outer membrane opacity proteins)	Adhesion and invasion of bacterium	Kupsch et al., (1993)
Rmp (Reduction modifiable protein)	Blocks the bactericidal antibodies against LOS and Por	Gulati et al., (2015)
Tbp (Transferrin binding protein)	Iron acquisition for growth and invasion	Ronpirin et al., (2001)
Lbp (Lactoferrin binding protein)	Iron acquisition for growth and invasion	Brooks et al., (2014)
IgA1 proteases	A serine protease that can aid in phagosomal escape	Pohlner et al., (1987)
LOS (Lipooligosaccharide)	Adherence, stimulates TNF	Plant et al., (2006)
FarAB	Efflux pump	Lee et al., (2003)
MtrCDE	Efflux pump	Ohneck et al., (2015)
Ghfp (gonococcal analog of fHbp of *N. meningitidis*)	Immune modulator	Rippa et al., (2015)
NspA	Immune modulator	Criss and Seifert (2012)
Type IV pili (T4P)	Adherence and aggregation	Giltner et al., (2012)

PATHOGENESIS

The virulence factors mentioned above are involved in the pathogenesis of the bacteria. Pathogenesis refers to both the mechanism by which infections are caused and the mechanism by which the disease develops by a chain of reactions. The *N. gonorrhoea* infection in women, although beginning at the cervix, can be seen to ascend further till the fallopian tubes (Lenz and Dillard, 2018).The bacterium gets attached to the non-ciliated epithelial cells of the fallopian tube by using pili, and/or opa proteins(major adherent factors). The Opa of one bacterium attaches to the lipooligosaccharides (LOS) of the neighboring bacterium forming colonies(LeVan et al., 2012), like a biofilm - communities of microorganisms that live attached to surfaces (Karatan and Watnick, 2009). The bacteria are then drawn in to enter the host epithelial cells (parasite mediated endocytosis) after their interaction with the mucosal membranes. Further, the mucosal cell pinches off as a vacuole containing the bacteria and they are released into the sub-epithelial tissue by a process called exocytosis(Edwards and Apicella, 2004).Porins and opacity-associated proteins (Opa) are important in the invasion of host tissue (Hung and Christodoulides, 2013).

It has also been studied that *N. gonorrhoeae* possess excellent iron acquisition system that is able to obtain iron from the host for their growth and development from iron group containing proteins such as lactoferrin (Lbp), transferrin (Tbp) and even from hemoglobin (Hb) (Desai et al., 2000). The bacteria also possess unique IgA proteases that can breakdown the antibodies thereby leading to an immune response that makes it to be in more of an unresponsive state even upon infection. The lipooligosaccharides (LOS) found in *N. gonorrhoeae*, just like any lipo-polysaccharide(Patrone and Stein, 2007)., behaves like a potent immunogen that causes the host to elicit an immune response by stimulating the production of tumor necrosis factor (TNF) (Mogensen, 2009). Eventually, the phagocytic cells are attracted to the site where they try to phagocytize the bacteria; some bacteria can escape the phagocytosis mechanism, possibly due to the presence of certain capsule proteins (Uribe-Querol and Rosales, 2017). Autolysis, or self-digestion, is a common mechanism that is seen in *N. gonorrhoeae* infections. It consists in the destruction (or lysis) of the cells by its own enzymes. By this, LOS and peptidoglycans are broken down by various self-enzymes, and this is responsible for causing severe immunogenic responses such as the activation of alternate complement pathway in the host (Janeway et al., 2001). Rmp (outer membrane protein 3) is found to be in association with LOS and Por and it deactivates the antibodies that are either secreted by the body upon *Neisserial* infection or the antibodies directed against the infection from external sources (e.g. Antibiotic drugs). Drug efflux by the efflux pumps is an important mechanism found in gram-negative bacteria and this property contributes to the antimicrobial resistance. It has been observed that the resistance to certain antimicrobial HAs (host-derived antimicrobial hydrophobic agents) has been attributed to the *mtrCDE.* Another system of efflux was found by the farAB system which was indirectly regulated by MtrR (Quillin and Seifert, 2018; Lenz and Dillard, 2018).

ANTIMICROBIAL RESISTANCE OF THE BACTERIUM

For several years now, *Neisseria gonorrhoeae* strains have developed severe antimicrobial resistance and are almost uncontrollable, and a major health care issue in many countries. They have developed resistance against sulfonamides, penicillin, tetracycline, spectinomycin, quinolones, macrolides and cephalosporins, one by one over the years in different parts of the world (Manju Bala, 2011). The antimicrobial resistance development in gonococcus has been categorized into three different eras as the pre-quinolone, quinolone and the post-quinolone era. These periods are when the bacterium gained resistance to a large spectrum of antibiotics by acquiring the resistance determinants that may lie on the chromosome or may exist as plasmids (Costa-Lourenço et al., 2017). Sulphonamides were the first antibiotics used to treat *N. gonorrhoeae* and this antibiotic gained resistance just about two years (Dunlop, 1949). Then, the prevalence of penicillin use was high, and this treatment lasted for several decades until even this antibiotic gained resistance (Unemo and Shafer, 2014). These isolates were termed Penicillinase producing *Neisseria gonorrhoeae* (PPNG). Penicillinases have a specific type of beta-lactamase that has specificity towards the penicillin and penicillin-derived antibiotics. These resistant strains of PPNG are gonococcus that gained an extrachromosomal element of plasmid that held the beta-lactamase gene. This lactamase enzyme destroys the beta-lactam ring of penicillin making it ineffective against bacterium. Of the resistant strains, PPNG has had the greatest impact on public health in the mid-1980s (CDC, 1987). Later, tetracycline resistant strains were also detected and were termed the tetracycline resistant *Neisseria gonorrhoeae* (TRNG). The other alternative antibiotics such as the spectinomycin, cephalosporins, fluoroquinolones, ciprofloxacin, norfloxacin, ofloxacin, trovafloxacin were sought after much. The bacterium began to become resistant to almost all of these antibiotics as well over the years. The quinolone resistant strains were termed as quinolone resistant *Neisseria gonorrhoeae* (QRNG) (Patel et al., 2011). The genetic factors that contribute to the resistance gained by bacteria against several antibiotics, and the genes associated can be chromosomal or of plasmid DNA (Unemo and Shafer, 2014).

Table 2. Antibiotics and the genes associated to N. gonorrheae treatment resistance which, can be chromosomal or plasmid DNA.

Antibiotic	Resistance Determinant Genes	References
Sulfonamides	folP gene (chromosomal)	Fiebelkorn et al., (2005)
Penicillin	blaTEM-1 *(plasmid)	Reema Singh et al., (2019)
Penicillin	Mutations in penA, penB, ponA, mtrRgenes (Chromosomal)	Ropp et al., (2002)
Tetracycline	tetM gene (Plasmid)	Młynarczyk-Bonikowska et al., (2016)
Tetracycline	tet-2, mtrR, penB genes (Plasmid)	Caladoa et al., (2019)
Spectinomycin	rpsEgene	Unemo et al., (2013)
Quinolone	gyrA and parC (occasionally parE and gyrB)	Lindbäck et al., (2002)
Macrolide	Ermgenes	Ng et al., (2002)
Cephalosporin	penA, penB, ponA, mtrR, pilQ genes	Lindberg et al., (2007)

Many antibiotics target the peptidoglycan layer, and the bacteria one way or another manage to produce enzymes such as amidases, endopeptidases and lytic transglycosylases for the remodeling of the peptidoglycan layer (Vermassen et al., 2019).Neisseria gonorrhoea encodes for basic 5 lytic transglycosylases which are important for normal growth, pathogenesis and gene transfer between the bacteria. (Schmidt and Hensel, 2004) and lytic transglycosylases fragment the peptidoglycan layer further leading to the manifestation of the disease by killing the ciliary cells of the fallopian tubes (Chan, et al., 2012).

It has been found that the antibiotic resistant *N. gonorrhoeae* are higher in homosexual host populations than heterosexual populations (Chen et al., 2009). Moreover, according to a recent mathematical study, it has been found that antibiotic resistant *N. gonorrhoea* spreads faster with more treatment (Fingerhuth et.al. 2016). The CDC had reported in 2016 that gonorrhea may become resistant to all antibiotics by the year 2020. In late 2016CDC reported the first highly resistant *N. gonorrhoeae* in the US with azithromycin and low susceptibility to ceftriaxone (Papp, et al., 2017).

ASSAYS FOR DIAGNOSIS OF NEISSERIA GONORRHOEAE

For the diagnosis of *Neisseria gonorrhoeae* in patients, first samples must be collected and transported in appropriate conditions, and then several assays can be performed to check the presence or absence of this bacterium. The samples can be collected as urethral specimens, urinal specimens, rectal specimens, oropharyngeal specimens, cervical specimens, conjunctiva specimens, vaginal specimens and other body fluids. These isolated specimens then need to be cultured in the laboratory and used for further assays (Ng and Martin, 2005).

N. gonorrhoeae is grown well on chocolate agar or a modification of chocolate agar called Thayer-Martin agar. The gonococcus is unable to grow on common blood agar. But the chocolate agar contains lysed RBCs and hemoglobin for enrichment. The Thayer-Martin agar is an altered medium that contains antimicrobials vancomycin, colistin, nystatin, and trimethoprim lactate, which makes it selective for the growth of gonococcus, specifically (Ng and Martin, 2005). Modified New York City Medium or agar is also used for the culture of *N. gonorrhoea*e (Dillon et al., 1988). The diagnosis of gonorrhea in the laboratory includes the following methods:

MIC, MBC and Disk Diffusion Assays

MIC (minimum inhibitory concentration) and MBC (minimum bactericidal concentration) of pathogens are usually determined by examining the effects of different antibiotics of various concentrations on the culture of bacterium adjusted to 10^8 CFU/ml (colony-forming unit *per* ml) at 0.5 McFarland standards (is a chemical solution of Barium chloride which is used as the standard to compare the turbidity of bacterial suspension in the test sample); either plated on agar media or in a liquid broth culture. However, the agar dilution method exists as the gold standard for the susceptibility testing of *N. gonorrhoeae*(CDC, 2005; Unemo et al., 2013; Lahra and Enriquez,2017). *N. gonorrhoeae* being fastidious in nature, direct colony suspension method is preferred for the determination of MIC (Balouiri et al., 2016).

The MIC and MBC determinations of penicillin, ampicillin, cefoxitin and cefuroxime were made for beta-lactamase (like penicillinase) negative *N. gonorrhoeae* strains (de Repentigny and Turgeon, 1981). The MIC of several 6 different antibiotics, Cefdinir, Cefetamet, CI-960, Fleroxacin, Lomefloxacin, and Temafloxacin was analyzed (Erwin et al., 1992). MIC and MBC determinations for *N. gonorrhoeae* were made for spectinomycin, ampicillin and penicillin and the ranges of their susceptibility were obtained (Levy et al., 1972).The MIC values of different antibiotics determined for *N. gonorrhoea* are Amoxycillin- 0.5mg/L, Co-amoxiclav-0.5mg/L, Telithromycin-0.03mg/L, ABT773-0.03mg/L, Clarithromycin-0.5mg/L, Erythromycin-0.5mg/L, Ciprofloxacin-0.004mg/L and Moxifloxacin-0.004mg/L. (Andrews, 2001). The disk diffusion method is essentially used for MIC and MBC determinations and its being less preferred for *N. gonorrhoeae* compared to agar dilution method. This is because the antibiotic susceptibility testing for *N. gonorrhoeae*is complex and requires specialized laboratorial conditions, thus it is not suited in clinical practice environment due to the time constraints for initiating the treatment (Bala et al., 2016). As per records MIC, MBC and Disk diffusion assays are cost effective method to determine the resistance and drug efficiencies properties of this microbes.

Microscopy

Microscopy is the first, go-to preliminary assay used for observing the presence of bacteria or its look-alikes in patients' collected specimens. First, gram staining method will be used to detect gram-negative bacteria. *N. gonorrhoeae* diplococcus has a characteristic kidney bean shaped structure that can easily be identified. When the specimens are stained and viewed under the microscope, the bacteria may be detected in the neutrophils, eosinophils or basophils (polymorphonuclear leukocytes). Colony morphology and pigmentation (pinkish-brown color) can also be a distinctive measure to check the presence of *N. gonorrhoeae* bacteria (Janda and Knapp, 2003).

Biochemical Assays

Oxidase Test

The oxidase test is essentially used to identify bacteria that possess the cytochrome c oxidase (COX) system. It catalyzes the transfer of electrons from ferrocytochrome c to molecular oxygen, converting the latter to water. *N. gonorrhoeae* is a prolific source of c-type cytochromes (Turner et al., 2005). The bacteria that possess the COX enzyme act upon the reagent tetramethyl-*p*-phenylene-diamine, oxidizing it to a blue or purple color (indophenols) (Ehret and Judson, 1991). The bacteria lacking the enzyme do not oxidize the reagent leaving it colorless. There are a number of reagents used for this test such as Kovac's Oxidase Reagent (tetramethyl-p-phenylenediamine dihydrochloride), Gordon and McLeod's Reagent, Gaby and Hadley (indophenol oxidase) Reagent. There are several methods to perform this assay such as, filter paper method, direct plate method, swab method, test tube method and impregnated oxidase strip method (Shields and Cathcart, 2013). Commercial 'easy-to-use' kits are also available. *N. gonorrhoeae* is an oxidase-positive bacterium.

Acid Detection Test

A metabolic process performed by almost all types of bacteria is known as fermentation. Carbohydrates may be fermented by various bacteria in order to obtain energy. Different bacteria produce acid from either the fermentative pathway or oxidative pathway. Neisseria species produce acid by the latter pathway and determination of acid production is possible by the using Cystine tryptic agar (CTA), conventionally. In this method, the carbohydrate solution is added along with phenol red indictor which, changes its color from red to yellow that results from changing the pH from alkaline to acid, respectively. There are several rapid acid identification tests also available. However, they are not exceptionally recommended because species such as *N. gonorrhoeae* do not grow well on the media (Kraus, 1979). But it has been found that *N. gonorrhoeae* produces acid from only glucose and not from lactose, sucrose, fructose or maltose(Dillon et al., 1988; Ng and Martin, 2005) and this fermentation assay alone not adequate to conclude results further experimentation required for the confirmation.

Catalase Test

Catalase enzyme protects the cells from oxidative damage; it catalyzes the release of oxygen from hydrogen peroxide. In this test, hydrogen peroxide (H_2O_2) is used to detect catalase.Generally,3% H_2O_2 is used for aerobes while 15% is used in anaerobes (Brooks et al., 2004). Usually this assay is performed using a test tube and a slide. The release of oxygen from catalase activity generates bubbles. *N. gonorrhoeae* should be catalase positive (Janda and Knapp, 2003).

Superoxol Tests

The Superoxol (Merck & Co., Inc., Rahway, N.J.) test (catalase test using 30% H_2O_2) (Saginur et al, 1982) is a specialized test very similar to that of the previously described catalase test and is used to identify *N. gonorrhoeae* from the other Neisserial species (Janda and Knapp, 2003). In this test, 30% hydrogen peroxide is used, and the *N. gonorrhoeae* are marked by immediate vigorous bubbling when the reagent is added to the bacterial colonies. Other Neisserial species produce delayed bubbling.

Nitrate Reduction Test

Nitrate is reduced by bacteria in two ways namely, the assimilatory nitrate reduction (aerobic) and the dissimilatory nitrate reduction (anaerobic). Many bacteria possess nitrate reductase enzymes which are able to convert nitrate to nitrite when the only source of nitrogen is nitrate which, may further be degraded to nitrogen oxide, nitrous oxide, ammonia, etc. depending on the enzyme system of the organism and its atmosphere. In this assay, the bacteria are inoculated and after 4 hours of incubation, sulfanilic acid reagent and α- naphthylamine are added. The sulfanilic acid might react with the produced nitrous acid and form diazotized sulfanilic acid, which further reacts with α- naphthylamine to form a red colored compound. If the red color was not produced, it suggests that the organism was unable to reduce nitrate and hence another step adding zinc is required for confirmation. *N. gonorrhoeae* has been found to be negative for the nitrate reduction test (Ng and Martin, 2005).

Colistin Resistance Test

Colistin, also known as polymyxin E, belongs to the class of polypeptide antibiotics. It's an effective antibiotic against multi-drug resistant gram-negative organisms(Gupta et al., 2009). It is susceptible to most gram-negative bacteria but not susceptible to gram-positive organisms(Trimble et al., 2016). This antibiotic was discovered in the 1940s(Ainsworth et al., 1947) and due to its serious toxic effects, it was stopped. But later in 1990s, it regained its position in the market for most gram-negative bacterial infections. Colistin is a mixture of cyclic polypeptides synthesized by *Bacillus polymyxa spp colistinus* ((Prazmowski 1880) Macé 1889),a gram-positive bacterium capable of fixing nitrogen. *N. gonorrhoeae*, although being gram-negative and multi-drug resistant, is highly resistant to even colistin (Exner et al., 2017).

Polysaccharide From Sucrose

Certain bacterial species produce polysaccharide from sucrose, and this can be detected by using iodine that turns blue-black color. This test is essentially performed on starch free medium with 1% or 5% sucrose depending on the strain used. After incubation period of about either 24 hours or 3-4 days, iodine can be added to detect the formation of polysaccharide by a distinct color change and that does not occur when there is no polysaccharide formation (Hehre, 1949). However, *N. gonorrheae* produce the distinctive color changes to confirm the occurrence.

Production of DNase

The enzyme DNase is an endonuclease that has the ability to hydrolyze DNA and utilize it as a source of carbon and energy (Pinchuk et al., 2008). This test allows detecting whether the enzyme is present in the microorganism or not. This test can be performed using the differential media or using commercial kits. While using the DNase agar, the media is pale green in color due to the indicator DNA methyl-green which is positively charged and, hence gets attached to the negatively charged DNA. When the organism possesses DNase, the DNA gets broken down by the enzyme and the DNA gets detached from the methyl-green. This causes a colorless zone to be formed around the colony. But if the organism does not possess DNase, there is no visible change around the colony. By using the commercial kits, the pH indicator present will exhibit changes in color from red (alkaline) to yellow (acid) when DNase is present in the organism. It has been found that *N. gonorrhoeae* is DNase negative (Janda et al., 1987).

Serological Testing

Fluorescent Antibody Tests

Fluorescence isothiocyanate labelled monoclonal antisera against porins and outer membrane proteins bind to the bacteria exhibiting antigens against these molecules and fluoresce under fluorescence microscopes. Despite some unspecific binding, this test holds almost 100% sensitivity and specificity to *N. gonorrhoeae* (Ng and Martin, 2005).

Coagulation Test

Cell suspensions of primary cultures are boiled, and monoclonal antibodies are combined with it to detect the heat stable epitopes of the bacterial proteins; the assay shows a positive result when the test reagents get coagulated. There are commercial assay kits available for coagulation testing. In this test, *N. gonorrhoeae* species is connected to species-dependent abilities to directly stimulate coagulation (Roth et al., 1992).

Colorimetric

The colorimetric assays eliminate the heat treatment step mentioned in the previous assay, and the antibody and bacterial proteins complex are passed through a filtration unit. The appearance of a red color indicates a positive result. Commercial kits are also available for this assay. For example, in immune caspase activity assays *N. gonorrhoeae* activates caspases in MDMs (monocyte-derived macrophages) being associated with macrophage cell death due to intracellular gonococci (Ritter and Genco, 2018)

Enzymatic Assays

Certain enzymes, other than the above mentioned (e.g. catalase and nitrate reductase), are used to detect *N. gonorrhoeae* such as, beta-galactosidase, gamma-glutamylaminopeptidase and prolylhydroxyprolyl aminopeptidase (Kulkarni et al., 2015). Commercially kits are available for these assays but they are not 100% specific or sensitive and, hence require additional testing for confirmation (Ng and Martin, 2005).

Nucleic Acid Tests

Commercial and automated/semi-automated processes are available for identification of bacteria. In non-amplification methods, as the name suggests, amplification of nucleic acids is not required whereas, a probe can be used to target the nucleic acid of the bacteria. There are commercial kits available specific for *N. gonorrhoeae* alone and *N. gonorrhoeae* with *Chlamydia trachomatis* (Ng and Martin, 2005).

Aptima^{tm} Assay

This is based in 'target capture technology' for *in vitro* detection of *N. gonorrhoeae.* It detects ribosomal RNA and there are specialized kits for these assays. The GenProbe TMA (Transcription-mediated amplification) works by replicating the 16s rRNA from *N. gonorrhoeae* and use of specific unique primers (Munson et al., 2013). Nucleic acid hybridization takes place for the identification of the specific rRNA from bacteria. Single-stranded chemiluminescent DNA probes complementary to the specific target then hybridizes to the RNA-DNA hybrids. The un-hybridized probes can be eliminated and, the exact signals obtained from the hybridized probes can be read by the luminometer thus, giving positive or negative results, accordingly. The GEN-PROBE APTIMA Combo® 2 Assay is an 'extension' of the Aptima assay which, replicates a specific region of the 23S rRNA from *C. trachomatis* and a specific region of the 16S rRNA from *N. gonorrhoeae* via DNA intermediates. By this, both STDs pathogens can be detected.

In Vitro Infection Models

It has become easier to study the effect of infections or drugs *in vitro*, at least initially and, then progress into *in vivo* studies. Obligate human pathogens do not need to be studied in human specimens; rather, *in vitro* cell line samples allow hypothesizing similar effects *in vivo*. Several cell lines have been used for the study of *N. gonorrhoeae.* Some of the most commonly used cell lines are immortal cell lines such as HeLa, Chang, HaCaT, ME180 etc.

Table 3. Cell lines used to study the pathogenic Neisseria gonorrhoeae

Cell Type	References
HeLa cells	Brodeur et al, 1977; Frenette, et al, 1984; Naumann, et al, 1997; Li, et al., 2013; Mavrogiorgos, et al., 2014
HeLa- CEACAM3 cells	McCaw et al., 2004
HaCaT cells	Naumann, et al, 1997
Chang	Naumann et al, 1997; Weel et al, 1991
ME180	Song et al, 2000; LeVan et al, 2012; Kim et al., 2019
End/E6E7	Follows et al, 2009; Fichorova et al, 2001
HL-60	Chen and Seifert, 2011; Châteauand Seifert, 2016
WI 38	Frenette, et al, 1984
Human urethral epithelium	Harvey et al., 1997; Almonacid-Mendoza et al., 2018
A431 Human epidermoid carcinoma	Higashi et al, 2009; Arvidson et al, 1999; Hopper, et al, 2000
HTB-33 cell	Wenxia Song, et al, 2000
Hs-68 cell	Li, et al., 2013
Beas2b cell	Li, et al., 2013
OEC-M1 cells	Li, et al., 2013
VK2/E6E7	Weyler et al. 2014; Fichorova et al, 2001

continues on following page

Table 3. Continued

Cell Type	References
Human colonic epithelial cells, T84	Stein et al., 2015; Hopper, et al, 2000
Human corneal epithelial cells	Long et al., 2001
HEp-2 cell	Brodeur et al, 1977
RE2 cell	Brodeur et al, 1977
HEC-1-B cell	Arvidson et al, 1999; Jarvis et al., 1999
RT112 cells	Scheuerpflug et al., 1999
Caco cells	Jarvis et al., 1999
HT29	Jarvis et al., 1999
Primary human ectocervical epithelial (pex) cells	Potter et al., 2009
HeLa229 cells	CDC, 2014
FRT tissues and epithelial cells	Wira et al., 2011
HEK 293 cells	Mavrogiorgos, et al., 2014
Monocytic cells - MonoMac-6 and THP-1	Hauck et al., 1997; Château and Seifert, 2016
Myelomonocytic cell line JOSK-M	Hauck et al., 1997
THUEC	Harvey et al., 2002
PMN cells	Soler-García and Jerse, 2007
Ect1/E6E7	Fichorova et al, 2001

In Vivo Infection Models

In vivo models include tissue culture models as well as, the use of animal models to study pathogens. Since *N. gonorrhoeae* is an obligate human pathogen, it would demand a human model for systematic data analysis and even for the development of a vaccine (Quillin and Seifert, 2018). But human experimentation been possible, easily performed in men because the experimentation with female specimens makes the investigation very complicated (Ng and Martin, 2005) due to the structural organ variations. Thus, the *in vivo* models such as organ culture and other animal models have been used extensively for obtaining similar data by which we can suffice the diagnostic and therapeutic ends.

Organ Culture

Animal organs are essentially used for the study of bacterial interactions for the extrapolation of molecular and pathological data and further analysis and inferences to be made. In the *N. gonorrhoeae* infection, the most used organ for culture in laboratory is the fallopian tubes (Lenz and Dillard, 2018). This organ has been obtained from rabbit, murine, rat and mouse and, inclusively women and has been studied extensively Carney et al., (1973).For example: fallopian tubes derived from several human women aged 45and still menstruating were collected and the MCW activity of *N. gonorrhoeae* and its endotoxin were studied (Mårdh et al.,1979). Human fallopian tubes were also collected from premenopausal, non-pregnant females and the significant increase in toxicity of modified *N. gonorrhoeae*, mutant gly1 locus was studied (Arvidson et al, 1999). Fallopian tubes were collected from 13 healthy female donors of different age groups and the Neisserialpil$^-$ and pil$^+$ (piliated organisms) strains were inoculated and, the effects of these different strains were studied for the attenuation of the cytokine response (Velasquez et al., 2011). Cervical endo and ecto-cells were obtained from biopsies and cultured to study the effect of the bacterial infection causing cytoskeletal rearrangements (Edwards et al, 2000).

Chicken tracheal organs and mammalian murine tracheal organs were cultured with gonococcus and the former was seen to survive little longer than the latter (Carney and Taylor-Robinson, 1973). Lactating and non-lactating goat mammary glands were used for study of inoculated gonococci and this organ culture was performed owing to its similarities with the lower urogenital tract of men (Pasieka, et al., 1976). A comparative study of the epithelial damage caused by *N. gonorrhoeae*tothe oviducts and fallopian tubes of white rabbit hybrids and humans was carried out (Taylor-Robinson et al, 1974). Subcutaneous chamber model of guinea pigs was used to study the role of pilus of *N. gonorrhoea in vivo* and the effect of anti-pilus antibodies (Lambden, et al., 1982). Chicken embryo obtained from White Leghorn chicken were inoculated with *N. gonorrhoea* via yolk sac (YS) and chorioallantoic membrane (CAM) routes and the differences in the infectivity and death rate of both these routes were studied (Foster and Vinson, 1977). The transmission of *N. gonorrhoeae* from infected pregnant Sprague-Dawley rats to the fetus was also evaluated (Nowicki, et al., 1999).

Animal Models

Several animal models are used for the study of *Neisseria gonorrhoeae*. A large number of studies of this bacterium have been performed upon animal models. Balb/C mice that were 7-8 weeks old were infected with streptomycin resistant *N. gonorrhoeae* and immunological studies were performed (Liu and Russell, 2011). Balb/c mice were used to find the role of IL-17 (Interleukin 17) and Th-17 (T helper 17) cells in the mice infected with *N. gonorrhoeae*. Antibiotic and estradiol treated mice were also used and in the same study, IL-17 was blocked or the IL-17 receptor was deleted by knockout mechanism in mice were found to have prolonged infection (Feinen, et al., 2010). Female balb/c mice that were 6-8 weeks old were treated with 17β-estradiol to test the local and humoral cell immune responses against the *N. gonorrhoeae*infections (Song, et al, 2008). Female BALB/c mice were infected via vagina and the enhancement of adaptive immunity was studied by the administration of microencapsulated IL-12 (Liu, et al., 2013). Male or female Balb/c mice that were 6-8 weeks old were obtained for the removal of spleenocytes to study the gonococcal infection that modulates the host immune response. Anti-pilusmonoclonal antibodies (mAbs) were produced by immunizing the BALB/c mice and polyclonal antibodies were produced by immunizing rabbits (Swanson, et al., 1987). Polyclonal antibodies were produced by immunizing rabbits and the production of monoclonal antibodies was obtained by immunizing BALB/c mice (Weel, et al., 1991).New Zealand red rabbits were used for obtaining antisera followed by the immune diffusion assays used for the serological classification of *N. gonorrhoeae*(Johnston, et al., 1976).

Young adult female mice were collected, and the gonococci were inoculated intra-nasally and the lungs were isolated for study. The effect of the gonococci causing pneumonia in mice in the presence or absence of cyclophosphamide was studied by Johnson, et al, (1977).One study was aimed to obtain IgE (Immunoglobulin E) antibodies against *N. gonorrhoeae* using outbred male wistar rats (Vijay, et al., 1977). Young adult female mice of strains C3H, CBA, TO and BALB/c were bred and the neisserial strains were tested *in vivo* and, the results showed that the bacteria were unable to adhere to the genital tract of mice (Johnson, et al., 1989).

Guinea pigs were injected subcutaneously with nine isolated strains of *N. gonorrhoeae* and this type of immunization could pave way for further drug and vaccine development. This study focused on the identification of immune-protective types and new immune types (Wong, et al., 1979).Adult Harley strain guinea pigs and adult swiss mice were inoculated with *N. gonorrhoeae* and the differences in the histopathological features of both were studied by Chandler, et al., (1976). New Zealand white outbred rabbits were inoculated with different strains of gonococci and antisera was obtained and immune-diffusion tests were performed to test the interactions between the antigen and antisera (Pierce, et al., 1975).Mice were used as an experimental model to test the efficacy of micro-biocides on genital infection caused by *N. gonorrhoeae*(Spencer, et al., 2004).

Endotoxin resistant and endotoxin susceptible strains of mice namely C3H/HeJ and C3H/HeN respectively were inoculated with the gonococci and comparative analyses of immune response were studied by Streeter and Corbei (1981).BALB/c mice were infected with *N. gonorrhoeae* and inflammation analyses were made along with the Opa protein expression and the effect of estradiol treated mice were studied by Jerse (1999).Chimpanzee models were used for the study of acquired and natural immunity by making pharyngeal, cervical and urethral inoculations of *N. gonorrhoeae* by Kraus, et al., (1975).Competitive infection analysis of lipid A PEA (lipid A phosphor ethanolamine transferase) enzymes of *N. gonorrhoeae* was studied in Balb/C mice and men. The mutant lacking PEA transferase was inoculated and the effects of non-host restricted interactions with host immune elements were studied (Hobbs et al., 2013).Finally, even *Rhesus* macaques were used as a model to study the molecular mechanisms of colonization, transmission, persistence, and horizontal gene transfer of *Neisseria gonorrhoeae* and could potentially be used as a model for pre-clinical studies for development of vaccines (Weyanda, et al., 2013).

FUTURE RESEARCH DIRECTIONS

- As the spread of this infection is a public health problem, there is a desperate requirement for social mindfulness and schooling on sex education on a continuous basis among people. Distinguishing and focusing on vulnerable and susceptible populaces could ensure the success and sustenance of efforts to control the spread of the disease.
- Development of a reliable vaccination for Neisseria gonorrhoeae is indispensable. Albeit immense research, there is little progress towards an effective vaccine that can protect populations. However, recent investigations light a hope in this arena. For these purposes, many in vitro and in vivo models are used, perhaps even genetically engineered to humanize a model and this will eventually enable the finding to stop the spread of the bacterium.

- The development of new antibiotics or new treatment alternatives requires high anti-gonococcal intensity, and additionally no cross-resistance with current antibiotics to guarantee their efficacy over the long haul.

CONCLUSION

The bacteria *Neisseria gonorrhoeae* is increasingly reported to be becoming multi-antimicrobial drug resistant at an alarming rate. The sexually transmitted disease gonorrhea is becoming almost untreatable these days being a huge source of worry and burden to the society as it damages the reproductive health of people. There has been a potent gonorrheal vaccine candidate (protein) that has been identified recent year (Jerse et al., 2014). A new antibiotic (Solithromycin) has also been identified as an anti-gonorrheal. Throughout the years, much research has been performed on various *in vitro* and *in vivo* models enabling us to extrapolate the data for the human case. Yet, the quest for new antibiotics has not ended due to the continuous mutations in the bacteria leading to antimicrobial resistance. Thus, it would be advantageous to look into the disease in a deeper perspective as the age-old proverb says 'prevention is better than cure'. It is better to prevent the disease by following moral and safe sexual practices which is primarily important as this would decrease the rate of further infection spread to other hosts. There have been however obstacles to this communication and prevention of societies. The information is not reaching people as much as it should, nor has it been clear, engaging and shocking enough for, especially the young generation, to change habits.

Thus, in a digital age such as this, we have access to the entire world in our gadgets through the internet and we can make use of this opportunity to communicate with people across the globe. Health activists, researchers, Governmental health bodies etc. can expand their reach to people by being extremely active on the social media or host free conferences/webinars online that can educate and raise awareness on STIs and prevention on a scientific basis. The necessity to communicate to people to be safe in sexual practices is pressing even though there is a stigma around the topic of STIs. But non-communication of this could lead to more devastating consequences.

N. gonorrhoea is not the only STI superbug, there are several others such as, chlamydia, syphilis, and recently, there has been a warning about a possible STI causing superbug called *Mycoplasma genitalium.* It has been found that the symptoms are very similar to that of chlamydia but if left untreated, it can lead to permanent infertility in women.

With so many sexually transmitted infections prevailing, it is definitely necessary to understand the importance of safe sexual practices and implement such campaigns creating awareness among sexually active men and women. People must be encouraged to speak to their partners about any STI contractions before sexual ventures so that the partners are also not at the risk of such dreadful communicable diseases.

Each and every human is at risk due to the increasing superbug infections. Research is already focused on continuous improvement of drugs that can exploit the potential weaknesses of multi-drug bacteria to provide a cure. The need to develop specific drugs, such as, for example nonmaterial's can be a major focus area for complete eradication of these superbugs. However, drugs are not the only source of STI management. There needs to be support from every government to enable people to rise above the stigma of STDs. Such stigma causes barriers to communicating about prevention and care. Today, communication is extending far beyond our possible imagination in the past. Social media influencers and celebrities have large fan following and exert a large influence in people across the globe. This influence can be exploited for marketing education and awareness among people of the world so that the world is a safer place.

ACKNOWLEDGMENT

This book chapter work was supported by the DST Science and Engineering Research Board (SERB, Grant No. SERB/LS-267/2014), India and Extra Mural Research Funding of AYUSH (Ayurveda, Yoga and Naturopathy, Unani, Siddha and Homoeopathy, Sanction Order No. Z. 28015/209 /2015-HPC), India.

REFERENCES

Ainsworth, G. C., Bisby, G. R., Brown, A. M., Marsden, P., Smith, P. A., & Spilsbury, J. F. (1947). A method for the large-scale production of penicillin by surface culture. *Journal of General Microbiology*, *1*(3), 335–343. doi:10.1099/00221287-1-3-335 PMID:20270632

Almonacid-Mendoza, H. L., Humbert, M. V., Dijokaite, A., Cleary, D. W., Soo, Y., Hung, M. C., Orr, C. M., Machelett, M. M., Tews, I., & Christodoulides, M. (2018). Structure of the Recombinant *Neisseria gonorrhoeae* Adhesin Complex Protein (rNg-ACP) and Generation of Murine Antibodies with Bactericidal Activity against Gonococci. *MSphere*, *3*(5), e00331–e18. doi:10.1128/mSphere.00331-18 PMID:30305317

Andrews, J. M. (2018). Determination of minimum inhibitory concentrations. *The Journal of Antimicrobial Chemotherapy*, *48*(1), 5–16. PMID:11420333

Arvidson, C. G., Kirkpatrick, R., Witkamp, M. T., Larson, J. A., Schipper, C. A., Waldbeser, L. S., O'Gaora, P., Cooper, M., & So, M. (1999). *Neisseria gonorrhoeae* mutants altered in toxicity to human fallopian tubes and molecular characterization of the genetic locus involved. *Infection and Immunity*, *67*(2), 643–652. doi:10.1128/IAI.67.2.643-652.1999 PMID:9916071

Ayala, P., Vasquez, B., Wetzler, L., & So, M. (2002). *Neisseria gonorrhoeae* porin P1.B induces endosome exocytosis and a redistribution of Lamp1 to the plasma membrane. *Infection and Immunity*, *70*(11), 5965–5971. doi:10.1128/IAI.70.11.5965-5971.2002 PMID:12379671

Bala, M. (2011). Antimicrobial resistance in *Neisseria gonorrhoeae* in South-East Asia. *Regional Health Forum*, *15*(1).

Bala, M., Mullick, J. B., Muralidhar, S., Kumar, J., & Ramesh, V. (2011). Gonorrhoea & its co-infection with other ulcerative, non-ulcerative sexually transmitted & HIV infection in a Regional STD Centre. *The Indian Journal of Medical Research*, *133*(3), 346–349. PMID:21441694

Bala, M., Singh, V., Philipova, I., Bhargava, A., Joshi, C., & Unemo, M. (2016). Gentamicin in vitro activity and tentative gentamicin interpretation criteria for the CLSI and calibrated dichotomous sensitivity disc diffusion methods for *Neisseria gonorrhoeae. The Journal of Antimicrobial Chemotherapy*, *71*(7), 1856–1859. doi:10.1093/jac/dkw102 PMID:27073269

Balloux, F., & van Dorp, L. (2017). Q&A: What are pathogens, and what have they done to and for us? *BMC Biology*, *15*(1), 91. doi:10.118612915-017-0433-z PMID:29052511

Balouiri, M., Sadiki, M., & Ibnsouda, S. K. (2016). Methods for *in vitro* evaluating antimicrobial activity: A review. *Journal of Pharmaceutical Analysis*, *6*(2), 71–79. doi:10.1016/j.jpha.2015.11.005 PMID:29403965

Barlow, D., & Phillips, I. (1978). Gonorrhoea in women.Diagnostic, clinical, and laboratory aspects. *Lancet*, *1*(8067), 761–764. doi:10.1016/S0140-6736(78)90870-X PMID:76760

Brodeur, B. R., Johnson, W. M., Johnson, K. G., & Diena, B. B. (1977). In vitro interaction of *Neisseria gonorrhoeae* type 1 and type 4 with tissue culture cells. *Infection and Immunity*, *15*(2), 560–567. doi:10.1128/IAI.15.2.560-567.1977 PMID:403139

Brooks, C. L., Arutyunova, E., & Lemieux, M. J. (2014). The structure of lactoferrin-binding protein B from Neisseria meningitidis suggests roles in iron acquisition and neutralization of host defences. *Acta Crystallographica. Section F, Structural Biology Communications*, *70*(Pt 10), 1312–1317. doi:10.1107/S2053230X14019372 PMID:25286931

Brooks, G. F., Butel, J. S., & Morse, S. A. (2004). Cultivation of Microorganisms. In Medical Microbiology (23rd ed.). McGraw-Hill Companies.

Brown, M. A., Potroz, M. G., Teh, S. W., & Cho, N. J. (2016). Natural Products for the Treatment of *Chlamydiaceae* Infections. *Microorganisms*, *4*(4), 39. doi:10.3390/microorganisms4040039 PMID:27754466

Caladoa, J., Castroa, R., Lopesa, A., Camposb, M. J., & Rochab, M. (2019). Filomena PereiraAntimicrobial resistance and molecular characteristics of *Neisseria gonorrhoeae* isolates from men who have sex with men. *International Journal of Infectious Diseases*, *79*, 116–122. doi:10.1016/j.ijid.2018.10.030 PMID:30412735

Carney, F. E. Jr, & Taylor-Robinson, D. (1973). Growth and effect of *Neisseria gonorrhoeae* in organ cultures. *The British Journal of Venereal Diseases*, *49*(5), 435–440. doi:10.1136ti.49.5.435 PMID:4201243

Centers for Disease Control and Prevention. (2014). Recommendations for the laboratory-based detection of Chlamydia trachomatis and Neisseria gonorrhoeae--2014. MMWR. Recommendations and reports: Morbidity and mortality weekly report. Recommendations and reports, 63(RR-02), 1–19.

Centers for Disease Control and Prevention Bulletin B88. (2005). *Neisseria Gonorrhoeae Reference Strains for Antimicrobial Susceptibility Testing.* Available at: https://www.cdc.gov/std/gonorrhea/arg/B88-Feb-2005.pdf

Centers for Disease Control (CDC). (1987). Antibiotic-resistant strains of *Neisseriagonorrhoeae*. Policy guidelines for detection, management, and control. *MMWR Supplements*, *36*(5), 1S–18S. https://www.cdc.gov/std/gonorrhea/arg/MMWR_AR-GC-PolicyGuidelinesDetectionManagementandControl_Vol36No5S.pdf PMID:3116397

Centers for Disease Control (CDC). (2007). Update to CDC's sexually transmitted diseases treatment guidelines, 2006: Fluoroquinolones no longer recommended for treatment of gonococcal infections. *MMWR. Morbidity and Mortality Weekly Report*, *56*(14), 332–336. PMID:17431378

Chan, Y. A., Hackett, K. T., & Dillard, J. P. (2012). The lytic transglycosylases of *Neisseria gonorrhoeae*. *Microbial Drug Resistance (Larchmont, N.Y.)*, *18*(3), 271–279. doi:10.1089/mdr.2012.0001 PMID:22432703

Chandler, F. W., Kraus, S. J., & Watts, J. C. (1976). Pathological features of experimental gonococcal infection in mice and guinea pigs. *Infection and Immunity*, *13*(3), 909–914. doi:10.1128/IAI.13.3.909-914.1976 PMID:818019

Château, A., & Seifert, H. S. (2016). *Neisseria gonorrhoeae* survives within and modulates apoptosis and inflammatory cytokine production of human macrophages. *Cellular Microbiology*, *18*(4), 546–560. doi:10.1111/cmi.12529 PMID:26426083

Chen, A., & Seifert, H. S. (2011). *Neisseria gonorrhoeae*-mediated inhibition of apoptotic signalling in polymorphonuclear leukocytes. *Infection and Immunity*, *79*(11), 4447–4458. doi:10.1128/IAI.01267-10 PMID:21844239

Chen, M. I., Ghani, A. C., & Edmunds, W. J. (2009). A metapopulation modelling framework for gonorrhoea and other sexually transmitted infections in heterosexual populations. *Journal of the Royal Society, Interface*, *6*(38), 775–791. doi:10.1098/rsif.2008.0394 PMID:18986961

Chesson, H. W., Mayaud, P., & Aral, S. O. (2017). Sexually Transmitted Infections: Impact and Cost-Effectiveness of Prevention. In *Major Infectious Diseases* (3rd ed.). The International Bank for Reconstruction and Development / The World Bank. doi:10.1596/978-1-4648-0524-0_ch10

Costa-Lourenço, A., Barros Dos Santos, K. T., Moreira, B. M., Fracalanzza, S., & Bonelli, R. R. (2017). Antimicrobial resistance in *Neisseria gonorrhoeae*: history, molecular mechanisms and epidemiological aspects of an emerging global threat. *Brazilian Journal of Microbiology*, *48*(4), 617–628. . doi:10.1016/j.bjm.2017.06.001

Cousin, S. Jr, Whittington, W. L., & Roberts, M. C. (2003). Acquired macrolide resistance genes in pathogenic Neisseria spp. isolated between 1940 and 1987. *Antimicrobial Agents and Chemotherapy*, *47*(12), 3877–3880. doi:10.1128/AAC.47.12.3877-3880.2003 PMID:14638497

Criss, A. K., & Seifert, H. S. (2012). A bacterial siren song: Intimate interactions between Neisseria and neutrophils. *Nature Reviews. Microbiology*, *10*(3), 178–190. doi:10.1038/nrmicro2713 PMID:22290508

de Repentigny, L., & Turgeon, P. L. (1981). Screening of *Neisseria gonorrhoeae* for tolerant response to beta-lactam antibiotics. *Antimicrobial Agents and Chemotherapy*, *19*(4), 645–648. doi:10.1128/AAC.19.4.645 PMID:6787980

Desai, P. J., Garges, E., & Genco, C. A. (2000). Pathogenic neisseriae can use hemoglobin, transferrin, and lactoferrin independently of the tonB locus. *Journal of Bacteriology, 182*(19), 5586–5591. doi:10.1128/JB.182.19.5586-5591.2000 PMID:10986265

Detels, R., Green, A. M., Klausner, J. D., Katzenstein, D., Gaydos, C., Handsfield, H., Pequegnat, W., Mayer, K., Hartwell, T. D., & Quinn, T. C. (2011). The incidence and correlates of symptomatic and asymptomatic Chlamydia trachomatis and *Neisseria gonorrhoeae* infections in selected populations in five countries. *Sexually Transmitted Diseases, 38*(6), 503–509. doi:10.1097/OLQ.0b013e318206c288 PMID:22256336

Dillon, J. R., Carballo, M., & Pauzé, M. (1988). Evaluation of eight methods for identification of pathogenic Neisseria species: Neisseria-Kwik, RIM-N, Gonobio-Test, Minitek, Gonochek II, GonoGen, Phadebact Monoclonal GC OMNI Test, and Syva MicroTrak Test. *Journal of Clinical Microbiology, 26*(3), 493–497. doi:10.1128/JCM.26.3.493-497.1988 PMID:3128578

Dunlop, E. M. (1949). Gonorrhoea and the sulphonamides. *The British Journal of Venereal Diseases, 25*(2), 81–83. PMID:18151908

Edwards, J. L., & Apicella, M. A. (2004). The molecular mechanisms used by *Neisseria gonorrhoeae* to initiate infection differ between men and women. *Clinical Microbiology Reviews, 17*(4), 965–981. doi:10.1128/CMR.17.4.965-981.2004 PMID:15489357

Edwards, J. L., Shao, J. Q., Ault, K. A., & Apicella, M. A. (2000). *Neisseria gonorrhoeae* elicits membrane ruffling and cytoskeletal rearrangements upon infection of primary human endocervical and ectocervical cells. *Infection and Immunity, 68*(9), 5354–5363. doi:10.1128/IAI.68.9.5354-5363.2000 PMID:10948165

Ehret, J. M., & Judson, F. N. (1991). Gonorrhea. In B. B. Wentworth (Ed.), *Laboratory Methods for the Diagnosis of Sexually Transmitted Disease* (2nd ed., pp. 53–94). American Public Health Association.

Erwin, M. E., Jones, R. N., Koontz, F. P., Gerlach, E. H., Murray, P. R., & Washington, J. A. (1992). MIC and disk diffusion quality control guidelines for *Neisseria gonorrhoeae* susceptibility tests of cefdinir, cefetamet, CI-960, fleroxacin, lomefloxacin, and temafloxacin. *Journal of Clinical Microbiology, 30*(5), 1317–1319. doi:10.1128/JCM.30.5.1317-1319.1992 PMID:1316371

European Centre for Disease Prevention and Control. (n.d.). *Annual epidemiological report for 2015 – Gonorrhoea.* Stockholm: ECDC. Available from: https://ecdc.europa.eu/sites/portal/files/documents/AER_for_2015-gonorrhoea.pdf

European Centre for Disease Prevention and Control. (2016). *Annual Epidemiological Report 2016 – Gonorrhoea.* ECDC.

Exner, M., Bhattacharya, S., Christiansen, B., Gebel, J., Goroncy-Bermes, P., Hartemann, P., ... Trautmann, M. (2017). Antibiotic resistance: What is so special about multidrug-resistant Gram-negative bacteria? *GMS Hygiene and Infection Control, 12*, Doc05. doi:10.3205/dgkh000290 PMID:28451516

Feinen, B., Jerse, A. E., Gaffen, S. L., & Russell, M. W. (2010). Critical role of Th17 responses in a murine model of *Neisseria gonorrhoeae* genital infection. *Mucosal Immunology, 3*(3), 312–321. doi:10.1038/mi.2009.139 PMID:20107432

Fichorova, R. N., Desai, P. J., Gibson, F. C. III, & Genco, C. A. (2001). Distinct proinflammatory host responses to *Neisseria gonorrhoeae* infection in immortalized human cervical and vaginal epithelial cells. *Infection and Immunity, 69*(9), 5840–5848. doi:10.1128/IAI.69.9.5840-5848.2001 PMID:11500462

Fiebelkorn, K. R., Crawford, S. A., & Jorgensen, J. H. (2005). Mutations in *folP* Associated with Elevated Sulfonamide MICs for *Neisseria meningitidis* Clinical Isolates from Five Continents. *Antimicrobial Agents and Chemotherapy, 49*(2), 536540. doi:10.1128/AAC.49.2.536-540.2005 PMID:15673729

Fingerhuth, S. M., Bonhoeffer, S., Low, N., & Althaus, C. L. (2016). Antibiotic-Resistant *Neisseria gonorrhoeae* Spread Faster with More Treatment, Not More Sexual Partners. *PLoS Pathogens, 12*(5), e1005611. doi:10.1371/journal.ppat.1005611 PMID:27196299

Follows, S. A., Murlidharan, J., Massari, P., Wetzler, L. M., & Genco, C. A. (2009). *Neisseria gonorrhoeae* infection protects human endocervical epithelial cells from apoptosis via expression of host antiapoptotic proteins. *Infection and Immunity, 77*(9), 3602–3610. doi:10.1128/IAI.01366-08 PMID:19546192

Foster, R. S., & Vinson, J. W. (1977). Chicken embryo as an animal model for gonorrhea. *Infection and Immunity, 16*(2), 568–574. doi:10.1128/IAI.16.2.568-574.1977 PMID:405324

Frenette, M., Beaudet, R., Bisaillon, J. G., Sylvestre, M., & Portelance, V. (1984). Chemical and biological characterization of a gonococcal growth inhibitor produced by Staphylococcus haemolyticus isolated from urogenital flora. *Infection and Immunity, 46*(2), 340–345. doi:10.1128/IAI.46.2.340-345.1984 PMID:6437979

Gesink Law, D., Rink, E., Mulvad, G., & Koch, A. (2008). Sexual health and sexually transmitted infections in the North American Arctic. *Emerging Infectious Diseases, 14*(1), 4–9. doi:10.3201/eid1401.071112 PMID:18258070

Ghanem, K. G. (n.d.). Clinical manifestations and diagnosis of *Neisseria gonorrhoeae* infection in adults and adolescents. *UpToDate*. www.uptodate.com/contents/clinical-manifestations-and-diagnosis-of-neisseria-gonorrhoeae-infection-in-adults-and-adolescents

Giltner, C. L., Nguyen, Y., & Burrows, L. L. (2012). Type IV pilin proteins: Versatile molecular modules. *Microbiology and molecular biology reviews. Microbiology and Molecular Biology Reviews, 76*(4), 740–772. doi:10.1128/MMBR.00035-12 PMID:23204365

Gulati, S., Mu, X., Zheng, B., Reed, G. W., Ram, S., & Rice, P. A. (2015). Antibody to reduction modifiable protein increases the bacterial burden and the duration of gonococcal infection in a mouse model. *The Journal of Infectious Diseases, 212*(2), 311–315. doi:10.1093/infdis/jiv024 PMID:25596304

Gupta, S., Govil, D., Kakar, P. N., Prakash, O., Arora, D., Das, S., ... Malhotra, A. (2009). Colistin and polymyxin B: A re-emergence. *Indian Journal of Critical Care Medicine: Peer-Reviewed, Official Publication of Indian Society of Critical Care Medicine*, *13*(2), 49–53. doi:10.4103/0972-5229.56048 PMID:19881183

Gurung, A., Prabhakar, P., Narayanan, P., Mehendale, S., Risbud, A., & Das, A. (2010). *Prevalence of asymptomatic gonorrhea and chlamydia among men having sex with men (MSM) in India and associated risk factors*. International AIDS Conference, Washington, DC.

Harvey, H. A., Post, D. M., & Apicella, M. A. (2002). Immortalization of human urethral epithelial cells: A model for the study of the pathogenesis of and the inflammatory cytokine response to *Neisseria gonorrhoeae* infection. *Infection and Immunity*, *70*(10), 5808–5815. doi:10.1128/IAI.70.10.5808-5815.2002 PMID:12228311

Hauck, C. R., Lorenzen, D., Saas, J., & Meyer, T. F. (1997). An in vitro-differentiated human cell line as a model system to study the interaction of *Neisseria gonorrhoeae* with phagocytic cells. *Infection and Immunity*, *65*(5), 1863–1869. doi:10.1128/IAI.65.5.1863-1869.1997 PMID:9125573

Hehre, E. J. (1949). Synthesis of a polysaccharide of the starch-glycogen class from sucrose by a cell free, bacterial enzyme system. *The Journal of Biological Chemistry*, *177*(1), 267–279. PMID:18107430

Higashi, D. L., Zhang, G. H., Biais, N., Myers, L. R., Weyand, N. J., Elliott, D. A., & So, M. (2009). Influence of type IV pilus retraction on the architecture of the *Neisseria gonorrhoeae*-infected cell cortex. *Microbiology (Reading, England)*, *155*(Pt 12), 4084–4092. doi:10.1099/mic.0.032656-0 PMID:19762436

Hobbs, M. M., Anderson, J. E., Balthazar, J. T., Kandler, J. L., Carlson, R. W., Ganguly, J., Begum, A. A., Duncan, J. A., Lin, J. T., Sparling, P. F., Jerse, A. E., & Shafer, W. M. (2013). Lipid A's structure mediates *Neisseria gonorrhoeae* fitness during experimental infection of mice and men. *mBio*, *4*(6), e00892–e13. doi:10.1128/mBio.00892-13 PMID:24255126

Hopper, S., Wilbur, J. S., Vasquez, B. L., Larson, J., Clary, S., Mehr, I. J., Seifert, H. S., & So, M. (2000). Isolation of *Neisseria gonorrhoeae* mutants that show enhanced trafficking across polarized T84 epithelial monolayers. *Infection and Immunity*, *68*(2), 896–905. doi:10.1128/IAI.68.2.896-905.2000 PMID:10639460

Hung, M. C., & Christodoulides, M. (2013). The biology of Neisseria adhesins. *Biology (Basel)*, *2*(3), 1054–1109. doi:10.3390/biology2031054 PMID:24833056

Janda, W. J., & Knapp, J. S. (2003). *Neisseria* and *Moraxella catarrhalis*. In P. R. Murray, E. J. Baron, M. A. Pfaller, J. H. Jorgensen, & R. H. Yolken (Eds.), *Manual of Clinical Microbiology* (8th ed., pp. 585–608). American Society Microbiology.

Janda, W. M., Zigler, K. L., & Bradna, J. J. (1987). API QuadFERM+ with rapid DNase for identification of Neisseria spp. and Branhamella catarrhalis. *Journal of Clinical Microbiology*, *25*(2), 203–206. doi:10.1128/JCM.25.2.203-206.1987 PMID:3102550

Janeway, C. A., Jr., Travers, P., Walport, M., & Shlomchik, M.J. (2001). *Immunobiology: The Immune System in Health and Disease* (5th ed.). New York: Garland Science. Available from: https://www.ncbi.nlm.nih.gov/books/NBK27100/

Jarvis, G. A., Li, J., & Swanson, K. V. (1999). Invasion of human mucosal epithelial cells by *Neisseria gonorrhoeae* upregulates expression of intercellular adhesion molecule 1 (ICAM-1). *Infection and Immunity*, *67*(3), 1149–1156. doi:10.1128/IAI.67.3.1149-1156.1999 PMID:10024555

Jerse, A. E. (1999). Experimental gonococcal genital tract infection and opacity protein expression in estradiol-treated mice. *Infection and Immunity*, *67*(11), 5699–5708. doi:10.1128/IAI.67.11.5699-5708.1999 PMID:10531218

Jerse, A. E., Bash, M. C., & Russell, M. W. (2014). Vaccines against gonorrhea: Current status and future challenges. *Vaccine*, *32*(14), 1579–1587. doi:10.1016/j.vaccine.2013.08.067 PMID:24016806

Johnson, A., Tuffrey, M., & Taylor-Robinson, D. (1989). Resistance of mice to genital infection with *Neisseria gonorrhoeae*. *Journal of Medical Microbiology*, *30*(1), 33–36. doi:10.1099/00222615-30-1-33 PMID:2506350

Johnson, A. P., Taylor-Robinson, D., & Slavin, G. (1977). Pneumonia in mice produced by *Neisseria gonorrhoeae*. *The British Journal of Venereal Diseases*, *53*(1), 26–30. doi:10.1136ti.53.1.26 PMID:843896

Johnson, M. B., & Criss, A. K. (2011). Resistance of *Neisseria gonorrhoeae* to neutrophils. *Frontiers in Microbiology*, *2*, 77. doi:10.3389/fmicb.2011.00077 PMID:21747795

Johnston, K. H., Holmes, K. K., & Gotschlich, E. C. (1976). The serological classification of *Neisseria gonorrhoeae*. I. Isolation of the outer membrane complex responsible for serotypic specificity. *The Journal of Experimental Medicine*, *143*(4), 741–758. doi:10.1084/jem.143.4.741 PMID:56416

Karatan, E., & Watnick, P. (2009). Signals, regulatory networks, and materials that build and break bacterial biofilms. Microbiology and molecular biology reviews. *Microbiology and Molecular Biology Reviews*, *73*(2), 310–347. doi:10.1128/MMBR.00041-08 PMID:19487730

Kim, W. J., Mai, A., Weyand, N. J., Rendón, M. A., Van Doorslaer, K., & So, M. (2019). *Neisseria gonorrhoeae* evades autophagic killing by downregulating CD46-cyt1 and remodeling lysosomes. *PLoS Pathogens*, *15*(2), e1007495. doi:10.1371/journal.ppat.1007495 PMID:30753248

Klimpel, G. R. (1996). Immune Defenses. In Med Microbiol. Galveston, TX: University of Texas Medical Branch at Galveston.

Kraus, S. J. (1979). Culture Methods for Neisseria Gonorrhoea. *Archives of Andrology*, *3*(4), 343–349. doi:10.3109/01485017908988426 PMID:119501

Kraus, S. J., Brown, W. J., & Arko, R. J. (1975). Acquired and natural immunity to gonococcal infection in chimpanzees. *The Journal of Clinical Investigation*, *55*(6), 1349–1356. doi:10.1172/JCI108054 PMID:805797

Kulkarni, S., Bala, M., & Risbud, A. (2015). Performance of tests for identification of *Neisseria gonorrhoeae*. *The Indian Journal of Medical Research*, *141*(6), 833–835. doi:10.4103/0971-5916.160721 PMID:26205027

Kupsch, E. M., Knepper, B., Kuroki, T., Heuer, I., & Meyer, T. F. (1993). Variable opacity (Opa) outer membrane proteins account for the cell tropisms displayed by *Neisseria gonorrhoeae* for human leukocytes and epithelial cells. *The EMBO Journal*, *12*(2), 641–650. doi:10.1002/j.1460-2075.1993.tb05697.x PMID:8440254

Lahra, M. M., & Enriquez, R. P. (2017). Australian Gonococcal Surveillance Programme, 1 July to 30 September 2016. *Communicable Diseases Intelligence*, *41*(1), 109–110. PMID:28385144

Lambden, P. R., Heckels, J. E., & Watt, P. J. (1982). Effect of anti-pilus antibodies on survival of gonococci within guinea pig subcutaneous chambers. *Infection and Immunity*, *38*(1), 27–30. doi:10.1128/IAI.38.1.27-30.1982 PMID:6128301

Lenz, J. D., & Dillard, J. P. (2018). Pathogenesis of *Neisseria gonorrhoeae* and the Host Defense in Ascending Infections of Human Fallopian Tube. *Frontiers in Immunology*, *9*, 2710. doi:10.3389/fimmu.2018.02710 PMID:30524442

LeVan, A., Zimmerman, L. I., Mahle, A. C., Swanson, K. V., DeShong, P., Park, J., Edwards, V. L., Song, W., & Stein, D. C. (2012). Construction and characterization of a derivative of *Neisseria gonorrhoeae* strain MS11 devoid of all opa genes. *Journal of Bacteriology*, *194*(23), 6468–6478. doi:10.1128/JB.00969-12 PMID:23002223

Levy, J., Wicher, K., & Rose, N. R. (1973). In vitro susceptibility of *Neisseria gonorrhoeae* to spectinomycin examined by a broth dilution method. *Antimicrobial Agents and Chemotherapy*, *3*(3), 335–337. doi:10.1128/AAC.3.3.335 PMID:4275225

Li, L. H., Yen, M. Y., Ho, C. C., Wu, P., Wang, C. C., Maurya, P. K., Chen, P.-S., Chen, W., Hsieh, W.-Y., & Chen, H. W. (2013). Non-cytotoxic nanomaterials enhance antimicrobial activities of cefmetazole against multidrug-resistant *Neisseria gonorrhoeae*. *PLoS One*, *8*(5), e64794. doi:10.1371/journal.pone.0064794 PMID:23705013

Ligon, B. E., Ludwig, A., & Neisser, S. (2005). Discoverer of the Cause of Gonorrhea. *Seminars in Pediatric Infectious Diseases*, *16*(4), 336–341. doi:10.1053/j.spid.2005.07.001 PMID:16210113

Lindbäck, E., Rahman, M., Jalal, S., & Wretlind, B. (2002). Mutations in *gyrA, gyrB, parC*, and *parE* in quinolone-resistant strains of *Neisseria gonorrhoeae*. *APMIS*, *110*(9), 651–657. doi:10.1034/j.1600-0463.2002.1100909.x PMID:12529019

Lindberg, R., Fredlund, H., Nicholas, R., & Unemo, M. (2007). *Neisseria gonorrhoeae* isolates with reduced susceptibility to cefixime and ceftriaxone: Association with genetic polymorphisms in penA, mtrR, porB1b, and ponA. *Antimicrobial Agents and Chemotherapy*, *51*(6), 2117–2122. doi:10.1128/AAC.01604-06 PMID:17420216

Liu, Y., Egilmez, N. K., & Russell, M. W. (2013). Enhancement of adaptive immunity to *Neisseria gonorrhoeae* by local intravaginal administration of microencapsulated interleukin 12. *The Journal of Infectious Diseases*, *208*(11), 1821–1829. doi:10.1093/infdis/jit354 PMID:24048962

Liu, Y., & Russell, M. W. (2011). Diversion of the immune response to *Neisseria gonorrhoeae* from Th17 to Th1/Th2 by treatment with anti-transforming growth factor β antibody generates immunological memory and protective immunity. *mBio*, *2*(3), e00095–e11. doi:10.1128/mBio.00095-11 PMID:21610119

Long, C. D., Hayes, S. F., van Putten, J. P., Harvey, H. A., Apicella, M. A., & Seifert, H. S. (2001). Modulation of gonococcal piliation by regulatable transcription of pilE. *Journal of Bacteriology*, *183*(5), 1600–1609. doi:10.1128/JB.183.5.1600-1609.2001 PMID:11160091

Lunzen, J. V., & Altfeld, M. (2014). Sex Differences in Infectious Diseases–Common but Neglected. *The Journal of Infectious Diseases*, *209*(3, suppl 3), S79–S80. doi:10.1093/infdis/jiu159 PMID:24966193

Mak, D. B., Smith, D. W., Harnett, G. B., & Plant, A. J. (2001). A large outbreak of conjunctivitis caused by a single genotype of *Neisseria gonorrhoeae* distinct from those causing genital tract infections. *Epidemiology and Infection*, *126*(3), 373–378. doi:10.1017/S0950268801005477 PMID:11467794

Mårdh, P. A., Weström, L., von Mecklenburg, C., & Hammar, E. (1976). Studies on ciliated epithelia of the human genital tract. I. Swelling of the cilia of Fallopian tube epithelium in organ cultures infected with Mycoplasma hominis. *The British Journal of Venereal Diseases*, *52*(1), 52–57. doi:10.1136ti.52.1.52 PMID:1260408

Matejcek, A., & Goldman, R. D. (2013). Treatment and prevention of ophthalmia neonatorum. *Canadian Family Physician Medecin de Famille Canadien*, *59*(11), 1187–1190. PMID:24235191

Mavrogiorgos, N., Mekasha, S., Yang, Y., Kelliher, M. A., & Ingalls, R. R. (2014). Activation of NOD receptors by *Neisseria gonorrhoeae* modulates the innate immune response. *Innate Immunity*, *20*(4), 377–389. doi:10.1177/1753425913493453 PMID:23884094

McCaw, S. E., Liao, E. H., & Gray-Owen, S. D. (2004). Engulfment of *Neisseria gonorrhoeae*: Revealing distinct processes of bacterial entry by individual carcinoembryonic antigen-related cellular adhesion molecule family receptors. *Infection and Immunity*, *72*(5), 2742–2752. doi:10.1128/IAI.72.5.2742-2752.2004 PMID:15102784

Mehta, S. D., Rothman, R. E., Kelen, G. D., Quinn, T. C., & Zenilman, J. M. (2001). Clinical Aspects of Diagnosis of Gonorrhea and *Chlamydia* Infection in an Acute Care Setting. *Clinical Infectious Diseases*, *32*(4), 655–659. doi:10.1086/318711 PMID:11181134

Młynarczyk-Bonikowska, B., Kujawa, M., Malejczyk, M., Młynarczyk, G., & Majewski, S. (2016). Plasmid-mediated resistance to tetracyclines among *Neisseria gonorrhoeae* strains isolated in Poland between 2012 and 2013. *Postepy Dermatologii i Alergologii*, *33*(6), 475–479. doi:10.5114/ada.2016.63887 PMID:28035227

Mogensen, T. H. (2009). Pathogen recognition and inflammatory signaling in innate immune defenses. *Clinical Microbiology Reviews*, *22*(2), 240–273. doi:10.1128/CMR.00046-08 PMID:19366914

Montano, M., Flanagan, J.N., Jiang, L., Sebastiani, P., Rarick, M., LeBrasseur, … Bhasin, S. (2007). Transcriptional Profiling of Testosterone-Regulated Genes in the Skeletal Muscle of Human Immunodeficiency Virus-Infected Men Experiencing Weight Loss. *The Journal of Clinical Endocrinology & Metabolism*, *92*(7), 2793–2802. doi:10.1210/jc.2006-2722

Munson, E., Wenten, D., Phipps, P., Gremminger, R., Schuknecht, M. K., Napierala, M., Hamer, D., Olson, R., Schell, R. F., & Hryciuk, J. E. (2013). Retrospective assessment of transcription-mediated amplification-based screening for Trichomonas vaginalis in male sexually transmitted infection clinic patients. *Journal of Clinical Microbiology*, *51*(6), 1855–1860. doi:10.1128/JCM.00455-13 PMID:23554208

Naumann, M., Wessler, S., Bartsch, C., Wieland, B., & Meyer, T. F. (1997). *Neisseria gonorrhoeae* epithelial cell interaction leads to the activation of the transcription factors nuclear factor kappaB and activator protein 1 and the induction of inflammatory cytokines. *The Journal of Experimental Medicine*, *186*(2), 247–258. doi:10.1084/jem.186.2.247 PMID:9221754

Newman, L., Rowley, J., Vander Hoorn, S., Wijesooriya, N. S., Unemo, M., Low, N., Stevens, G., Gottlieb, S., Kiarie, J., & Temmerman, M. (2015). Global Estimates of the Prevalence and Incidence of Four Curable Sexually Transmitted Infections in 2012 Based on Systematic Review and Global Reporting. *PLoS One*, *10*(12), e0143304. doi:10.1371/journal.pone.0143304 PMID:26646541

Ng, L. K., Martin, I., Liu, G., & Bryden, L. (2002). Mutation in 23S rRNA associated with macrolide resistance in *Neisseria gonorrhoeae*. *Antimicrobial Agents and Chemotherapy*, *46*(9), 3020–3025. doi:10.1128/AAC.46.9.3020-3025.2002 PMID:12183262

Ng, L. K., & Martin, I. E. (2005). The laboratory diagnosis of *Neisseria gonorrhoeae*. *The Canadian journal of infectious diseases & medical microbiology =. The Canadian Journal of Infectious Diseases & Medical Microbiology*, *16*(1), 15–25. doi:10.1155/2005/323082 PMID:18159523

Nowicki, S., Selvarangan, R., & Anderson, G. (1999). Experimental transmission of *Neisseria gonorrhoeae* from pregnant rat to fetus. *Infection and Immunity*, *67*(9), 4974–4976. doi:10.1128/IAI.67.9.4974-4976.1999 PMID:10456962

Ohneck, E. A., Goytia, M., Rouquette-Loughlin, C. E., Joseph, S. J., Read, T. D., Jerse, A. E., & Shafer, W. M. (2015). Overproduction of the MtrCDE efflux pump in *Neisseria gonorrhoeae* produces unexpected changes in cellular transcription patterns. *Antimicrobial Agents and Chemotherapy*, *59*(1), 724–726. doi:10.1128/AAC.04148-14 PMID:25367915

Papp, J. R., Abrams, A. J., Nash, E., Katz, A. R., Kirkcaldy, R. D., O'Connor, N. P., O'Brien, P. S., Harauchi, D. H., Maningas, E. V., Soge, O. O., Kersh, E. N., Komeya, A., Tomas, J. E., Wasserman, G. M., Kunimoto, G. Y., Trees, D. L., & Whelen, A. C. (2017). Azithromycin Resistance and Decreased Ceftriaxone Susceptibility in *Neisseria gonorrhoeae*, Hawaii, USA. *Emerging Infectious Diseases*, *23*(5), 830–832. doi:10.3201/eid2305.170088 PMID:28418303

Parra, A., Ponte, C., Cenjor, C., García-Olmos, M., Giménez, M. J., Aguilar, L., & Soriano, F. (2004). In vivo activity of amoxicillin/clavulanic acid and erythromycin in experimental otitis media caused by Streptococcus pneumoniae plus Haemophilus influenzae. *International Journal of Antimicrobial Agents*, *23*(1), 25–31. doi:10.1016/j.ijantimicag.2003.05.016 PMID:14732310

Pasieka, A. E., Ota, F., Ryan, A., Ashton, F. E., Wallace, R., Perusse, C., & Diena, B. B. (1976). The goat mammary gland as a model infection site for *Neisseria gonorrhoeae. The British Journal of Venereal Diseases*, *52*(3), 170–171. doi:10.1136ti.52.3.170 PMID:819088

Patel, A. L., Chaudhry, U., Sachdev, D., Sachdeva, P. N., Bala, M., & Saluja, D. (2011). An insight into the drug resistance profile & mechanism of drug resistance in *Neisseria gonorrhoeae. The Indian Journal of Medical Research*, *134*(4), 419–431. PMID:22089602

Patrone, J. B., & Stein, D. C. (2007). Effect of gonococcal lipooligosaccharide variation on human monocytic cytokine profile. *BMC Microbiology*, *7*(1), 7. doi:10.1186/1471-2180-7-7 PMID:17257430

Patton, M. E., Kidd, S., Llata, E., Stenger, M., Braxton, J., Asbel, L., Bernstein, K., Gratzer, B., Jespersen, M., Kerani, R., Mettenbrink, C., Mohamed, M., Pathela, P., Schumacher, C., Stirland, A., Stover, J., Tabidze, I., Kirkcaldy, R. D., & Weinstock, H. (2014). Extragenital gonorrhea and chlamydia testing and infection among men who have sex with men—STD Surveillance Network, United States, 2010-2012. *Nephrology, Dialysis, Transplantation*, *58*(11), 1564–1570. doi:10.1093/cid/ciu184 PMID:24647015

Peterson, J. W. (1996). Bacterial Pathogenesis. In S. Baron (Ed.), *Medical Microbiology* (4th ed.). University of Texas Medical Branch at Galveston. Available from https://www.ncbi.nlm.nih.gov/books/NBK8526/

Pierce, W. A. Jr, Leong, J. K., & Hough, D. M. (1975). Strain-specific virulence-associated antigen of *Neisseria gonorrhoeae. Infection and Immunity*, *11*(5), 898–903. doi:10.1128/IAI.11.5.898-903.1975 PMID:804445

Pinchuk, G. E., Ammons, C., Culley, D. E., Li, S. W., McLean, J. S., Romine, M. F., Nealson, K. H., Fredrickson, J. K., & Beliaev, A. S. (2008). Utilization of DNA as a Sole Source of Phosphorus, Carbon, and Energy by *Shewanella* spp.: Ecological and Physiological Implications for Dissimilatory Metal Reduction. *Applied and Environmental Microbiology*, *74*(4), 1198–1208. doi:10.1128/AEM.02026-07 PMID:18156329

Plant, L., Sundqvist, J., Zughaier, S., Lövkvist, L., Stephens, D. S., & Jonsson, A. B. (2006). Lipooligosaccharide structure contributes to multiple steps in the virulence of Neisseria meningitidis. *Infection and Immunity*, *74*(2), 1360–1367. doi:10.1128/IAI.74.2.1360-1367.2006 PMID:16428785

Pohlner J, Halter R, Beyreuther K & Meyer TF. (1987).Gene structure and extracellular secretion of *Neisseria gonorrhoeae* IgA protease. *Nature*, *325*(6103), 458-62.

Potter, A. J., Kidd, S. P., Edwards, J. L., Falsetta, M. L., Apicella, M. A., Jennings, M. P., & McEwan, A. G. (2009). Thioredoxin reductase is essential for protection of *Neisseria gonorrhoeae* against killing by nitric oxide and for bacterial growth during interaction with cervical epithelial cells. *The Journal of Infectious Diseases*, *199*(2), 227–235. doi:10.1086/595737 PMID:19032106

Quillin, S. J., & Seifert, H. S. (2018). *Neisseria gonorrhoeae* host adaptation and pathogenesis. *Nature Reviews. Microbiology*, *16*(4), 226–240. doi:10.1038/nrmicro.2017.169 PMID:29430011

Rahal, A., Kumar, A., Singh, V., Yadav, B., Tiwari, R., Chakraborty, S., & Dhama, K. (2014). Oxidative stress, prooxidants, and antioxidants: The interplay. *BioMed Research International*, *2014*, 761264. doi:10.1155/2014/761264 PMID:24587990

Rippa, V., Santini, L., Lo Surdo, P., Cantini, F., Veggi, D., Gentile, M. A., Grassi, E., Iannello, G., Brunelli, B., Ferlicca, F., Palmieri, E., Pallaoro, M., Aricò, B., Banci, L., Pizza, M., & Scarselli, M. (2015). Molecular Engineering of Ghfp, the Gonococcal Orthologue of Neisseria meningitidis Factor H Binding Protein. *Clinical and Vaccine Immunology; CVI*, *22*(7), 769–777. doi:10.1128/CVI.00794-14 PMID:25947148

Ritter, J. L., & Genco, C. A. (2018). *Neisseria gonorrhoeae*-Induced Inflammatory Pyroptosis in Human Macrophages is Dependent on Intracellular Gonococci and Lipooligosaccharide. *Journal of Cell Death*, *11*, 1179066017750902. doi:10.1177/1179066017750902 PMID:29434478

Ronpirin, C., Jerse, A. E., & Cornelissen, C. N. (2001). Gonococcal genes encoding transferrin-binding proteins A and B are arranged in a bicistronic operon but are subject to differential expression. *Infection and Immunity*, *69*(10), 6336–6347. doi:10.1128/IAI.69.10.6336-6347.2001 PMID:11553578

Ropp, P. A., Hu, M., Olesky, M., & Nicholas, R. A. (2002). Mutations in ponA, the gene encoding penicillin-binding protein 1, and a novel locus, penC, are required for high-level chromosomally mediated penicillin resistance in *Neisseria gonorrhoeae. Antimicrobial Agents and Chemotherapy*, *46*(3), 769–777. doi:10.1128/AAC.46.3.769-777.2002 PMID:11850260

Roth, R. I., Yamasaki, R., Mandrell, R. E., & Griffiss, J. M. (1992). Ability of gonococcal and meningococcal lipooligosaccharides to clot Limulus amebocyte lysate. *Infection and Immunity*, *60*(3), 762–767. doi:10.1128/IAI.60.3.762-767.1992 PMID:1541549

Rouphael, N. G., & Stephens, D. S. (2012). Neisseria meningitidis: Biology, microbiology, and epidemiology. *Methods in Molecular Biology (Clifton, N.J.)*, *799*, 1–20. doi:10.1007/978-1-61779-346-2_1 PMID:21993636

Saginur, R., Clecner, B., Portnoy, J., & Mendelson, J. (1982). Superoxol(catalase)test for identification of *Neisseria gonorrhoeae. Journal of Clinical Microbiology*, *15*(3), 475–477. doi:10.1128/JCM.15.3.475-477.1982 PMID:6804487

Satterwhite, C. L., Torrone, E., Meites, E., Dunne, E. F., Mahajan, R., Ocfemia, M. C., Su, J., Xu, F., & Weinstock, H. (2013). Sexually transmitted infections among US women and men: Prevalence and incidence estimates, 2008. *Sexually Transmitted Diseases*, *40*(3), 187–193. doi:10.1097/OLQ.0b013e318286bb53 PMID:23403598

Scheenstra, M. R. (2010). *Antiphagocytosis - a bacterial mechanism to inhibit phagocytosis* (Unpublished master thesis). Department of Immunology, UMC Utrecht, Netherlands.

Scheuerpflug, I., Rudel, T., Ryll, R., Pandit, J., & Meyer, T. F. (1999). Roles of PilC and PilE proteins in pilus-mediated adherence of *Neisseria gonorrhoeae* and Neisseria meningitidis to human erythrocytes and endothelial and epithelial cells. *Infection and Immunity*, *67*(2), 834–843. doi:10.1128/IAI.67.2.834-843.1999 PMID:9916098

Schmidt, H., & Hensel, M. (2004). Pathogenicity islands in bacterial pathogenesis. *Clinical Microbiology Reviews*, *17*(1), 14–56. doi:10.1128/CMR.17.1.14-56.2004 PMID:14726454

Shields, P., & Cathcart, L. (2013). *Oxidase Test Protocol.* American Society for Microbiology.

Shim, B. S. (2011). Current concepts in bacterial sexually transmitted diseases. *Korean Journal of Urology*, *52*(9), 589–597. doi:10.4111/kju.2011.52.9.589 PMID:22025952

Simons, M. P., Nauseef, W. M., & Apicella, M. A. (2005). Interactions of *Neisseria gonorrhoeae* with adherent polymorphonuclear leukocytes. *Infection and Immunity*, *73*(4), 1971–1977. doi:10.1128/IAI.73.4.1971-1977.2005 PMID:15784537

Singh, R., Perera, S. R., Katselis, G. S., Chumala, P., Martin, I., Kusalik, A., Mitzel, K. M., & Dillon, J.-A. R. (2019). A β-lactamase-producing plasmid from *Neisseria gonorrhoeae* carrying a unique 6 bp deletion in $bla_{TEM\text{-}1}$ encoding a truncated 24 kDa TEM-1 penicillinase that hydrolyses ampicillin slowly. *The Journal of Antimicrobial Chemotherapy*, *74*(10), 2904–2912. doi:10.1093/jac/dkz306 PMID:31335939

Smith, J. C., Mailman, T., & Macdonald, N. E. (2013). How to get and get rid of gonorrhea. *Advances in Experimental Medicine and Biology*, *764*, 219–239. doi:10.1007/978-1-4614-4726-9_19 PMID:23654071

Soler-García, A. A., & Jerse, A. E. (2007). *Neisseria gonorrhoeae* catalase is not required for experimental genital tract infection despite the induction of a localized neutrophil response. *Infection and Immunity*, *75*(5), 2225–2233. doi:10.1128/IAI.01513-06 PMID:17296753

Song, W., Condron, S., Mocca, B. T., Veit, S. J., Hill, D., Abbas, A., & Jerse, A. E. (2008). Local and humoral immune responses against primary and repeat *Neisseria gonorrhoeae* genital tract infections of 17beta-estradiol-treated mice. *Vaccine*, *26*(45), 5741–5751. doi:10.1016/j.vaccine.2008.08.020 PMID:18762223

Song, W., Ma, L., Chen, R., & Stein, D. C. (2000). Role of lipooligosaccharide in Opa-independent invasion of *Neisseria gonorrhoeae* into human epithelial cells. *The Journal of Experimental Medicine*, *191*(6), 949–960. doi:10.1084/jem.191.6.949 PMID:10727457

Speers-Roesch, B., & Ballantyne, J. S. (2005). Activities of antioxidant enzymes and cytochrome c oxidase in liver of Arctic and temperate teleosts. *Comparative Biochemistry and Physiology*, *140*(4), 487–494. doi:10.1016/j.cbpb.2005.02.014 PMID:15936709

Spencer, S. E., Valentin-Bon, I. E., Whaley, K., & Jerse, A. E. (2004). Inhibition of *Neisseria gonorrhoeae*Genital Tract Infection by Leading-Candidate Topical Microbicides in a Mouse Model. *The Journal of Infectious Diseases*, *189*(3), 410–419. doi:10.1086/381125 PMID:14745698

Spinosa, M. R., Progida, C., Talà, A., Cogli, L., Alifano, P., & Bucci, C. (2007). The Neisseria meningitidis capsule is important for intracellular survival in human cells. *Infection and Immunity*, *75*(7), 3594–3603. doi:10.1128/IAI.01945-06 PMID:17470547

Stein, D. C., LeVan, A., Hardy, B., Wang, L. C., Zimmerman, L., & Song, W. (2015). Expression of Opacity Proteins Interferes with the Transmigration of *Neisseria gonorrhoeae*across Polarized Epithelial Cells. *PLoS One*, *10*(8), e0134342. doi:10.1371/journal.pone.0134342 PMID:26244560

Streeter, P. R., & Corbeil, L. B. (1981). Gonococcal infection in endotoxin-resistant and endotoxin-susceptible mice. *Infection and Immunity*, *32*(1), 105–110. doi:10.1128/IAI.32.1.105-110.1981 PMID:6783547

Swanson, J., Robbins, K., Barrera, O., Corwin, D., Boslego, J., Ciak, J., Blake, M., & Koomey, J. M. (1987). Gonococcal pilin variants in experimental gonorrhea. *The Journal of Experimental Medicine*, *165*(5), 1344–1357. doi:10.1084/jem.165.5.1344 PMID:3106555

Taylor-Robinson, D., Whytock, S., Green, C. J., & Carney, F. E. Jr. (1974). Effect of *Neisseria gonorrhoeae* on human and rabbit oviducts. *The British Journal of Venereal Diseases*, *50*(4), 279–288. doi:10.1136ti.50.4.279 PMID:4213729

Trimble, M. J., Mlynárčik, P., Kolář, M., & Hancock, R. E. (2016). Polymyxin: Alternative Mechanisms of Action and Resistance. *Cold Spring Harbor Perspectives in Medicine*, *6*(10), a025288. doi:10.1101/cshperspect.a025288 PMID:27503996

Turner, S. M., Moir, J. W., Griffiths, L., Overton, T. W., Smith, H., & Cole, J. A. (2005). Mutational and biochemical analysis of cytochrome c′, a nitric oxide-binding lipoprotein important for adaptation of *Neisseria gonorrhoeae* to oxygen-limited growth. *The Biochemical Journal*, *388*(Pt 2), 545–553. doi:10.1042/BJ20041766 PMID:15689189

Tzeng, Y. L., Datta, A., Kolli, V. K., Carlson, R. W., & Stephens, D. S. (2002). Endotoxin of Neisseria meningitidis composed only of intact lipid A: Inactivation of the meningococcal 3-deoxy-D-manno-octulosonic acid transferase. *Journal of Bacteriology*, *184*(9), 2379–2388. doi:10.1128/JB.184.9.2379-2388.2002 PMID:11948150

Unemo, M., Ballard, R., Ison, C., Lewis, D., Ndowa, F., & Peeling, R. (2013). Laboratory Diagnosis of Sexually Transmitted Infections, including human immunodeficiency virus. *World Health Organisation Manual*. Available at: https://www.who.int/reproductivehealth/publications/rtis/9789241505840/en/

Unemo, M., Del Rio, C., & Shafer, W. M. (2016). Antimicrobial Resistance Expressed by *Neisseria gonorrhoeae*: A Major Global Public Health Problem in the 21st Century. *Microbiology Spectrum, 4*(3), doi:10.1128/microbiolspec

Unemo, M., Golparian, D., Skogen, V., Olsen, A. O., Moi, H., Syversen, G., & Hjelmevoll, S. O. (2013). *Neisseria gonorrhoeae* strain with high-level resistance to spectinomycin due to a novel resistance mechanism (mutated ribosomal protein S5) verified in Norway. *Antimicrobial Agents and Chemotherapy, 57*(2), 1057–1061. doi:10.1128/AAC.01775-12 PMID:23183436

Unemo, M., & Shafer, W. M. (2014). Antimicrobial resistance in *Neisseria gonorrhoeae* in the 21st century: Past, evolution, and future. *Clinical Microbiology Reviews, 27*(3), 587–613. doi:10.1128/CMR.00010-14 PMID:24982323

Uribe-Querol, E., & Rosales, C. (2017). Control of Phagocytosis by Microbial Pathogens. *Frontiers in Immunology, 8*, 1368. doi:10.3389/fimmu.2017.01368 PMID:29114249

Velasquez, L., García, K., Morales, F., Heckels, J. E., Orihuela, P., Rodas, P. I., Christodoulides, M., & Cardenas, H. (2012). *Neisseria gonorrhoeae* pilus attenuates cytokine response of human fallopian tube explants. *Journal of Biomedicine & Biotechnology, 491298*, 1–7. Advance online publication. doi:10.1155/2012/491298 PMID:22318778

Vermassen, A., Leroy, S., Talon, R., Provot, C., Popowska, M., & Desvaux, M. (2019). Cell Wall Hydrolases in Bacteria: Insight on the Diversity of Cell Wall Amidases, Glycosidases and Peptidases Toward Peptidoglycan. *Frontiers in Microbiology, 10*, 331. doi:10.3389/fmicb.2019.00331 PMID:30873139

Vijay, H. M., Lavergne, G., Ashton, F. E., Ryan, A., & Diena, B. B. (1977). Homocytotropic antibodies (IgE) to *Neisseria gonorrhoeae* in the rat and a cross-reactivity of heterologous gonococcal strains. *The British Journal of Venereal Diseases, 53*(2), 106–108. doi:10.1136ti.53.2.106 PMID:66964

Weel, J. F., Hopman, C. T., & van Putten, J. P. (1991). In situ expression and localization of *Neisseria gonorrhoeae* opacity proteins in infected epithelial cells: Apparent role of Opa proteins in cellular invasion. *The Journal of Experimental Medicine, 173*(6), 1395–1405. doi:10.1084/jem.173.6.1395 PMID:1903430

Weyand, N. J., Wertheimer, A. M., Hobbs, T. R., Sisko, J. L., Taku, N. A., Gregston, L. D., Clary, S., Higashi, D. L., Biais, N., Brown, L. M., Planer, S. L., Legasse, A. W., Axthelm, M. K., Wong, S. W., & So, M. (2013). Neisseria infection of rhesus macaques as a model to study colonization, transmission, persistence, and horizontal gene transfer. *Proceedings of the National Academy of Sciences of the United States of America, 110*(8), 3059–3064. doi:10.1073/pnas.1217420110 PMID:23382234

Weyler, L., Engelbrecht, M., Mata Forsberg, M., Brehwens, K., Vare, D., Vielfort, K., Wojcik, A., & Aro, H. (2014). Restriction endonucleases from invasive *Neisseria gonorrhoeae* cause double-strand breaks and distort mitosis in epithelial cells during infection. *PLoS One, 9*(12), e114208. doi:10.1371/journal.pone.0114208 PMID:25460012

Wira, C. R., Ghosh, M., Smith, J. M., Shen, L., Connor, R. I., Sundstrom, P., Frechette, G. M., Hill, E. T., & Fahey, J. V. (2011). Epithelial cell secretions from the human female reproductive tract inhibit sexually transmitted pathogens and Candida albicans but not Lactobacillus. *Mucosal Immunology*, *4*(3), 335–342. doi:10.1038/mi.2010.72 PMID:21048705

Wong, K. H., Arko, R. J., Schalla, W. O., & Steurer, F. J. (1979). Immunological and serological diversity of *Neisseria gonorrhoeae*: Identification of new immunotypes and highly protective strains. *Infection and Immunity*, *23*(3), 717–722. doi:10.1128/IAI.23.3.717-722.1979 PMID:88414

Woods, C. R. (2005). Gonococcal Infections in Neonates and Young Children. *Seminars in Pediatric Infectious Diseases*, *16*(4), 258–270. doi:10.1053/j.spid.2005.06.006 PMID:16210106

Workowski, K. A., Bolan, G. A., & Centers for Disease Control and Prevention. (2015). Sexually transmitted diseases treatment guidelines, 2015. *MMWR. Recommendations and reports: Morbidity and mortality weekly report. Recommendations and reports*, *64*(RR-03), 1–137.

Xiong, M., Lan, L., Feng, T., Zhao, G., Wang, F., Hong, F., Wu, X., Zhang, C., Wen, L., Liu, A., Best, J. M. C., & Tang, W. (2016). Analysis of the sex ratio of reported gonorrhoea incidence in Shenzhen, China. *BMJ Open*, *6*(3), e009629. doi:10.1136/bmjopen-2015-009629 PMID:26975933

KEY TERMS AND DEFINITIONS

Antibiotics: A type of antimicrobial substance that actively fight bacterial infections.

Diagnosis: Identification of the nature and cause of a certain phenomenon and distinguishing it from others, such as a disease.

Ectopic Pregnancy: A condition in which a fertilized egg implants and grows outside the main cavity of the uterus, such as in the fallopian tubes, ovaries, or cervix.

Epidemiology: A study of incidence, distribution, and determinants in causing diseases in specified populations.

Models: Systems used to carry out experiments in isolated cells, cell cultures, biological molecules, organs, or tissues (in vitro) and those used for whole animal investigations (in vivo).

Resistance: A force, such as that of microbes that stops the progress of or acceptance of antimicrobial agents.

Superbug: An informal term given to microorganisms that are resistant to most antibiotics and medications prescribed to treat them.

Susceptibility: A state of being pre-disposed to or sensitive to, for example an infection or even a drug.

Chapter 9
Hepatitis E:
Overview and Management in Namibia

Daniel Opotamutale Ashipala
University of Namibia, Rundu, Namibia

Nestor Tomas
University of Namibia, Namibia

Medusalem Hangula Joel
https://orcid.org/0000-0003-3886-0367
MoHSS, Intermediate Hospital, Rundu, Namibia

ABSTRACT

Hepatitis E (HEV) remains one of the foremost public health problems globally and it is estimated to have affected one-third of the human population. Usually, symptoms appear 2 to 9 weeks after exposure to the virus and include fever, fatigue, lack of appetite, abdominal pain, and jaundice. While the government has a duty to provide access to clean water, communities, and individuals can equally play an important role in practicing and maintaining good physical and environmental hygiene. In Namibia, the spread of HEV has been a public health concern since it's outbreak in 2017. Before then, the country had two outbreaks in 1983 and 1995-1996 which affected mainly areas lacking potable water and waste disposal facilities in Kavango region. This chapter ought to provide an overview and different prevention measures and supportive management approaches used to contain and prevent the spread of HEV. The above statistic calls for plans and actions from national, regional, district management teams to implement effective active surveillance interventions in place that are geared towards curbing the spread of HEV.

INTRODUCTION

HEV is an inflammation of the liver that can be caused by HEV virus, chemicals, drugs, alcohol, inherited diseases, or patient's own immune system characterized by diffuse inflammatory changes and necrosis of the liver.

DOI: 10.4018/978-1-7998-4414-3.ch009

Hepatitis E virus (HEV) forms part of Orthohepevirus genus belonging to a family Hepeviridae, under four species being A to D with an infection believed to be caused by strains of species A (Smith et al., 2020). In addition, species A is further divided into 8 genotypes, two (HEV1 and HEV2) of which are endemic in various animal species (Ouoba, 2019), however, HEV3 and HEV4 can still spread causing zoonotic human infections. On the other hand, other genotypes appear to affect mainly wild boar (HEV5, HEV6) and camels (HEV7, HEV8) despite a HEV7 human infection being reported (Purdy et al, 2017; van Tong et al, 2016). In addition, HEV 1 and 2 have so far only been found have been contracted by human from fecal contaminated drinking water.

HEV is a waterborne emergent infection and thus a source-originated epidemic of acute disease with a case fatality rate deemed to vary by age and pregnancy status (Rein, Stevens, Theaker, Wittenborn, & Wiersma, 2012). In addition, the virus usually spread by the fecal-oral route with fecal contaminated drinking water known to be the main source of the virus. However, each of about four HEV genotypes that cause illness in humans presents with unique epidemiological and clinical features in developing as compared to developed countries. In an area where HEV is endemic, case(s) typically present either as a large outbreak and sporadic cases (WHO, 2017). Even so, various new HEV-like viruses have been detected in numerous animal species, inclusive of carnivores; however, the phylogenetic conjunctions amongst these viruses remain poorly resolved, as parts of them were known to be rodent-related (Lanszki, et al., 2020). In addition, the red fox which is a universal well known carnivore is known to be a host of numerous viruses that transmit from wildlife to humans or domestic animals which has a potential to transmit and circulate rodent-borne HEV.

Objectives

Upon completion of the chapter reader must be able to:

- Demonstrate understanding on the term "HEV"
- Define different case definitions
- List the signs and symptoms of HEV Virus
- Explain different measures to prevent HEV transmission
- Explain different levels of case management
- Discuss the current public health actions / response interventions
- Outline the effective priority interventions taken to scale down the spread of HEV in Namibia.

BACKGROUND

A male patient in Hong Kong became the first person in the world to be confirmed with a strain of HEV virus which was previously found only in rats and other animals (Medical express, 2018). Despite the unknown mode of contraction, the man is believed to have accidentally ingested droppings which were contaminated with HEV. In India however, the first HEV patient was discovered in Kashmir Valley during the 1978 epidemic, which further infected approximately 52,000 persons, causing a total of 1700 fatalities (Purdy& Khudyakov, 2011). Since then, the world recorded a wide spread of HEV causing approximately 20-million infections worldwide each year, of which 17.7-millions were asymptomatic resulting into 44,000 deaths in 2015. Despite being rare in developed countries, locally acquired HEV infection can result in acute Hepatitis with tendency to progress to chronic HEV mainly among solid organ transplant recipients (WHO, 2017; WHOa, 2020).

To date, HEV became the most common cause of acute viral hepatitis among adults throughout the Africa continent (Kaba, 2009). The is however an increase in the number of HEV cases in 28 of 56 African countries as a result of poor sanitation as well as lack of safe drinking water. The virus cases are mainly attributed to pregnant mothers, fetuses as well as to those who are immune compromised. Since 1979, a total of 17 HEV outbreaks have been so far recorded in Africa.

In Namibia, the spread of HEV has been a public health concern since 2017. Before then, the country had two outbreaks in 1983 and 1995-1996 which affected mainly area lacking potable water and waste disposal facilities in Kavango region (WHO, 2017). The 1983 outbreak affected mainly 72% of male which further resulted into 7 fatalities of which 6 were pregnant mothers. Towards the end of 2018, the country recorded an alarming spread of the HEV, with a total of 2748 cumulative HEV case as well as 34 deaths (including 16 maternal deaths) whereas 634 suspected cases awaited confirmation. Pregnant women, particularly those in the second semester and third trimester of pregnancy were the most at risk of acute HEV. Acute HEV is often severe, and results in fulminant hepatitis (acute river failure) which often led to maternal mortality.

Figure 1. Clinical signs of HEV
Source: WHOb (2020)

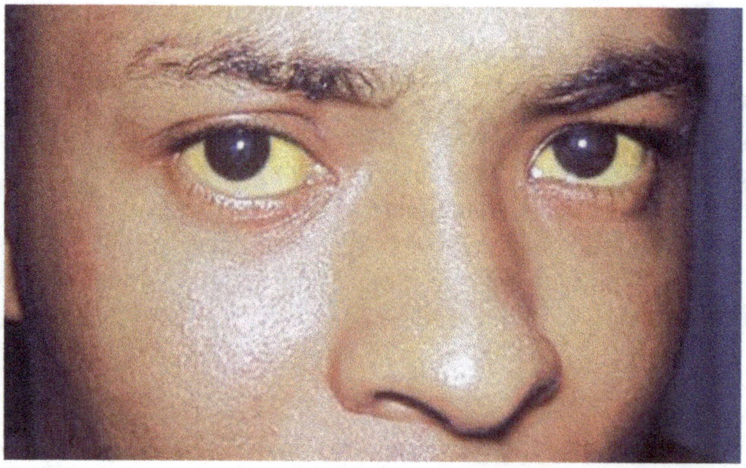

Typical signs and symptoms of HEV include (WHOa, 2020; WHO, 2014):

- Jaundice (yellow discoloration of the skin and sclera of the eyes),
- An initial phase of mild fever,
- Fatigue
- Anorexia (reduced appetite),
- Nausea and vomiting, lasting for a few days;
- Some patients may present with abdominal pain,
- Dark urine
- Joints pain.
- Itching (without skin rash for few days)
- A slightly enlarged, tender liver (hepatomegaly)

Figure 2. Hepatomegaly
Source: Hauston Reginal Gastroeterology(2020)

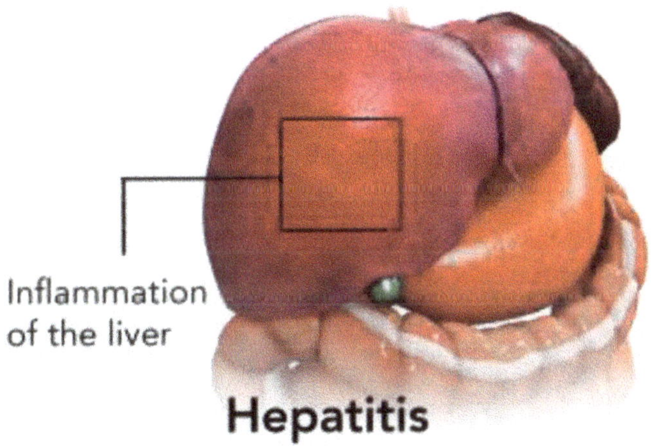

Mode of Transmission and People at Risk

HEV is transmitted mainly through the fecal-oral due to fecal contamination of drinking water/ untreated water (Genotype 1 and 2) and consuming uncooked meat (Genotype 3 and 4).

Incubation Period

- Infected persons shows signs and symptoms between 2 to 10, with most victims showing signs and symptoms between 4-6 weeks post exposure to HEV.

High Risk Groups

According to (WHOa, 2020; WHO, 2014) vulnerable groups include:

- Younger adults between the age of 15-40 years
- Children under the age of 5 years
- Elderly people over the age of 65 years
- Pregnant and postpartum within 6 weeks of delivery
- Immuno-compromised individuals, (people living with HIV/AIDS, TB patients, diabetic patients).
- Chronic underlying medical conditions (liver diseases).

Figure 3. HEV preventions
Source: MedicalNewsToday (2020)

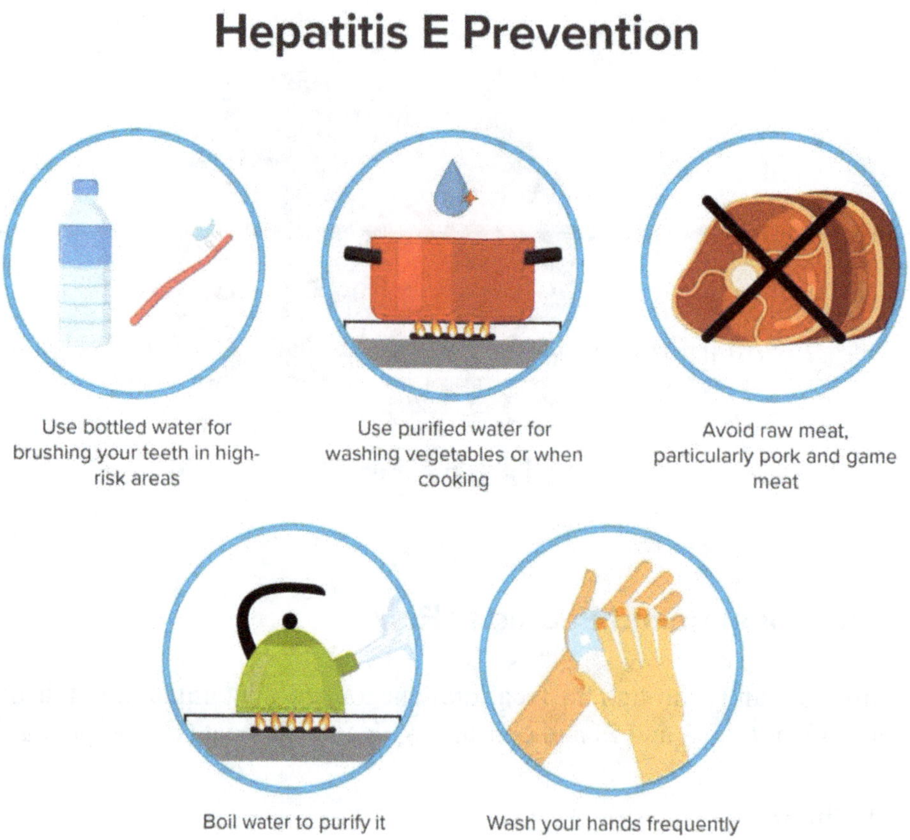

Preventative Methods of HEV

WHO (2020) recommended the following preventative methods:

- Practice good hygiene
- Avoid shaking hands at public gathering such as funerals
- Washing hands before meals
- Washing hands after using toilet
- Boiling water or drink bottled water in the areas with risk of hepatitis contamination.
- Eating cooked food.
- Eat fruits that can peel or always wash fruits before eating
- Avoid raw or steamed shellfish that live in contaminated water.

BURDEN OF HEPATITIS E VIRUS IN NAMIBIA

The first case of HEV in Namibia was reportedly identified in 13 October 2017 in Windhoek state hospital (MOHSS, 2017). As by the end of July 2017 a number of 16 cases were recorded, with 13 cases been laboratory confirmed countrywide. Ministry of Health and Social Services (MoHSS) declared HEV outbreak on 14 December 2017 in Windhoek, Khomas region. Genotye 1 and 2 were the common cause of HEV infection in Namibia. The outbreak continued in Windhoek, and spread to other regions around April 2018, eventually involving Erongo, Kavango, Ohangwena, Omusati, Oshana, Oshikoto, Omaheke, Hardap and Otjozondjupa regions amounting to 10 regions and all are carrying out the response activities. Cases have been reported mainly from informal settlements such as Havana and Goreangab in Windhoek, DRC in Swakopmund and similar settings in other regions where access to safe water, sanitation, and hygiene is limited. Most cases from less affected regions have a travel history to the above-mentioned informal settlements in Windhoek or Swakopmund (MoHSS, 2017).

According to MoHSS (2019) report sporadic cases have also been reported during 2018-2019 (to date) as follow:

In Kunene region, all district reported more than 9 confirmed cases. Luderitz in Karas region reported 5 sporadic confirmed cases while Otjozondjupa region recently confirmed an outbreak during week 30 with a total of 20 lab confirmed cases of which 10 are from Okahandja district during week 24-30. All the above cases have a history of travel to outbreak affected regions, especially Khomas and Erongo. Cumulatively, as of 11 August 2019, a total of 6151 HEV cases were reported. This includes 1390 laboratory confirmed, 3966 Epi-linked and 795 Suspected/ probable cases. Since the outbreak was confirmed, 964 specimens tested negative for HEV and were therefore discarded. Khomas region remains the most affected region, accounting for 3894 (63%) of the confirmed cases, followed by Erongo 1393 (23%) since the outbreak began. The remaining regions account for 864 (14%) of the reported cases. Among the total HEV cases 20 (0.3%) are residence of Angola. The national Case Fatality Rate (CFR) is 56 (0.9%), female are 36 (64%); male 20 (46%). Of the 56 deaths, 23 (41%) are maternal deaths, of which pregnant are 12 (52%), postpartum 10 (43%) and miscarriage 1 (4%). Majority (73%) of cases are among those in the age-group 20-29 (39%) and 30-39 (34%) respectively and the lowest is children under 1 year, whereas males are more affected than their female counterparts.

The latest HEV outbreak in Namibia was recorded cases in October 2017 with Khomas region having the highest number of cases than other 6 regions (MOHSS, 2017). According to the MOHSS rapid assessment survey (2018), the total 3973 HEV cumulative cases were reported at the end of 2018 of which 2748 were from Khomas region. Other 6 region with HEV cases were Erongo, Oshana, Ohangwena, Omusati, Oshikoto and Kavango with the lowest cumulative of 37 cases. Patients screened presented with the following signs and symptoms jaundices, abdominal pain, dark urine, pale stool, mild temperature and liver enlargements. The survey further indicated the risk group were people living informal settlement, with limited access to safe drinking and poor sanitation such lack toilets. Other risk groups include children less than 5 years, pregnant women elderly and people with immune compromised. There is no specific HEV in Namibia but its treatment is self-limiting except giving immune booster to the patient. The table (below) was extract from the rapid assessment HEV per region for MOHSS (2018). The graph below indicates number of HEV cases per region in the years 2018. It has shown had that highest number of HEV cumulative case of 2748 and 26 death cases. Moreover Erongo was the second region to hit HEV 879 cumulative case and 3 deaths respectively. Additionally two regions namely Kavango and Ohangwena had recorded zero death.

Figure 4. HEV Cases Fractuation for 2018

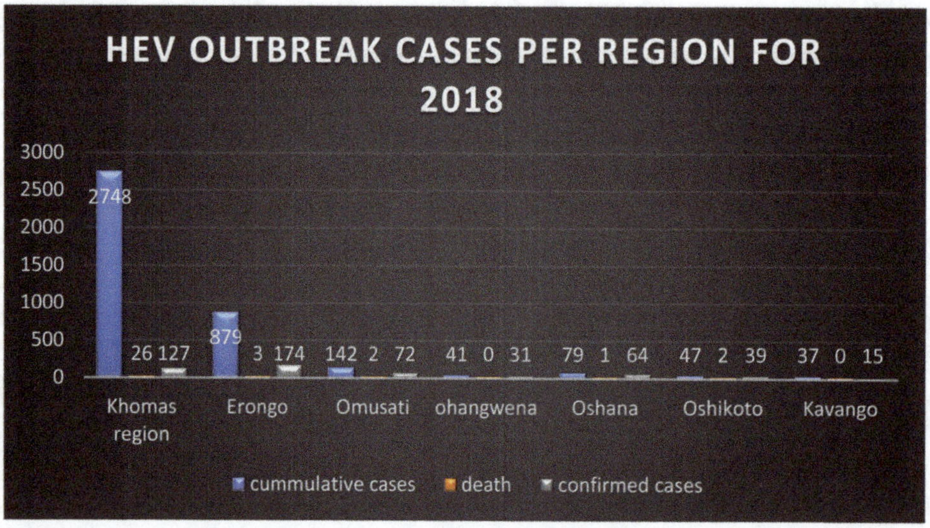

World Health Organization (WHO) Risk Assessment in Namibia

Although hepatitis A, B, and C are common in Namibia, HEV is rarely diagnosed in the country. As a result, the country has limited capacity for HEV laboratory diagnosis. Additionally, the majority of HEV cases have been reported from informal settlements within the capital district, Windhoek, where living conditions are poor. These areas are overcrowded, and have limited access to safe drinking water, sanitation, and hygiene. Moreover, the holiday season will likely increase the movement of people within the country. All of these could be major contributing factors to this outbreak.

Additionally, during the rainy season, people often use rainwater or other surface water for drinking and domestic uses. This likely increases the risk of HEV infection. Therefore, the above-mentioned factors might lead to the propagation of the cases from this area to other informal settlements and its distribution to other towns or districts, with similar poor environmental health conditions. Thus, the overall risk is assessed as high at the national level and low at regional and global levels.

CHALLENGES AND GAPS

According to (WHO, 2018) the following gaps and challenges have been observed:

- The outbreak has become protracted and had spread to other locations in Windhoek and to all regions in the country, with the exception of Zambezi.
- Suboptimal coordination of the outbreak response at all levels
- Inadequate WASH interventions and sanitation facilities including portable water, latrines and hand washing facilities, among others, in informal.
- Inadequate risk communication activities to facilitate behaviour change and enforce hygiene and sanitation practices, early health seeking behaviours and sense of ownership among community members.
- Sub-optimal updates and involvements from thematic leads of the technical working groups

NAMIBIA HEV RESPONSE PLAN

Despite limited resources Namibia adhered to WHO steps in responding to the unexpected disease event of HEV outbreak. The response plan included the following plans:

Coordination

Partner organizations continue to provide in-country technical assistance (WHO and CDC). The Overall coordinator continues to support the setting up of the Public Health Operation Centre (PHEOC) located at the National Health Training Centre (NHTC, Windhoek). The National Costed

Activity Plan for HEV response has been finalized; following incorporation of UNDP sponsored activities. However, this response plan is yet to be endorsed by the financial advisor of MoHSS. On 14 December 2017, the national, regional, and district Health Emergency Management Committees were activated and the government of the city of Windhoek was informed of the outbreak. Five different working groups were formed to strengthen coordination and plan response activities under the following thematic areas; surveillance and laboratory, case management, coordination and logistics, WASH, environmental health, and social mobilization (WHO, 2018)..

Surveillance, Laboratory, and Case Management

MoHSS took a lead in case management and all suspected cases have been referred to hospitals for treatment. Regional and District surveillance teams started to conduct health education, case tracing, mapping and reporting of HEV cases on a weekly basis. National Institute of Pathology (NIP) responsibility is HEV testing at district laboratories; however the expansion of RDTs to other facilities within Windhoek and all part of the country has been slow. To further strengthen surveillance and laboratory response activities, data collection and reporting tools have been distributed to health facilities. Case reporting and investigation, and line listing of cases have been enhanced. As a result, field epidemiologist from MoHSS were deployed to support the community engagement teams to ensure active case search and coordinated. In addition, Red Cross volunteers and community health workers were trained to implement community sensitization and mobilization activities in areas at high risk to HEV (WHO, 2017; WHO, 2018).

Social Mobilization & Risk communication

Community meetings were used as a platform to sensitize communities on occasional basis. HEV information was shared in local radios on a bi-weekly basis by the affected municipalities/councils. The call emphasized by the coordinator was for the additional volunteers from the community to strengthen the health education, social mobilization and referral of cases at a community level. The involvement of the Minister of Health on media briefings was directed to educate the public about the outbreak with the participation of WHO and partners. In addition, national radio campaign to sensitize the affected communities to the risk of HEV were campaign to sensitize the affected communities to the risk of HEV was ongoing along with regular briefings on the outbreak (WHO, 2017;WHO, 2018).

Water, Sanitation, and Hygiene (WASH)

The affected municipalities/Councils UNICEF, MAWF and partners came together, to facilitate the Community-Led Total Sanitation in affected areas. Mapping of sanitation centers was done in Samora Machel and Moses Garoeb constituencies. CLTS task force committees that were identified, involving the councilors, were orientated on HEV and sanitation by UNICEF and MoHSS. An environmental health team from the Ministry of Health and Social Services along with municipalities/councils got involved in environmental investigations to identify exposures that led to the outbreak, with the focus to test water quality of the affected areas (Shikongo, 2020).

PRIORITY INTERVENTIONS TAKEN TO SCALE DOWN THE SPREAD OF HEV IN NAMIBIA

- Adoption of the Incident Management System (IMS) at all levels and the orientation of sub national incident managers and the response committees.
- Expedite the identification/assignment of the Incident Manager
- Intensification of outbreak response through effective coordination and use of available resources (financial, human).
- MoHSS to develop a plan and schedule for the training of additional health facility staff to further strengthen HEV testing capacity using RDTs in Khomas, Erongo and other regions, in collaboration with NIP.
- Endorsement and implementation the cost national response plan by MoHSS executive
- Massive scaling up of WASH activities including CLTS and active community involvement to ensure ownership and reduce vandalism and theft of provided sanitation facilities.
- Strengthened social mobilisation for behavioural changes
- Improved data quality through use of standardized line list and timely reporting.
- Regional management teams to ensure accountability regarding the outbreak response and timely reporting.
- Continuation of case tracing, additional case search and laboratory testing of high-risk populations.
- Resource mobilization to support response activities.

SOLUTIONS AND RECOMMENDATIONS

It is recommended that Namibia and other countries develop responsive plan to way before any outbreak to minimize contraction of communicable diseases including HEV. Furthermore, the situation requires that municipalities, town councils and village councils take the wellbeing of the residents seriously by providing accessible clean water to the residents and by employing epidemiologists, environmentalist and other candle of public health expertise in mitigating further spread of communicable diseases including HEV in Namibia.

FUTURE RESEARCH DIRECTIONS

Further studies are needed to determine the epidemiological triads of HEV and other types of Hepatitis in Namibia. Furthermore, a study needs to be done to determine economic viability of having public health experts employed by municipalities, town councils and village councils in Namibia.

CONCLUSION

It is concluded that a lot needs to be done in Namibia in the fight against HEV. Despite political will to ensure health for all in Namibia, lack of public health coordination in most institutions in Namibia remains a gray area that needs attention.

REFERENCES

Boslaugh, S. (2008). *Encyclopedia of epidemiology* (Vol. 1-2). Sage Publications, Inc. doi:10.4135/9781412953948

Centers for Disease Control and Prevention (CDC). (2014). *Introduction to Public Health. In: Public Health 101 Series.* Atlanta, GA: U.S. Department of Health and Human Services, CDC. Retrieved: https://www.cdc.gov/publichealth101/surveillance.html

Houston Regional Gastroenterology. (2020). Retrieved: Https://www.hrgastro.com/hepatitis-gastroenterology-hepatology-sugar-land-humble-kingwood-tx.html

Kaba, M., Davoust, B., Marié, J. L., Barthet, M., Henry, M., Tamalet, C., Raoult, D., & Colson, P. (2009). Frequent transmission of hepatitis E virus among piglets in farms in Southern France. *Journal of Medical Virology*, *81*(10), 1750–1759. doi:10.1002/jmv.21553 PMID:19697419

Khuroo, M. S., Khuroo, M. S., & Khuroo, N. S. (2016). Hepatitis E: Discovery, global impact, control and cure. *World Journal of Gastroenterology*, *22*(31), 7030–7045. doi:10.3748/wjg.v22.i31.7030 PMID:27610014

Lanszki, Z., Kurucz, K., Zeghbib, S., Kemenesi, G., Lanszki, J., & Jakab, F. (2020). Identification of Hepatitis E Virus in the Feces of Red Foxes (Vulpes vulpes). Animals. *MDPI Journal.*, *10*(10), 1841. doi:10.3390/ani10101841 PMID:33050408

Lanszki, Z., Kurucz, K., Zeghbib, S., Kemenesi, G., Lanszki, J., & Jakab, F. (2020). Identification of Hepatitis E Virus in the Feces of Red Foxes (*Vulpes vulpes*). *Animals (Basel)*, *10*(10), 1841. doi:10.3390/ani10101841 PMID:33050408

Lee, G. H., Tan, B. H., Teo, E. C., Lim, S. G., Dan, Y. Y., Wee, A., Aw, P. P., Zhu, Y., Hibberd, M. L., Tan, C. K., Purdy, M. A., & Teo, C. G. (2016). Chronic Infection With Camelid Hepatitis E Virus in a Liver Transplant Recipient Who Regularly Consumes Camel Meat and Milk. *Gastroenterology*, *150*(2), 355–7.e3. doi:10.1053/j.gastro.2015.10.048 PMID:26551551

Medical Express. (2018). *World's first human case of rat disease found in Hong Kong*. Retrieved: https://medicalxpress.com/news/2018-09-world-human-case-rat-disease.html

Medical News Today. (2020). Retrieved: https://www.medicalnewstoday.com/articles/324204

MoHSS. (2017). *Outbreak of Hepatitis E Virus (HEV) in Namibia Situation Report* (SITREP No. 64). Retrieved: https://www.afro.who.int/sites/default/files/2019-08/National%20SITREP%2064%20on%20Hepatitis%20E%20%20%20outbreak%20Final.pdf

Ouoba, J. B., Traore, K. A., Rouamba, H., Setondji, K. V. M., Minoungou, G. L., Ouoba, B. L., Ouedraogo, A., Moctar, S., M'Bengue, A. K., Kakou, S. N., Doumbia, M., Traore, A. S., Roques, P., & Barro, N. (2019). Prevalence of anti-hepatitis E virus antibodies in domestic animal from three representative provinces of Burkina Faso. *Journal of Veterinary & Animal Sciences (Lahore)*, *7*, 1–7. doi:10.1016/j.vas.2019.100059 PMID:32734080

Purdy, M. A., Harrison, T. J., Jameel, S., Meng, X. J., Okamoto, H., Van der Poel, W., & Smith, D. B.Ictv Report Consortium. (2017). ICTV Virus Taxonomy Profile: Hepeviridae. *The Journal of General Virology*, *98*(11), 2645–2646. doi:10.1099/jgv.0.000940 PMID:29022866

Rein, D. B., Stevens, G. A., Theaker, J., Wittenborn, J. S., & Wiersma, S. T. (2012). The global burden of hepatitis E virus genotypes 1 and 2 in 2005. *Hepatology (Baltimore, Md.)*, *55*(4), 988–997. doi:10.1002/hep.25505 PMID:22121109

Rein, D. B., Stevens, G. A., Theaker, J., Wittenborn, J. S., & Wiersma, S. T. (2012). The global burden of hepatitis E virus genotypes 1 and 2 in 2005. *Journal of American Association for the Study of Liver Diseases.*, *55*(4), 988–997. doi:10.1002/hep.25505 PMID:22121109

Shikongo, A. The Namibian newspaper. (2020). *Hepatitis-E continues to spread.* Retrieved: https://www.namibian.com.na/198938/archive-read/Hepatitis-E-continues-to-spread

Smith, D. B., Izopet, J., Nicot, F., Simmonds, P., Jameel, S., Meng, X. J., Norder, H., Okamoto, H., van der Poel, W. H. M., Reuter, G., & Purdy, M. A. (2020). Update: Proposed reference sequences for subtypes of hepatitis E virus (species Orthohepevirus A). *The Journal of General Virology*, *101*(7), 692–698. doi:10.1099/jgv.0.001435 PMID:32469300

Smith, D. B., Simmonds, P., Jameel, S., Emerson, S. U., Harrison, T. J., Meng, X.-J., Okamoto, H., Van der Poel, W. H. M., & Purdy, M. A.Members Of The International Committee On The Taxonomy Of Viruses Study Group. (2014). Consensus proposals for classification of the family Hepeviridae. *The Journal of General Virology*, *95*(Pt 10), 2223–2232. doi:10.1099/vir.0.068429-0 PMID:24989172

van Tong, H., Hoan, N.X., Wang, B., Wedemeyer, H., Bock, C.T., & Velavan, T.P. (2016). Hepatitis E Virus Mutations: Functional and Clinical Relevance. *EBioMedicine Journal, 11*, 41-42. doi:10.1016/j.ebiom.2016.07.039

WHO. (2014). *Waterborne outbreaks of hepatitis E: recognition, investigation and control technical report.* Retrieved: https://apps.who.int/iris/bitstream/handle/10665/129448/9789241507608_eng.pdf;jsessionid=500CBD02380CD28F6956B10FCABEC63B?sequence=1

WHO. (2016). *Report on the 9th Global Conference for Health Promotion: All for Health, Health for All.* https://www.who.int/healthpromotion/conferences/9gchp/shanghai-conference-report/en/

WHO. (2017). *Global hepatitis report.* Retrieved https://apps.who.int/iris/bitstream/handle/10665/255016/9789241565455 eng.pdf?sequence=1

WHO. (2018). *Hepatitis E-Namibia. Emergencies preparedness, response*. Retrieved: https://www.who.int/csr/don/15-january-2018-hepatitis-e-namibia/en/

WHO. (2020a). *Hepatitis E*. Retrieved: https://www.who.int/news-room/fact-sheets/detail/hepatitis-e

WHO. (2020b). *Hepatitis*. Retrieved: http://www.emro.who.int/health-topics/hepatitis/index.html

KEY TERMS AND DEFINITIONS

Case Fatality Rate: In epidemiology, the proportion of people who die from a specified disease among all individuals diagnosed with the disease over a certain period of time compared to the total number of people diagnosed with the disease for a particular period Boslaugh (2008).

Hepatitis E: Is a liver disease caused by infection with a virus known as hepatitis E virus (HEV) (WHOa, 2020).

Jaundice: Is a condition in which the skin, whites of the eyes and mucous membranes turn yellow because of a high level of bilirubin, a yellow-orange bile pigment (WHO, 2020).

Sanitation: Refers to public health conditions related to clean drinking water and adequate treatment and disposal of human excreta and sewage (WHOa, 2020).

Social Mobilization: Is the process of bringing together all societal and personal influences to raise awareness of and demand for health care, assist in the delivery of resources and services, and cultivate sustainable individual and community involvement (WHO, 2016).

Surveillance: Is "the ongoing, systematic collection, analysis, and interpretation of health-related data essential to planning, implementation, and evaluation of public health practice" (CDC, 2014).

Zoonotic: Diseases is an infectious disease caused by a pathogen (an infectious agent, such as a bacterium, virus, parasite or prion) that has jumped from a non-human animal (usually a vertebrate) to a human (CDC, 2014).

Glossary

Antibiotics: A type of antimicrobial substance that actively fight bacterial infections.

Automated Auditory Brainstem Response (AABR): This is a test of how well the brain and the hearing nerve react to the sound.

Caregivers: This is a salaried or un-paid family member of an individual who supports them with everyday life activities.

Case Definition: It is a set of common criteria for classifying a person with a specific illness, disease, or other health condition.

Case Fatality Rate: In epidemiology, the proportion of people who die from a specified disease among all individuals diagnosed with the disease over a certain period of time compared to the total number of people diagnosed with the disease for a particular period Boslaugh (2008).

Confirmed Case: A person/s who tested positive that is confirmed by one or more of the laboratory methods listed in the case definition.

Congenital Hearing Loss: This is loss of hearing at birth or hearing loss that can occur subsequently but is attributable to hereditary factors or other conditions that have affected the fetus while in the womb.

Contact Tracing: The process of identifying, assessing, and managing people who might have come in contact and been exposed to a virus in order to prevent transmission.

Counseling: A process in which two people meet to explore personal problems and to identify solutions through meaningful discussions and well-informed choices.

COVID-19: The pandemic situation due to spreading SARS-CoV-2, a pandemic occurs in 2019 and still continue.

COVID-19: An infectious disease caused by coronavirus. It is the acronym for the full name coronavirus of 2019. It means "the coronavirus disease of 2019, which is caused by severe acute respiratory syndrome coronavirus 2" (SARS-CoV-2) (WHO, 2020).

Diagnosis: Identification of the nature and cause of a certain phenomenon and distinguishing it from others, such as a disease.

Ectopic Pregnancy: A condition in which a fertilized egg implants and grows outside the main cavity of the uterus, such as in the fallopian tubes, ovaries, or cervix.

Endemic: It is the infectious disease present in a certain geographic region, or in a certain race of people.

Epidemic Curve: It is a vertical column bar chart showing the number of new cases of a specific disease that arise over a period of time.

Epidemiology: It is the approach used to classify the causes of illnesses and health outcomes in populations. The patient is the group of epidemiology, and is treated collectively by individuals.

Epidemiology: A scientific study process where a data driven systematically to find out the risk factor and causes of healthcare-oriented conditions and facts in definite inhabitants.

Epidemiology: A study of incidence, distribution, and determinants in causing diseases in specified populations.

Health Access Livelihood Framework: The framework links social science and public health research with broader development approaches to improve health system development. Access becomes an issue once illness is recognized and treatment seeking is initiated. Five dimensions of access influence the course of the health-seeking process: Availability, Accessibility, Affordability, Adequacy, and Acceptability.

Hepatitis E: Is a liver disease caused by infection with a virus known as hepatitis E virus (HEV) (WHOa, 2020).

Illness Episode: It is nothing but the illness stories of patients.

Infection: This is the penetration of the body by infectious micro-organisms or parasites.

Isolation Facility: The public health practice of separating sick people with a contagious disease from people who are not sick.

Jaundice: Is a condition in which the skin, whites of the eyes and mucous membranes turn yellow because of a high level of bilirubin, a yellow-orange bile pigment (WHO, 2020).

Loneliness: An unpleasant emotional response to perceived isolation that causes a person/s to feel empty, alone and unwanted due to lack of connection with other people.

Meningitis: This is an infection of the brain and spinal cord membranes, commonly triggered by disease.

Models: Systems used to carry out experiments in isolated cells, cell cultures, biological molecules, organs, or tissues (in vitro) and those used for whole animal investigations (in vivo).

Otoacoustic Emission (OAE): This is sound that is produced from inside the inner ear.

Outbreak: It is exactly the same as an epidemic, i.e., an elevated incidence of a disease in a given population or geographic area above the normal (endemic rate).

Outbreak Investigation: It is a series of techniques used to determine the cause of the disease, the people affected, the circumstances and manner of disease transmission and other relevant factors involved in epidemic propagation.

Pandemic: It refers to epidemics that occur in multiple locations around the globe at the same time.

Popular, Folk, and Professional Sectors: These are available health care options that the community people frequently used in response to their multiple health hazards. Popular sector deals with the experiences of aged family members to treat illness. Folk sectors deal with the community healers in response to diagnose multiple illness in the community where professional sectors mainly touches the modern medical facilities.

Psychosocial Support: Psychosocial support is a process of facilitating resilience within individual, families, and communities by respecting the independence, dignity and coping mechanisms of individuals and communities. It promotes restoration of social cohesion and infrastructure.

Quarantine Facility: The public health practice of separating and limiting the movement of people who were exposed to a contagious disease to see if they become sick during a given period.

Recovery: A person who was infected with the virus and has survived a virus with no long-term health effects. This simply means that one's immune system has found and destroyed the virus in the body.

Resistance: A force, such as that of microbes that stops the progress of or acceptance of anti-microbial agents.

Sanitation: Refers to public health conditions related to clean drinking water and adequate treatment and disposal of human excreta and sewage (WHOa, 2020).

SARS-CoV-2: A virus which effects human bodies and extremely transmittable also pathogenic viral infection which first spread from the seafood market of Wuhan, China from 12th Dec 2019; now spreads worldwide.

Social Mobilization: Is the process of bringing together all societal and personal influences to raise awareness of and demand for health care, assist in the delivery of resources and services, and cultivate sustainable individual and community involvement (WHO, 2016).

Stigma: This involves negative attitudes and beliefs toward someone or group of people based on their health status which lead to prejudice and discrimination. For example, some people who tested positive with Covid-19 were stigmatized and discriminated against as people perceived to spread the virus.

Superbug: An informal term given to micro-organisms that are resistant to most antibiotics and medications prescribed to treat them.

Surveillance: Is "the ongoing, systematic collection, analysis, and interpretation of health-related data essential to planning, implementation, and evaluation of public health practice" (CDC, 2014).

Susceptibility: A state of being pre-disposed to or sensitive to, for example an infection or even a drug.

Therapeutic Decision Making: It is a comprehensive process in which people usually make decision to response any physical, psychological, and social illness.

Transient-Evoked Otoacoustic Emissions (TEOAE): This is are Sounds that are produced by the outer hair cells of the cochlea in reaction to a temporary click.

Treatment: A process where a patient is given medical facilities to recover or fight against the disease or illness.

Universal Newborn Hearing Screening (UNHS): This is an approach that assists in recognising the inherited deafness and earshot damage in new babies before leaving the hospital.

WHO: World Health Organization is a statutory organization of the United Nations that observes the main health related issues worldwide.

World Health Assembly: This is a platform in which the World Health Organization is regulated by its 190 countries and territories and also the highest health policy setting body in the world.

World Health Organization: The specialist body United Nations that is accountable for global public health.

Zoonotic: Diseases is an infectious disease caused by a pathogen (an infectious agent, such as a bacterium, virus, parasite or prion) that has jumped from a non-human animal (usually a vertebrate) to a human (CDC, 2014).

Compilation of References

Abdul-Majid, A., Zakaria, M., Abdullah, N. A. C., Hamzah, S., & Mukari, S. S. (2017). Current development, issues and challenges of universal newborn hearing screening program in Malaysia. *International Educational Scientific Journal*, *3*(4), 1–27.

Agostini, M. L., Andres, E. L., Sims, A. C., Graham, R. L., Sheahan, T. P., Lu, X., Smith, E. C., Case, J. B., Feng, J. Y., Jordan, R., Ray, A. S., Cihlar, T., Siegel, D., Mackman, R. L., Clarke, M. O., Baric, R. S., & Denison, M. R. (2018). Coronavirus susceptibility to the antiviral remdesivir (gs-5734) is mediated by the viral polymerase and the proofreading exoribonuclease. *mBio*, *9*(2), e00221–e18. doi:10.1128/mBio.00221-18 PMID:29511076

Ahmad, A., Mohamad, I., Mansor, S., Daud, M. K., & Sidek, D. (2011). Outcome of a newborn hearing screening program in a tertiary hospital in Malaysia: The first five years. *Annals of Saudi Medicine*, *31*(1), 24–28. doi:10.4103/0256-4947.75774 PMID:21245595

Ainsworth, G. C., Bisby, G. R., Brown, A. M., Marsden, P., Smith, P. A., & Spilsbury, J. F. (1947). A method for the large-scale production of penicillin by surface culture. *Journal of General Microbiology*, *1*(3), 335–343. doi:10.1099/00221287-1-3-335 PMID:20270632

Akram, P., & Liao, L. (2017). Prediction of missing common genes for disease pairs using network based module separation on incomplete human interactome. *BMC Genomics*, *18*(10), 902. doi:10.118612864-017-4272-7 PMID:29244004

Alessa, A., & Faezipour, M. (2018). A review of influenza detection and prediction through social networking sites. *Theoretical Biology & Medical Modelling*, *15*(1), 2. doi:10.118612976-017-0074-5 PMID:29386017

Almonacid-Mendoza, H. L., Humbert, M. V., Dijokaite, A., Cleary, D. W., Soo, Y., Hung, M. C., Orr, C. M., Machelett, M. M., Tews, I., & Christodoulides, M. (2018). Structure of the Recombinant *Neisseria gonorrhoeae* Adhesin Complex Protein (rNg-ACP) and Generation of Murine Antibodies with Bactericidal Activity against Gonococci. *MSphere*, *3*(5), e00331–e18. doi:10.1128/mSphere.00331-18 PMID:30305317

Andrews, J. M. (2018). Determination of minimum inhibitory concentrations. *The Journal of Antimicrobial Chemotherapy*, *48*(1), 5–16. PMID:11420333

Arabi, Y. M., Asiri, A. Y., Assiri, A. M., Aziz Jokhdar, H. A., Alothman, A., Balkhy, H. H., AlJohani, S., Al Harbi, S., Kojan, S., Al Jeraisy, M., Deeb, A. M., Memish, Z. A., Ghazal, S., Al Faraj, S., Al-Hameed, F., AlSaedi, A., Mandourah, Y., Al Mekhlafi, G. A., Sherbeeni, N. M., ... Hussein, M. A. (2020). Treatment of Middle East respiratory syndrome with a combination of lopinavir/ritonavir and interferon-β1b (MIRACLE trial): Statistical analysis plan for a recursive two-stage group sequential randomized controlled trial. *Trials*, *21*(1), 8. doi:10.118613063-019-3846-x PMID:31900204

Arvidson, C. G., Kirkpatrick, R., Witkamp, M. T., Larson, J. A., Schipper, C. A., Waldbeser, L. S., O'Gaora, P., Cooper, M., & So, M. (1999). *Neisseria gonorrhoeae* mutants altered in toxicity to human fallopian tubes and molecular characterization of the genetic locus involved. *Infection and Immunity, 67*(2), 643–652. doi:10.1128/IAI.67.2.643-652.1999 PMID:9916071

Asif, M., Martiniano, H. F., Vicente, A. M., & Couto, F. M. (2018). Identifying disease genes using machine learning and gene functional similarities, assessed through Gene Ontology. *PLoS One, 13*(12), e0208626. doi:10.1371/journal.pone.0208626 PMID:30532199

Assiri, A., Al-Tawfiq, J. A., Al-Rabeeah, A. A., Al-Rabiah, F. A., Al-Hajjar, S., Al-Barrak, A., Flemban, H., Al-Nassir, W. N., Balkhy, H. H., Al-Hakeem, R. F., Makhdoom, H. Q., Zumla, A. I., & Memish, Z. A. (2013). Epidemiological, demographic, and clinical characteristics of 47 cases of Middle East respiratory syndrome coronavirus disease from Saudi Arabia: A descriptive study. *The Lancet. Infectious Diseases, 13*(9), 752–761. doi:10.1016/S1473-3099(13)70204-4 PMID:23891402

Atkinson, K. M., Westeinde, J., Ducharme, R., Wilson, S. E., Deeks, S. L., Crowcroft, N., & Wilson, K. (2016). Can mobile technologies improve on-time vaccination? A study piloting maternal use of ImmunizeCA, a Pan-Canadian immunization app. *Human Vaccines & Immunotherapeutics, 12*(10), 2654–2661. doi:10.1080/21645515.2016.1194146 PMID:27322109

Ayala, P., Vasquez, B., Wetzler, L., & So, M. (2002). *Neisseria gonorrhoeae* porin P1.B induces endosome exocytosis and a redistribution of Lamp1 to the plasma membrane. *Infection and Immunity, 70*(11), 5965–5971. doi:10.1128/IAI.70.11.5965-5971.2002 PMID:12379671

Babbidge Jr, H. D. (1965). *Education of the deaf.* A report to the secretary of health, education, and welfare by his advisory committee on the education of the deaf.

Bala, M. (2011). Antimicrobial resistance in *Neisseria gonorrhoeae* in South-East Asia. *Regional Health Forum, 15*(1).

Bala, M., Mullick, J. B., Muralidhar, S., Kumar, J., & Ramesh, V. (2011). Gonorrhoea & its co-infection with other ulcerative, non-ulcerative sexually transmitted & HIV infection in a Regional STD Centre. *The Indian Journal of Medical Research, 133*(3), 346–349. PMID:21441694

Bala, M., Singh, V., Philipova, I., Bhargava, A., Joshi, C., & Unemo, M. (2016). Gentamicin in vitro activity and tentative gentamicin interpretation criteria for the CLSI and calibrated dichotomous sensitivity disc diffusion methods for *Neisseria gonorrhoeae. The Journal of Antimicrobial Chemotherapy, 71*(7), 1856–1859. doi:10.1093/jac/dkw102 PMID:27073269

Balloux, F., & van Dorp, L. (2017). Q&A: What are pathogens, and what have they done to and for us? *BMC Biology, 15*(1), 91. doi:10.118612915-017-0433-z PMID:29052511

Balouiri, M., Sadiki, M., & Ibnsouda, S. K. (2016). Methods for *in vitro* evaluating antimicrobial activity: A review. *Journal of Pharmaceutical Analysis, 6*(2), 71–79. doi:10.1016/j.jpha.2015.11.005 PMID:29403965

Banerjee, A., Kulcsar, K., Misra, V., Frieman, M., & Mossman, K. (2019). Bats and coronaviruses. *Viruses, 11*(1), E41. doi:10.3390/v11010041 PMID:30634396

Barlow, D., & Phillips, I. (1978). Gonorrhoea in women.Diagnostic, clinical, and laboratory aspects. *Lancet, 1*(8067), 761–764. doi:10.1016/S0140-6736(78)90870-X PMID:76760

Bender, A. P., Williams, A. N., Johnson, R. A., & Jagger, H. G. (1990). Appropriate public health responses to clusters: The art of being responsibly responsive. *American Journal of Epidemiology, 132*(suppl), S48–S52. doi:10.1093/oxfordjournals.aje.a115788 PMID:2356835

Bosch, B. J., van der Zee, R., de Haan, C. A., & Rottier, P. J. (2003). The coronavirus spike protein is a class I virus fusion protein: Structural and functional characterization of the fusion core complex. *Journal, 77*(16), 8801–8811. doi:10.1128/JVI.77.16.8801-8811.2003 PMID:12885899

Boslaugh, S. (2008). *Encyclopedia of epidemiology* (Vol. 1-2). Sage Publications, Inc. doi:10.4135/9781412953948

Bragazzi, N. L. (2013). A Google Trends-based approach for monitoring NSSI. *Psychology Research and Behavior Management, 7*, 1–8. doi:10.2147/PRBM.S44084 PMID:24376364

Brodeur, B. R., Johnson, W. M., Johnson, K. G., & Diena, B. B. (1977). In vitro interaction of *Neisseria gonorrhoeae* type 1 and type 4 with tissue culture cells. *Infection and Immunity, 15*(2), 560–567. doi:10.1128/IAI.15.2.560-567.1977 PMID:403139

Brooks, G. F., Butel, J. S., & Morse, S. A. (2004). Cultivation of Microorganisms. In Medical Microbiology (23rd ed.). McGraw-Hill Companies.

Brooks, C. L., Arutyunova, E., & Lemieux, M. J. (2014). The structure of lactoferrin-binding protein B from Neisseria meningitidis suggests roles in iron acquisition and neutralization of host defences. *Acta Crystallographica. Section F, Structural Biology Communications, 70*(Pt 10), 1312–1317. doi:10.1107/S2053230X14019372 PMID:25286931

Brooks, S. K., Webster, R. K., Smith, L. E., Woodland, L., Wessely, S., Greenberg, N., & Rubin, G. J. (2020). The psychological impact of quarantine and how to reduce it: Rapid review of the evidence. *Lancet, 395*(10227), 912–920. doi:10.1016/S0140-6736(20)30460-8 PMID:32112714

Brown, M. A., Potroz, M. G., Teh, S. W., & Cho, N. J. (2016). Natural Products for the Treatment of *Chlamydiaceae* Infections. *Microorganisms, 4*(4), 39. doi:10.3390/microorganisms4040039 PMID:27754466

Caladoa, J., Castroa, R., Lopesa, A., Camposb, M. J., & Rochab, M. (2019). Filomena PereiraAntimicrobial resistance and molecular characteristics of *Neisseria gonorrhoeae* isolates from men who have sex with men. *International Journal of Infectious Diseases, 79*, 116–122. doi:10.1016/j.ijid.2018.10.030 PMID:30412735

Caldera, M., Buphamalai, P., Müller, F., & Menche, J. (2017). Interactome-based approaches to human disease. *Current Opinion in Systems Biology, 3*, 88–94. doi:10.1016/j.coisb.2017.04.015

Caldwell, G. G. (1990). Twenty-two years of cancer cluster investigations at the Centers for Disease Control. *American Journal of Epidemiology, 132*(suppl1), S43–S47. doi:10.1093/oxfordjournals.aje.a115787 PMID:2162625

Carney, F. E. Jr, & Taylor-Robinson, D. (1973). Growth and effect of *Neisseria gonorrhoeae* in organ cultures. *The British Journal of Venereal Diseases, 49*(5), 435–440. doi:10.1136ti.49.5.435 PMID:4201243

Cartwright, R. A. (1999). Cluster investigations: Are they worth it? *The Medical Journal of Australia, 171*(4), 172. doi:10.5694/j.1326-5377.1999.tb123590.x PMID:10494229

Centers for Disease Control (CDC). (1987). Antibiotic-resistant strains of *Neisseriagonorrhoeae*.Policy guidelines for detection, management, and control. *MMWR Supplements, 36*(5), 1S–18S. https://www.cdc.gov/std/gonorrhea/arg/MMWR_AR-GC-PolicyGuidelinesDetectionManagementandControl_Vol36No5S.pdf PMID:3116397

Centers for Disease Control (CDC). (2007). Update to CDC's sexually transmitted diseases treatment guidelines, 2006: Fluoroquinolones no longer recommended for treatment of gonococcal infections. *MMWR. Morbidity and Mortality Weekly Report, 56*(14), 332–336. PMID:17431378

Centers for Disease Control and Prevention (CDC). (2014). *Introduction to Public Health. In: Public Health 101 Series.* Atlanta, GA: U.S. Department of Health and Human Services, CDC. Retrieved: https://www.cdc.gov/publichealth101/surveillance.html

Centers for Disease Control and Prevention Bulletin B88. (2005). *Neisseria Gonorrhoeae Reference Strains for Antimicrobial Susceptibility Testing.* Available at: https://www.cdc.gov/std/gonorrhea/arg/B88-Feb-2005.pdf

Centers for Disease Control and Prevention. (2000). *NIOSH health hazard evaluation program.* Cincinnati, OH: Department of Health and Human Services (NIOSH). *Publication No., 132*, 3.

Centers for Disease Control and Prevention. (2014). Recommendations for the laboratory-based detection of Chlamydia trachomatis and Neisseria gonorrhoeae--2014. MMWR. Recommendations and reports: Morbidity and mortality weekly report. Recommendations and reports, 63(RR-02), 1–19.

Centron, M., & Landwirth, J. (2005). Public health and ethical considerations in planning for quarantine. *The Yale Journal of Biology and Medicine*, *78*(5), 329. PMID:17132339

Cervellin, G., Comelli, I., & Lippi, G. (2017). Is Google Trends a reliable tool for digital epidemiology? Insights from different clinical settings. *Journal of Epidemiology and Global Health*, *7*(3), 185–189. doi:10.1016/j.jegh.2017.06.001 PMID:28756828

Chandler, F. W., Kraus, S. J., & Watts, J. C. (1976). Pathological features of experimental gonococcal infection in mice and guinea pigs. *Infection and Immunity*, *13*(3), 909–914. doi:10.1128/IAI.13.3.909-914.1976 PMID:818019

Chan, Y. A., Hackett, K. T., & Dillard, J. P. (2012). The lytic transglycosylases of *Neisseria gonorrhoeae. Microbial Drug Resistance (Larchmont, N.Y.)*, *18*(3), 271–279. doi:10.1089/mdr.2012.0001 PMID:22432703

Château, A., & Seifert, H. S. (2016). *Neisseria gonorrhoeae* survives within and modulates apoptosis and inflammatory cytokine production of human macrophages. *Cellular Microbiology*, *18*(4), 546–560. doi:10.1111/cmi.12529 PMID:26426083

Chen, A., & Seifert, H. S. (2011). *Neisseria gonorrhoeae*-mediated inhibition of apoptotic signalling in polymorphonuclear leukocytes. *Infection and Immunity*, *79*(11), 4447–4458. doi:10.1128/IAI.01267-10 PMID:21844239

Cheng, L., Li, J., Ju, P., Peng, J., & Wang, Y. (2014). SemFunSim: A new method for measuring disease similarity by integrating semantic and gene functional association. *PLoS One*, *9*(6), e99415. doi:10.1371/journal.pone.0099415 PMID:24932637

Chen, H. M., Liou, Y. Z., Chen, S. Y., & Li, J. S. (2013, June). Design of mobile healthcare service with health records format evaluation. In *2013 IEEE International Symposium on Consumer Electronics (ISCE)* (pp. 257-258). IEEE. 10.1109/ISCE.2013.6570215

Chen, M. I., Ghani, A. C., & Edmunds, W. J. (2009). A metapopulation modelling framework for gonorrhoea and other sexually transmitted infections in heterosexual populations. *Journal of the Royal Society, Interface*, *6*(38), 775–791. doi:10.1098/rsif.2008.0394 PMID:18986961

Chesson, H. W., Mayaud, P., & Aral, S. O. (2017). Sexually Transmitted Infections: Impact and Cost-Effectiveness of Prevention. In *Major Infectious Diseases* (3rd ed.). The International Bank for Reconstruction and Development / The World Bank. doi:10.1596/978-1-4648-0524-0_ch10

Chu, C. M., Cheng, V. C., Hung, I. F., Wong, M. M., Chan, K. H., & Chan, K. S. (2004). Role of lopinavir/ritonavir in the treatment of SARS: Initial virological and clinical findings. *Thorax*, *59*(3), 252–256. doi:10.1136/thorax.2003.012658 PMID:14985565

Communicable Diseases Module: 42. Epidemic Investigation and Management. (n.d.). Retrieved from https://www.open.edu/openlearncreate/mod/oucontent/view.php?id=128&printable=1

Costa-Lourenço, A., Barros Dos Santos, K. T., Moreira, B. M., Fracalanzza, S., & Bonelli, R. R. (2017). Antimicrobial resistance in *Neisseria gonorrhoeae*: history, molecular mechanisms and epidemiological aspects of an emerging global threat. *Brazilian Journal of Microbiology, 48*(4), 617–628. . doi:10.1016/j.bjm.2017.06.001

Cousin, S. Jr, Whittington, W. L., & Roberts, M. C. (2003). Acquired macrolide resistance genes in pathogenic Neisseria spp. isolated between 1940 and 1987. *Antimicrobial Agents and Chemotherapy*, *47*(12), 3877–3880. doi:10.1128/AAC.47.12.3877-3880.2003 PMID:14638497

Criss, A. K., & Seifert, H. S. (2012). A bacterial siren song: Intimate interactions between Neisseria and neutrophils. *Nature Reviews. Microbiology*, *10*(3), 178–190. doi:10.1038/nrmicro2713 PMID:22290508

Cui, J., Li, F., & Shi, Z. L. (2019). Origin and evolution of pathogenic coronaviruses. *Nature Reviews. Microbiology*, *17*(3), 181–192. doi:10.103841579-018-0118-9 PMID:30531947

Das, A., Manickam, P., Hutin, Y., Pattanaik, B., Pal, B. B., Chhotray, G. P., Kar, S. K., & Gupte, M. D. (2009). Two sequential outbreaks in two villages illustrate the various modes of transmission of cholera. *Epidemiology and Infection*, *137*(6), 906–912. doi:10.1017/S0950268808001611 PMID:19171080

Das, J., Fragoza, R., Lee, H. R., Cordero, N. A., Guo, Y., Meyer, M. J., & Yu, H. (2014). Exploring mechanisms of human disease through structurally resolved protein interactome networks. *Molecular BioSystems*, *10*(1), 9–17. doi:10.1039/C3MB70225A PMID:24096645

Davis, J. R., & Lederberg, J. (2000). *Public Health Systems and Emerging Infections: Assessing the Capabilities of the Public and Private Sectors*. National Academies Press (US).

de Repentigny, L., & Turgeon, P. L. (1981). Screening of *Neisseria gonorrhoeae* for tolerant response to beta-lactam antibiotics. *Antimicrobial Agents and Chemotherapy*, *19*(4), 645–648. doi:10.1128/AAC.19.4.645 PMID:6787980

de Wit, E., van Doremalen, N., Falzarano, D., & Munster, V. J. (2016). SARS and MERS: Recent insights into emerging coronaviruses. *Nature Reviews. Microbiology*, *14*(8), 523–534. doi:10.1038/nrmicro.2016.81 PMID:27344959

Department of Agriculture Extension. S. U. (2011). Village Profile 2010, Sariakandi Upazila. Dhaka: Ministry of Agriculture, The People's Republic of Bangladesh.

Desai, P. J., Garges, E., & Genco, C. A. (2000). Pathogenic neisseriae can use hemoglobin, transferrin, and lactoferrin independently of the tonB locus. *Journal of Bacteriology*, *182*(19), 5586–5591. doi:10.1128/JB.182.19.5586-5591.2000 PMID:10986265

Detels, R., Green, A. M., Klausner, J. D., Katzenstein, D., Gaydos, C., Handsfield, H., Pequegnat, W., Mayer, K., Hartwell, T. D., & Quinn, T. C. (2011). The incidence and correlates of symptomatic and asymptomatic Chlamydia trachomatis and *Neisseria gonorrhoeae* infections in selected populations in five countries. *Sexually Transmitted Diseases*, *38*(6), 503–509. doi:10.1097/OLQ.0b013e318206c288 PMID:22256336

DFID. (1997). *Sustainable Livelihood Guidance Sheets'*. Retrieved from http:// www.eldis.org/vfile/upload/1/document/0901/section2.pdf

Dillon, J. R., Carballo, M., & Pauzé, M. (1988). Evaluation of eight methods for identification of pathogenic Neisseria species: Neisseria-Kwik, RIM-N, Gonobio-Test, Minitek, Gonochek II, GonoGen, Phadebact Monoclonal GC OMNI Test, and Syva MicroTrak Test. *Journal of Clinical Microbiology*, *26*(3), 493–497. doi:10.1128/JCM.26.3.493-497.1988 PMID:3128578

Doherty, M., Buchy, P., Standaert, B., Giaquinto, C., & Prado-Cohrs, D. (2016). Vaccine impact: Benefits for human health. *Vaccine*, *34*(52), 6707–6714. doi:10.1016/j.vaccine.2016.10.025 PMID:27773475

Dong, Y., Mo, X., Hu, Y., Qi, X., Jiang, F., Jiang, Z., & Tong, S. (2020). *Epidemiological characteristics of 2143 Pediatric patients with 2019 coronavirus disease in China.* Journal., doi:10.1542/peds.2020-0702

Dubey, S., Biswas, P., Ghosh, R., Chatterjee, S., Dubey, M. J., Chatterjee, S., Lahiri, D., & Lavie, C. (2020). Psychosocial impact of COVID-19. *Diabetes & Metabolic Syndrome, 14*(5), 779–788. doi:10.1016/j.dsx.2020.05.035 PMID:32526627

Dunlop, E. M. (1949). Gonorrhoea and the sulphonamides. *The British Journal of Venereal Diseases, 25*(2), 81–83. PMID:18151908

Edwards, J. L., & Apicella, M. A. (2004). The molecular mechanisms used by *Neisseria gonorrhoeae* to initiate infection differ between men and women. *Clinical Microbiology Reviews, 17*(4), 965–981. doi:10.1128/CMR.17.4.965-981.2004 PMID:15489357

Edwards, J. L., Shao, J. Q., Ault, K. A., & Apicella, M. A. (2000). *Neisseria gonorrhoeae* elicits membrane ruffling and cytoskeletal rearrangements upon infection of primary human endocervical and ectocervical cells. *Infection and Immunity, 68*(9), 5354–5363. doi:10.1128/IAI.68.9.5354-5363.2000 PMID:10948165

Ehret, J. M., & Judson, F. N. (1991). Gonorrhea. In B. B. Wentworth (Ed.), *Laboratory Methods for the Diagnosis of Sexually Transmitted Disease* (2nd ed., pp. 53–94). American Public Health Association.

Erwin, M. E., Jones, R. N., Koontz, F. P., Gerlach, E. H., Murray, P. R., & Washington, J. A. (1992). MIC and disk diffusion quality control guidelines for *Neisseria gonorrhoeae* susceptibility tests of cefdinir, cefetamet, CI-960, fleroxacin, lomefloxacin, and temafloxacin. *Journal of Clinical Microbiology, 30*(5), 1317–1319. doi:10.1128/JCM.30.5.1317-1319.1992 PMID:1316371

European Centre for Disease Prevention and Control. (2016). *Annual Epidemiological Report 2016 – Gonorrhoea.* ECDC.

European Centre for Disease Prevention and Control. (n.d.). *Annual epidemiological report for 2015 – Gonorrhoea.* Stockholm: ECDC. Available from: https://ecdc.europa.eu/sites/portal/files/documents/AER_for_2015-gonorrhoea.pdf

Exner, M., Bhattacharya, S., Christiansen, B., Gebel, J., Goroncy-Bermes, P., Hartemann, P., ... Trautmann, M. (2017). Antibiotic resistance: What is so special about multidrug-resistant Gram-negative bacteria? *GMS Hygiene and Infection Control, 12*, Doc05. doi:10.3205/dgkh000290 PMID:28451516

Feinen, B., Jerse, A. E., Gaffen, S. L., & Russell, M. W. (2010). Critical role of Th17 responses in a murine model of *Neisseria gonorrhoeae* genital infection. *Mucosal Immunology, 3*(3), 312–321. doi:10.1038/mi.2009.139 PMID:20107432

Ferguson, N. M., Cummings, D. A., Cauchemez, S., Fraser, C., Riley, S., Meeyai, A., Iamsirithaworn, S., & Burke, D. S. (2005). Strategies for containing an emerging influenza pandemic in Southeast Asia. *Nature, 437*(7056), 209–214. doi:10.1038/nature04017 PMID:16079797

Fichorova, R. N., Desai, P. J., Gibson, F. C. III, & Genco, C. A. (2001). Distinct proinflammatory host responses to *Neisseria gonorrhoeae* infection in immortalized human cervical and vaginal epithelial cells. *Infection and Immunity, 69*(9), 5840–5848. doi:10.1128/IAI.69.9.5840-5848.2001 PMID:11500462

Fiebelkorn, K. R., Crawford, S. A., & Jorgensen, J. H. (2005). Mutations in *folP* Associated with Elevated Sulfonamide MICs for *Neisseria meningitidis* Clinical Isolates from Five Continents. *Antimicrobial Agents and Chemotherapy, 49*(2), 536540. doi:10.1128/AAC.49.2.536-540.2005 PMID:15673729

Fingerhuth, S. M., Bonhoeffer, S., Low, N., & Althaus, C. L. (2016). Antibiotic-Resistant *Neisseria gonorrhoeae* Spread Faster with More Treatment, Not More Sexual Partners. *PLoS Pathogens, 12*(5), e1005611. doi:10.1371/journal.ppat.1005611 PMID:27196299

Fiore, B. J., Hanrahan, L. P., & Anderson, H. A. (1990). State health department response to disease cluster reports: A protocol for investigation. *American Journal of Epidemiology, 132*(suppl), S14–S22. doi:10.1093/oxfordjournals.aje.a115776 PMID:2356826

Fischer, T. K., Gentsch, J., & Ashley, D. (2004) *Evaluation and utility of a novel diagnostic method in the investigation of an unusual outbreak of rotavirus diarrhea among children.* Presented at: *53rd Annual EIS Conference*, CDC, Atlanta, GA.

Follows, S. A., Murlidharan, J., Massari, P., Wetzler, L. M., & Genco, C. A. (2009). *Neisseria gonorrhoeae* infection protects human endocervical epithelial cells from apoptosis via expression of host antiapoptotic proteins. *Infection and Immunity, 77*(9), 3602–3610. doi:10.1128/IAI.01366-08 PMID:19546192

Foster, R. S., & Vinson, J. W. (1977). Chicken embryo as an animal model for gonorrhea. *Infection and Immunity, 16*(2), 568–574. doi:10.1128/IAI.16.2.568-574.1977 PMID:405324

Frenette, M., Beaudet, R., Bisaillon, J. G., Sylvestre, M., & Portelance, V. (1984). Chemical and biological characterization of a gonococcal growth inhibitor produced by Staphylococcus haemolyticus isolated from urogenital flora. *Infection and Immunity, 46*(2), 340–345. doi:10.1128/IAI.46.2.340-345.1984 PMID:6437979

Galil, K., Lee, B., Strine, T., Carraher, C., Baughman, A. L., Eaton, M., Montero, J., & Seward, J. (2002). Outbreak of varicella at a day-care center despite vaccination. *The New England Journal of Medicine, 347*(24), 1909–1915. doi:10.1056/NEJMoa021662 PMID:12477940

Garcia Alonso, L., Jiménez Almazán, J., Carbonell Caballero, J., Vela Boza, A., Santoyo López, J., Antiñolo, G., & Dopazo, J. (2014). The role of the interactome in the maintenance of deleterious variability in human populations. *Molecular Systems Biology, 10*(9), 752. doi:10.15252/msb.20145222 PMID:25261458

Gesink Law, D., Rink, E., Mulvad, G., & Koch, A. (2008). Sexual health and sexually transmitted infections in the North American Arctic. *Emerging Infectious Diseases, 14*(1), 4–9. doi:10.3201/eid1401.071112 PMID:18258070

Ghanem, K. G. (n.d.). Clinical manifestations and diagnosis of *Neisseria gonorrhoeae* infection in adults and adolescents. *UpToDate*. www.uptodate.com/contents/clinical-manifestations-and-diagnosis-of-neisseria-gonorrhoeae-infection-in-adults-and-adolescents

Ghiassian, S. D., Menche, J., & Barabási, A. L. (2015). A DIseAse MOdule Detection (DIAMOnD) algorithm derived from a systematic analysis of connectivity patterns of disease proteins in the human interactome. *PLoS Computational Biology, 11*(4), e1004120. doi:10.1371/journal.pcbi.1004120 PMID:25853560

Giltner, C. L., Nguyen, Y., & Burrows, L. L. (2012). Type IV pilin proteins: Versatile molecular modules. *Microbiology and molecular biology reviews. Microbiology and Molecular Biology Reviews, 76*(4), 740–772. doi:10.1128/MMBR.00035-12 PMID:23204365

Ginsberg, J., Mohebbi, M. H., Patel, R. S., Brammer, L., Smolinski, M. S., & Brilliant, L. (2009). Detecting influenza epidemics using search engine query data. *Nature, 457*(7232), 1012–1014. doi:10.1038/nature07634 PMID:19020500

Giovanetti, M., Benvenuto, D., Angeletti, S., & Ciccozzi, M. (2020). The first two cases of 2019-nCoV in Italy: Where they come from? *Journal of Medical Virology, 1–4*(5), 518–521. Advance online publication. doi:10.1002/jmv.25699 PMID:32022275

Goodman, R. A., Buehler, J. W., & Koplan, J. P. (1990). The epidemiologic field investigation: Science and judgment in public health practice. *American Journal of Epidemiology, 132*(1), 9–16. doi:10.1093/oxfordjournals.aje.a115647 PMID:2356818

Government Gazette of the Republic of Namibia. (2020). *Proclamation No.9. State of Emergency-COVID-19 Regulations*. Namibian Constitution.

Guan, W. J., Ni, Z. Y., Hu, Y., Liang, W. H., Ou, C. Q., He, J. X., Liu, L., Shan, H., Lei, C., Hui, D. S. C., Du, B., Li, L., Zeng, G., Yuen, K.-Y., Chen, R., Tang, C., Wang, T., Chen, P., Xiang, J., ... Zhong, N. (2020). Clinical characteristics of coronavirus disease 2019 in China. *The New England Journal of Medicine*, *382*(18), 1708–1720. Advance online publication. doi:10.1056/NEJMoa2002032 PMID:32109013

Gulati, S., Mu, X., Zheng, B., Reed, G. W., Ram, S., & Rice, P. A. (2015). Antibody to reduction modifiable protein increases the bacterial burden and the duration of gonococcal infection in a mouse model. *The Journal of Infectious Diseases*, *212*(2), 311–315. doi:10.1093/infdis/jiv024 PMID:25596304

Gupta, S., Govil, D., Kakar, P. N., Prakash, O., Arora, D., Das, S., ... Malhotra, A. (2009). Colistin and polymyxin B: A re-emergence. *Indian Journal of Critical Care Medicine: Peer-Reviewed, Official Publication of Indian Society of Critical Care Medicine*, *13*(2), 49–53. doi:10.4103/0972-5229.56048 PMID:19881183

Gurung, A., Prabhakar, P., Narayanan, P., Mehendale, S., Risbud, A., & Das, A. (2010). *Prevalence of asymptomatic gonorrhea and chlamydia among men having sex with men (MSM) in India and associated risk factors*. International AIDS Conference, Washington, DC.

Hampton, T. (2005). Bats may be SARS reservoir. *Journal of the American Medical Association*, *294*(18), 2291. doi:10.1001/jama.294.18.2291 PMID:16278351

Hardt, K., Bonanni, P., King, S., Santos, J. I., El-Hodhod, M., Zimet, G. D., & Preiss, S. (2016). Vaccine strategies: Optimising outcomes. *Vaccine*, *34*(52), 6691–6699. doi:10.1016/j.vaccine.2016.10.078 PMID:27887796

Harvey, H. A., Post, D. M., & Apicella, M. A. (2002). Immortalization of human urethral epithelial cells: A model for the study of the pathogenesis of and the inflammatory cytokine response to *Neisseria gonorrhoeae* infection. *Infection and Immunity*, *70*(10), 5808–5815. doi:10.1128/IAI.70.10.5808-5815.2002 PMID:12228311

Hauck, C. R., Lorenzen, D., Saas, J., & Meyer, T. F. (1997). An in vitro-differentiated human cell line as a model system to study the interaction of *Neisseria gonorrhoeae* with phagocytic cells. *Infection and Immunity*, *65*(5), 1863–1869. doi:10.1128/IAI.65.5.1863-1869.1997 PMID:9125573

Hawryluck, G., & Robinson, P. (2004). SARS control and psychological effects of quarantine, Toronto, Canada. *Emerging Infectious Diseases*, *10*(7), 1206–1212. doi:10.3201/eid1007.030703 PMID:15324539

Healthcare in India. (n.d.). Available: https://en.wikipedia.org/wiki/Healthcare_in_India

Hehre, E. J. (1949). Synthesis of a polysaccharide of the starch-glycogen class from sucrose by a cell free, bacterial enzyme system. *The Journal of Biological Chemistry*, *177*(1), 267–279. PMID:18107430

Helman, C. G. (1994). Culture, health and illness: An introduction for health professionals (3rd ed.). Butterworth Heinemann.

Higashi, D. L., Zhang, G. H., Biais, N., Myers, L. R., Weyand, N. J., Elliott, D. A., & So, M. (2009). Influence of type IV pilus retraction on the architecture of the *Neisseria gonorrhoeae*-infected cell cortex. *Microbiology (Reading, England)*, *155*(Pt 12), 4084–4092. doi:10.1099/mic.0.032656-0 PMID:19762436

Hobbs, M. M., Anderson, J. E., Balthazar, J. T., Kandler, J. L., Carlson, R. W., Ganguly, J., Begum, A. A., Duncan, J. A., Lin, J. T., Sparling, P. F., Jerse, A. E., & Shafer, W. M. (2013). Lipid A's structure mediates *Neisseria gonorrhoeae* fitness during experimental infection of mice and men. *mBio*, *4*(6), e00892–e13. doi:10.1128/mBio.00892-13 PMID:24255126

Hopkins, R. S., & Juranek, D. D. (1991). Acute giardiasis: An improved clinical case definition for epidemiologic studies. *American Journal of Epidemiology*, *133*(4), 402–407. doi:10.1093/oxfordjournals.aje.a115894 PMID:1994703

Hopper, S., Wilbur, J. S., Vasquez, B. L., Larson, J., Clary, S., Mehr, I. J., Seifert, H. S., & So, M. (2000). Isolation of *Neisseria gonorrhoeae* mutants that show enhanced trafficking across polarized T84 epithelial monolayers. *Infection and Immunity*, *68*(2), 896–905. doi:10.1128/IAI.68.2.896-905.2000 PMID:10639460

Houston Regional Gastroenterology. (2020). Retrieved: Https://www.hrgastro.com/hepatitis-gastroenterology-hepatology-sugar-land-humble-kingwood-tx.html

Huang, C., Wang, Y., Li, X., Ren, L., Zhao, J., Hu, Y., Zhang, L., Fan, G., Xu, J., Gu, X., Cheng, Z., Yu, T., Xia, J., Wei, Y., Wu, W., Xie, X., Yin, W., Li, H., Liu, M., ... Cao, B. (2020). Clinical features of patients infected with 2019 novel coronavirus in Wuhan, China. *Lancet*, *395*(10223), 497–506. doi:10.1016/S0140-6736(20)30183-5 PMID:31986264

Hung, M. C., & Christodoulides, M. (2013). The biology of Neisseria adhesins. *Biology (Basel)*, *2*(3), 1054–1109. doi:10.3390/biology2031054 PMID:24833056

Investigating an Outbreak: Principles of Epidemiology in Public Health Practice, An Introduction to Applied Epidemiology and Biostatistics Lesson 6. (2001). (3rd ed.). Retrieved from https://www.cdc.gov/csels/dsepd/ss1978/lesson6/section1.html

Ismail, A. I., Abdul Majid, A., Zakariab, M. N., Abdullah, N. A. C., Hamzah, S., & Mukarid, S. Z. (2018). Factors predicting health practitioners' awareness of UNHS program in Malaysian non-public hospitals. *International Journal of Pediatric Otorhinolaryngology*, *109*, 78–84. doi:10.1016/j.ijporl.2018.03.030 PMID:29728190

Janda, W. J., & Knapp, J. S. (2003). *Neisseria* and *Moraxella catarrhalis*. In P. R. Murray, E. J. Baron, M. A. Pfaller, J. H. Jorgensen, & R. H. Yolken (Eds.), *Manual of Clinical Microbiology* (8th ed., pp. 585–608). American Society Microbiology.

Janda, W. M., Zigler, K. L., & Bradna, J. J. (1987). API QuadFERM+ with rapid DNase for identification of Neisseria spp. and Branhamella catarrhalis. *Journal of Clinical Microbiology*, *25*(2), 203–206. doi:10.1128/JCM.25.2.203-206.1987 PMID:3102550

Janeway, C. A., Jr., Travers, P., Walport, M., & Shlomchik, M.J. (2001). *Immunobiology: The Immune System in Health and Disease* (5th ed.). New York: Garland Science. Available from: https://www.ncbi.nlm.nih.gov/books/NBK27100/

Jarrett, C., Wilson, R., O'Leary, M., Eckersberger, E., & Larson, H. J. (2015). Strategies for addressing vaccine hesitancy– A systematic review. *Vaccine*, *33*(34), 4180–4190. doi:10.1016/j.vaccine.2015.04.040 PMID:25896377

Jarvis, G. A., Li, J., & Swanson, K. V. (1999). Invasion of human mucosal epithelial cells by *Neisseria gonorrhoeae* upregulates expression of intercellular adhesion molecule 1 (ICAM-1). *Infection and Immunity*, *67*(3), 1149–1156. doi:10.1128/IAI.67.3.1149-1156.1999 PMID:10024555

Jerse, A. E. (1999). Experimental gonococcal genital tract infection and opacity protein expression in estradiol-treated mice. *Infection and Immunity*, *67*(11), 5699–5708. doi:10.1128/IAI.67.11.5699-5708.1999 PMID:10531218

Jerse, A. E., Bash, M. C., & Russell, M. W. (2014). Vaccines against gonorrhea: Current status and future challenges. *Vaccine*, *32*(14), 1579–1587. doi:10.1016/j.vaccine.2013.08.067 PMID:24016806

Jin, Y. H., Cai, L., Cheng, Z. S., Cheng, H., Deng, T., Fan, Y. P., Fang, C., Huang, D., Huang, L.-Q., Huang, Q., Han, Y., Hu, B., Hu, F., Li, B.-H., Li, Y.-R., Liang, K., Lin, L.-K., Luo, L.-S., Ma, J., ... Wang, X.-H. (2020). A rapid advice guideline for the diagnosis and treatment of 2019 novel coronavirus (2019-nCoV) infected pneumonia (standard version). *Military Medical Research*, *7*(1), 4. doi:10.118640779-020-0233-6 PMID:32029004

Johnson, A. P., Taylor-Robinson, D., & Slavin, G. (1977). Pneumonia in mice produced by *Neisseria gonorrhoeae. The British Journal of Venereal Diseases*, *53*(1), 26–30. doi:10.1136ti.53.1.26 PMID:843896

Johnson, A., Tuffrey, M., & Taylor-Robinson, D. (1989). Resistance of mice to genital infection with *Neisseria gonorrhoeae*. *Journal of Medical Microbiology*, *30*(1), 33–36. doi:10.1099/00222615-30-1-33 PMID:2506350

Johnson, M. B., & Criss, A. K. (2011). Resistance of *Neisseria gonorrhoeae* to neutrophils. *Frontiers in Microbiology*, *2*, 77. doi:10.3389/fmicb.2011.00077 PMID:21747795

Johnston, K. H., Holmes, K. K., & Gotschlich, E. C. (1976). The serological classification of *Neisseria gonorrhoeae*. I. Isolation of the outer membrane complex responsible for serotypic specificity. *The Journal of Experimental Medicine*, *143*(4), 741–758. doi:10.1084/jem.143.4.741 PMID:56416

Joint Committee on Infant Hearing. (1982). Joint Committee on Infant Hearing 1982 Position Statement. *Ear and Hearing*, *4*, 3–4. PMID:6832505

Joint Committee on Infant Hearing. (1994). Joint Committee on Infant Hearing Year 1994 position statement: Principles and guidelines for early hearing detection and intervention programs. *Pediatrics*, *95*, 152–156.

Joint Committee on Infant Hearing. (1995). Joint committee on infant hearing 1994 position statement. *Pediatrics*, *95*(1), 152–156. PMID:7770297

Kaba, M., Davoust, B., Marié, J. L., Barthet, M., Henry, M., Tamalet, C., Raoult, D., & Colson, P. (2009). Frequent transmission of hepatitis E virus among piglets in farms in Southern France. *Journal of Medical Virology*, *81*(10), 1750–1759. doi:10.1002/jmv.21553 PMID:19697419

Karatan, E., & Watnick, P. (2009). Signals, regulatory networks, and materials that build and break bacterial biofilms. Microbiology and molecular biology reviews. *Microbiology and Molecular Biology Reviews*, *73*(2), 310–347. doi:10.1128/MMBR.00041-08 PMID:19487730

Kemp, A. A. T., Delecrode, C. R., da Silva, G. C., Martins, F., Frizzo, A. C. F., & Cardoso, A. C. V. (2015). Neonatal hearing screening in a low-risk maternity in São Paulo state. *Revista Brasileira de Otorrinolaringologia (English Ed.)*, *81*(5), 505–513. doi:10.1016/j.bjorl.2015.07.010 PMID:26277836

Khuroo, M. S., Khuroo, M. S., & Khuroo, N. S. (2016). Hepatitis E: Discovery, global impact, control and cure. *World Journal of Gastroenterology*, *22*(31), 7030–7045. doi:10.3748/wjg.v22.i31.7030 PMID:27610014

Kim, W. J., Mai, A., Weyand, N. J., Rendón, M. A., Van Doorslaer, K., & So, M. (2019). *Neisseria gonorrhoeae* evades autophagic killing by downregulating CD46-cyt1 and remodeling lysosomes. *PLoS Pathogens*, *15*(2), e1007495. doi:10.1371/journal.ppat.1007495 PMID:30753248

Klimpel, G. R. (1996). Immune Defenses. In Med Microbiol. Galveston, TX: University of Texas Medical Branch at Galveston.

Kluge, H. N. P. (2020). *Statement-physical and mental health key to resilience during COVID-19 pandemic*. Academic Press.

Kraus, S. J. (1979). Culture Methods for Neisseria Gonorrhoea. *Archives of Andrology*, *3*(4), 343–349. doi:10.3109/01485017908988426 PMID:119501

Kraus, S. J., Brown, W. J., & Arko, R. J. (1975). Acquired and natural immunity to gonococcal infection in chimpanzees. *The Journal of Clinical Investigation*, *55*(6), 1349–1356. doi:10.1172/JCI108054 PMID:805797

Kulkarni, S., Bala, M., & Risbud, A. (2015). Performance of tests for identification of *Neisseria gonorrhoeae*. *The Indian Journal of Medical Research*, *141*(6), 833–835. doi:10.4103/0971-5916.160721 PMID:26205027

Kumari, S., Haripriya, A., Aruna, A., Vidya, D. S., & Nithy, M. N. (2017). Immunize—Baby steps for smart healthcare: Smart solutions to child vaccination. In *2017 International Conference on Innovations in Green Energy and Healthcare Technologies (IGEHT)* (pp. 1-4). IEEE. 10.1109/IGEHT.2017.8094048

Kupsch, E. M., Knepper, B., Kuroki, T., Heuer, I., & Meyer, T. F. (1993). Variable opacity (Opa) outer membrane proteins account for the cell tropisms displayed by *Neisseria gonorrhoeae* for human leukocytes and epithelial cells. *The EMBO Journal*, *12*(2), 641–650. doi:10.1002/j.1460-2075.1993.tb05697.x PMID:8440254

Kuusi, M., Nuorti, J. P., Maunula, L., Miettinen, I., Pesonen, H., & von Bonsdorff, C.-H. (2004). Internet use and epidemiologic investigation of gastroenteritis outbreak. *Emerging Infectious Diseases*, *10*(3), 447–450. doi:10.3201/eid1003.020607 PMID:15109411

Lage, K. (2014). Protein–protein interactions and genetic diseases: The interactome. *Biochimica et Biophysica Acta (BBA)-. Molecular Basis of Disease*, *1842*(10), 1971–1980. doi:10.1016/j.bbadis.2014.05.028 PMID:24892209

Lahra, M. M., & Enriquez, R. P. (2017). Australian Gonococcal Surveillance Programme, 1 July to 30 September 2016. *Communicable Diseases Intelligence*, *41*(1), 109–110. PMID:28385144

Lai, C. C., Shih, T. P., Ko, W. C., Tang, H. J., & Hsueh, P. R. (2020). Severe acute respiratory syndrome coronavirus 2 (SARS-CoV-2) and coronavirus disease-2019 (COVID-19): The epidemic and the challenges. *International Journal of Antimicrobial Agents*, 55.

Lambden, P. R., Heckels, J. E., & Watt, P. J. (1982). Effect of anti-pilus antibodies on survival of gonococci within guinea pig subcutaneous chambers. *Infection and Immunity*, *38*(1), 27–30. doi:10.1128/IAI.38.1.27-30.1982 PMID:6128301

Lanszki, Z., Kurucz, K., Zeghbib, S., Kemenesi, G., Lanszki, J., & Jakab, F. (2020). Identification of Hepatitis E Virus in the Feces of Red Foxes (Vulpes vulpes). Animals. *MDPI Journal.*, *10*(10), 1841. doi:10.3390/ani10101841 PMID:33050408

Lauridsen, J., & Pradhan, J. (2011). Socio-economic inequality of immunization coverage in India. *Health Economics Review*, *1*(1), 11. doi:10.1186/2191-1991-1-11 PMID:22828353

Lee, G. H., Tan, B. H., Teo, E. C., Lim, S. G., Dan, Y. Y., Wee, A., Aw, P. P., Zhu, Y., Hibberd, M. L., Tan, C. K., Purdy, M. A., & Teo, C. G. (2016). Chronic Infection With Camelid Hepatitis E Virus in a Liver Transplant Recipient Who Regularly Consumes Camel Meat and Milk. *Gastroenterology*, *150*(2), 355–7.e3. doi:10.1053/j.gastro.2015.10.048 PMID:26551551

Lee, N., Hui, D., Wu, A., Chan, P., Cameron, P., Joynt, G. M., Ahuja, A., Yung, M. Y., Leung, C. B., To, K. F., Lui, S. F., Szeto, C. C., Chung, S., & Sung, J. J. Y. (2003). A major outbreak of severe acute respiratory syndrome in Hong Kong. *The New England Journal of Medicine*, *348*(20), 1986–1994. doi:10.1056/NEJMoa030685 PMID:12682352

Lenz, J. D., & Dillard, J. P. (2018). Pathogenesis of *Neisseria gonorrhoeae* and the Host Defense in Ascending Infections of Human Fallopian Tube. *Frontiers in Immunology*, *9*, 2710. doi:10.3389/fimmu.2018.02710 PMID:30524442

Letko, M., Marzi, A., & Munster, V. (2020). Functional assessment of cell entry and receptor usage for SARS-CoV-2 and other lineage B betacoronaviruses. *Journal*, *5*(4), 562–569. doi:10.103841564-020-0688-y PMID:32094589

LeVan, A., Zimmerman, L. I., Mahle, A. C., Swanson, K. V., DeShong, P., Park, J., Edwards, V. L., Song, W., & Stein, D. C. (2012). Construction and characterization of a derivative of *Neisseria gonorrhoeae* strain MS11 devoid of all opa genes. *Journal of Bacteriology*, *194*(23), 6468–6478. doi:10.1128/JB.00969-12 PMID:23002223

Levy, J., Wicher, K., & Rose, N. R. (1973). In vitro susceptibility of *Neisseria gonorrhoeae* to spectinomycin examined by a broth dilution method. *Antimicrobial Agents and Chemotherapy*, *3*(3), 335–337. doi:10.1128/AAC.3.3.335 PMID:4275225

Ligon, B. E., Ludwig, A., & Neisser, S. (2005). Discoverer of the Cause of Gonorrhea. *Seminars in Pediatric Infectious Diseases*, *16*(4), 336–341. doi:10.1053/j.spid.2005.07.001 PMID:16210113

Li, L. H., Yen, M. Y., Ho, C. C., Wu, P., Wang, C. C., Maurya, P. K., Chen, P.-S., Chen, W., Hsieh, W.-Y., & Chen, H. W. (2013). Non-cytotoxic nanomaterials enhance antimicrobial activities of cefmetazole against multidrug-resistant *Neisseria gonorrhoeae*. *PLoS One*, *8*(5), e64794. doi:10.1371/journal.pone.0064794 PMID:23705013

Lim, J., Jeon, S., Shin, H. Y., Kim, M. J., Seong, Y. M., & Lee, W. J. (2020). Case of the index patient who caused tertiary transmission of COVID-19 infection in Korea: The application of lopinavir/ritonavir for the treatment of COVID-19 infected pneumonia monitored by quantitative RT-PCR. *Journal of Korean Medical Science*, *35*(6), e79. doi:10.3346/jkms.2020.35.e79 PMID:32056407

Lindbäck, E., Rahman, M., Jalal, S., & Wretlind, B. (2002). Mutations in *gyrA, gyrB, parC*, and *parE* in quinolone-resistant strains of *Neisseria gonorrhoeae*. *APMIS*, *110*(9), 651–657. doi:10.1034/j.1600-0463.2002.1100909.x PMID:12529019

Lindberg, R., Fredlund, H., Nicholas, R., & Unemo, M. (2007). *Neisseria gonorrhoeae* isolates with reduced susceptibility to cefixime and ceftriaxone: Association with genetic polymorphisms in penA, mtrR, porB1b, and ponA. *Antimicrobial Agents and Chemotherapy*, *51*(6), 2117–2122. doi:10.1128/AAC.01604-06 PMID:17420216

Liu, Y., Egilmez, N. K., & Russell, M. W. (2013). Enhancement of adaptive immunity to *Neisseria gonorrhoeae* by local intravaginal administration of microencapsulated interleukin 12. *The Journal of Infectious Diseases*, *208*(11), 1821–1829. doi:10.1093/infdis/jit354 PMID:24048962

Liu, Y., & Russell, M. W. (2011). Diversion of the immune response to *Neisseria gonorrhoeae* from Th17 to Th1/Th2 by treatment with anti-transforming growth factor β antibody generates immunological memory and protective immunity. *mBio*, *2*(3), e00095–e11. doi:10.1128/mBio.00095-11 PMID:21610119

Livingston, E., & Bucher, K. (2020). *Coronavirus disease 2019 (COVID-19) in Italy*. Journal., doi:10.1001/jama.2020.4344

Li, W., Shi, Z., Yu, M., Ren, W., Smith, C., & Epstein, J. H. (2005). Bats are natural reservoirs of SARS-like coronaviruses. *Science*, *310*(5748), 676–679. doi:10.1126cience.1118391 PMID:16195424

Li, Y., Liu, Z., & Zhang, Z. (2020). Progression of mental health services during the COVID-19 outbreak in China. *International Journal of Biological Sciences*, *16*, 1732–1738.

Long, C. D., Hayes, S. F., van Putten, J. P., Harvey, H. A., Apicella, M. A., & Seifert, H. S. (2001). Modulation of gonococcal piliation by regulatable transcription of pilE. *Journal of Bacteriology*, *183*(5), 1600–1609. doi:10.1128/JB.183.5.1600-1609.2001 PMID:11160091

Longini, I. M. Jr, Nizam, A., Xu, S., Ungchusak, K., Hanshaoworakul, W., & Cummings, D. A. (2005). Containing pandemic influenza at the source. *Science*, *309*(5737), 1083–1087. doi:10.1126cience.1115717 PMID:16079251

Lunzen, J. V., & Altfeld, M. (2014). Sex Differences in Infectious Diseases–Common but Neglected. *The Journal of Infectious Diseases*, *209*(3, suppl 3), S79–S80. doi:10.1093/infdis/jiu159 PMID:24966193

Lu, R., Zhao, X., Li, J., Niu, P., Yang, B., Wu, H., Wang, W., Song, H., Huang, B., Zhu, N., Bi, Y., Ma, X., Zhan, F., Wang, L., Hu, T., Zhou, H., Hu, Z., Zhou, W., Zhao, L., ... Tan, W. (2020). Genomic characterisation and epidemiology of 2019 novel coronavirus: Implications for virus origins and receptor binding. *Lancet*, *395*(10224), 565–574. doi:10.1016/S0140-6736(20)30251-8 PMID:32007145

Madhur Verma, M. D. (2018). Google Search Trends Predicting Disease Outbreaks: An Analysis from India. *Healthcare Informatics Research*, *24*(4), 300–308. doi:10.4258/hir.2018.24.4.300 PMID:30443418

Mak, D. B., Smith, D. W., Harnett, G. B., & Plant, A. J. (2001). A large outbreak of conjunctivitis caused by a single genotype of *Neisseria gonorrhoeae* distinct from those causing genital tract infections. *Epidemiology and Infection, 126*(3), 373–378. doi:10.1017/S0950268801005477 PMID:11467794

Mårdh, P. A., Weström, L., von Mecklenburg, C., & Hammar, E. (1976). Studies on ciliated epithelia of the human genital tract. I. Swelling of the cilia of Fallopian tube epithelium in organ cultures infected with Mycoplasma hominis. *The British Journal of Venereal Diseases, 52*(1), 52–57. doi:10.1136ti.52.1.52 PMID:1260408

Matejcek, A., & Goldman, R. D. (2013). Treatment and prevention of ophthalmia neonatorum. *Canadian Family Physician Medecin de Famille Canadien, 59*(11), 1187–1190. PMID:24235191

Mathur, S., & Dinakarpandian, D. (2012). Finding disease similarity based on implicit semantic similarity. *Journal of Biomedical Informatics, 45*(2), 363–371. doi:10.1016/j.jbi.2011.11.017 PMID:22166490

Mavrogiorgos, N., Mekasha, S., Yang, Y., Kelliher, M. A., & Ingalls, R. R. (2014). Activation of NOD receptors by *Neisseria gonorrhoeae* modulates the innate immune response. *Innate Immunity, 20*(4), 377–389. doi:10.1177/1753425913493453 PMID:23884094

May, C., Finch, T., Mair, F., Ballini, L., Dowrick, C., Eccleset, M., & … . (2007). Understanding the implementation of complex interventions in health care: The normalization process model. *BMC Health Services Research, 7*(1), 148. doi:10.1186/1472-6963-7-148 PMID:17880693

McCaw, S. E., Liao, E. H., & Gray-Owen, S. D. (2004). Engulfment of *Neisseria gonorrhoeae*: Revealing distinct processes of bacterial entry by individual carcinoembryonic antigen-related cellular adhesion molecule family receptors. *Infection and Immunity, 72*(5), 2742–2752. doi:10.1128/IAI.72.5.2742-2752.2004 PMID:15102784

Medical Express. (2018). *World's first human case of rat disease found in Hong Kong*. Retrieved: https://medicalxpress.com/news/2018-09-world-human-case-rat-disease.html

Medical News Today. (2020). Retrieved: https://www.medicalnewstoday.com/articles/324204

Mehta, S. D., Rothman, R. E., Kelen, G. D., Quinn, T. C., & Zenilman, J. M. (2001). Clinical Aspects of Diagnosis of Gonorrhea and *Chlamydia* Infection in an Acute Care Setting. *Clinical Infectious Diseases, 32*(4), 655–659. doi:10.1086/318711 PMID:11181134

Menche, J., Sharma, A., Kitsak, M., Ghiassian, S. D., Vidal, M., Loscalzo, J., & Barabási, A. L. (2015). Uncovering disease-disease relationships through the incomplete interactome. *Science, 347*(6224), 1257601. doi:10.1126cience.1257601 PMID:25700523

Ministry of Health and Social Services. (2020). *Namibia COVID-19 situation report No.46*. Windhoek: Author.

Młynarczyk-Bonikowska, B., Kujawa, M., Malejczyk, M., Młynarczyk, G., & Majewski, S. (2016). Plasmid-mediated resistance to tetracyclines among *Neisseria gonorrhoeae* strains isolated in Poland between 2012 and 2013. *Postepy Dermatologii i Alergologii, 33*(6), 475–479. doi:10.5114/ada.2016.63887 PMID:28035227

Mogensen, T. H. (2009). Pathogen recognition and inflammatory signaling in innate immune defenses. *Clinical Microbiology Reviews, 22*(2), 240–273. doi:10.1128/CMR.00046-08 PMID:19366914

MoHSS. (2017). *Outbreak of Hepatitis E Virus (HEV) in Namibia Situation Report* (SITREP No. 64). Retrieved: https://www.afro.who.int/sites/default/files/2019-08/National%20SITREP%2064%20on%20Hepatitis%20E%20%20%20outbreak%20Final.pdf

Montano, M., Flanagan, J.N., Jiang, L., Sebastiani, P., Rarick, M., LeBrasseur, … Bhasin, S. (2007). Transcriptional Profiling of Testosterone-Regulated Genes in the Skeletal Muscle of Human Immunodeficiency Virus-Infected Men Experiencing Weight Loss. *The Journal of Clinical Endocrinology & Metabolism*, *92*(7), 2793–2802. doi:10.1210/jc.2006-2722

Munson, E., Wenten, D., Phipps, P., Gremminger, R., Schuknecht, M. K., Napierala, M., Hamer, D., Olson, R., Schell, R. F., & Hryciuk, J. E. (2013). Retrospective assessment of transcription-mediated amplification-based screening for Trichomonas vaginalis in male sexually transmitted infection clinic patients. *Journal of Clinical Microbiology*, *51*(6), 1855–1860. doi:10.1128/JCM.00455-13 PMID:23554208

Murhekar, M., Moolenaar, R., Hutin, Y., & Broome, C. (2009). Investigating outbreaks: Practical guidance in the Indian scenario. *The National Medical Journal of India*, *22*(5). PMID:20334049

Muse, C., Harrison, J., Yoshinaga-Itano, C., Grimes, A., Brookhouser, P. E., Epstein, S., Buchman, C., Mehl, A., Vohr, B., Moeller, M. P., Martin, P., Benedict, B. S., Scoggins, B., Crace, J., King, M., Sette, A., & Martin, B. (2013). Joint Committee on Infant Hearing of the American Academy of Pediatrics. Supplement to the JCIH 2007 position statement: Principles and guidelines for early intervention after confirmation that a child is deaf or hard of hearing. *Pediatrics*, *131*(4), e1324–e1349. doi:10.1542/peds.2013-0008 PMID:23530178

Namibia, W. H. O. (2020). *COVID-19: Namibia WCO Bulletin*. Windhoek: Author.

Naumann, M., Wessler, S., Bartsch, C., Wieland, B., & Meyer, T. F. (1997). *Neisseria gonorrhoeae* epithelial cell interaction leads to the activation of the transcription factors nuclear factor kappaB and activator protein 1 and the induction of inflammatory cytokines. *The Journal of Experimental Medicine*, *186*(2), 247–258. doi:10.1084/jem.186.2.247 PMID:9221754

Newman, L., Rowley, J., Vander Hoorn, S., Wijesooriya, N. S., Unemo, M., Low, N., Stevens, G., Gottlieb, S., Kiarie, J., & Temmerman, M. (2015). Global Estimates of the Prevalence and Incidence of Four Curable Sexually Transmitted Infections in 2012 Based on Systematic Review and Global Reporting. *PLoS One*, *10*(12), e0143304. doi:10.1371/journal.pone.0143304 PMID:26646541

Ng, L. K., & Martin, I. E. (2005). The laboratory diagnosis of *Neisseria gonorrhoeae. The Canadian journal of infectious diseases & medical microbiology =. The Canadian Journal of Infectious Diseases & Medical Microbiology*, *16*(1), 15–25. doi:10.1155/2005/323082 PMID:18159523

Ng, L. K., Martin, I., Liu, G., & Bryden, L. (2002). Mutation in 23S rRNA associated with macrolide resistance in *Neisseria gonorrhoeae. Antimicrobial Agents and Chemotherapy*, *46*(9), 3020–3025. doi:10.1128/AAC.46.9.3020-3025.2002 PMID:12183262

Nguyen, V. A., & Lió, P. (2009, December). Measuring similarity between gene expression profiles: A Bayesian approach. *BMC Genomics*, *10*(3), S14. doi:10.1186/1471-2164-10-S3-S14 PMID:19958477

Niwattanakul, S., Singthongchai, J., Naenudorn, E., & Wanapu, S. (2013, March). Using of Jaccard coefficient for keywords similarity. In *Proceedings of the international multiconference of engineers and computer scientists* (*Vol. 1*, No. 6, pp. 380-384). Academic Press.

Noor, H. A. (2013). Implementation of Universal Newborn Hearing Screening programme to be expanded. *The Malaysian Borneo Post*. Retrieved on the July 18, 2018 from http://www.theborneopost.com/2013/05/17/implementation-of-universal-newborn-hearing-screening-programme-to-be-expanded/

Nowicki, S., Selvarangan, R., & Anderson, G. (1999). Experimental transmission of *Neisseria gonorrhoeae* from pregnant rat to fetus. *Infection and Immunity*, *67*(9), 4974–4976. doi:10.1128/IAI.67.9.4974-4976.1999 PMID:10456962

Obrist, B., Iteba, N., Lengeler, C., Makemba, A., Mshana, C., Nathan, R., ... Schulze, A. (2007). Access to health care in contexts of livelihood insecurity: A framework for analysis and action. *PLoS Medicine*, *4*(10), e308. doi:10.1371/journal.pmed.0040308 PMID:17958467

Ogundipe, S., Obinna, C., & Olawale, G. (2016). With advancing age, ear infections are inevitable. *The Nigerian Vanguard*. Retrieved on the April 23, 2018 from https://www.vanguardngr.com/2016/06/with-advancing-age-ear-infections-are-inevitable-professor-julius-ademokoya/

Ohneck, E. A., Goytia, M., Rouquette-Loughlin, C. E., Joseph, S. J., Read, T. D., Jerse, A. E., & Shafer, W. M. (2015). Overproduction of the MtrCDE efflux pump in *Neisseria gonorrhoeae* produces unexpected changes in cellular transcription patterns. *Antimicrobial Agents and Chemotherapy*, *59*(1), 724–726. doi:10.1128/AAC.04148-14 PMID:25367915

Okhakhu, A. L., Ibekwe, T. S., Sadoh, A. S., & Ogisi, F. O. (2010). Neonatal hearing screening in Benin City. *International Journal of Pediatric Otorhinolaryngology*, *74*(11), 1323–1326. doi:10.1016/j.ijporl.2010.08.017 PMID:20863576

Olusanya, B. O. (2007). Addressing the global neglect of childhood hearing impairment in developing countries. *PLoS Medicine*, *4*(4), 74. doi:10.1371/journal.pmed.0040074 PMID:17407384

Olusanya, B. O. (2009). Newborns at risk of sensorineural hearing loss in low-income countries. *Archives of Disease in Childhood*, *94*(3), 227–230. doi:10.1136/adc.2008.144550 PMID:18786955

Olusanya, B. O., Luxon, L. M., & Wirz, S. L. (2005a). Screening for early childhood hearing loss in Nigeria. *Journal of Medical Screening*, *12*(3), 115–118. doi:10.1258/0969141054855274 PMID:16156940

Olusanya, B. O., Luxon, L. M., & Wirz, S. L. (2005b). Childhood deafness poses problems in developing countries. *BMJ (Clinical Research Ed.)*, *330*(7489), 480. doi:10.1136/bmj.330.7489.480-c PMID:15731158

Olusanya, B. O., & Newton, V. E. (2007). Global burden of childhood hearing impairment and disease control priority project for developing countries. *Lancet*, *369*(9569), 1314–1317. doi:10.1016/S0140-6736(07)60602-3 PMID:17434407

Olusanya, B. O., & Somefun, A. O. (2009). Sensorineural hearing loss in infants with neonatal jaundice in Lagos: A community-based study. *Annals of Tropical Paediatrics*, *29*(2), 119–128. doi:10.1179/146532809X440734 PMID:19460265

Olusanya, B. O., Wirz, S. L., & Luxon, L. M. (2008). Community-based infant hearing screening for early detection of permanent hearing loss in Lagos, Nigeria: A cross-sectional study. *Bulletin of the World Health Organization*, *86*(12), 956–963. doi:10.2471/BLT.07.050005 PMID:19142296

Onder, G., Rezza, G., & Brusaferro, S. (2020). Case-fatality rate and characteristics of patients dying in relation to COVID-19 in Italy. *Journal of the American Medical Association*. Advance online publication. doi:10.1001/jama.2020.4683 PMID:32203977

Ouoba, J. B., Traore, K. A., Rouamba, H., Setondji, K. V. M., Minoungou, G. L., Ouoba, B. L., Ouedraogo, A., Moctar, S., M'Bengue, A. K., Kakou, S. N., Doumbia, M., Traore, A. S., Roques, P., & Barro, N. (2019). Prevalence of anti-hepatitis E virus antibodies in domestic animal from three representative provinces of Burkina Faso. *Journal of Veterinary & Animal Sciences (Lahore)*, *7*, 1–7. doi:10.1016/j.vas.2019.100059 PMID:32734080

Outbreak Investigation: National Health Portal of India. (n.d.). Retrieved from https://www.nhp.gov.in/outbreak-investigation_pg

Palmer, S. R. (1989). Epidemiology in search of infectious diseases: Methods in outbreak investigation. *Journal of Epidemiology and Community Health*, *43*(4), 311–314. doi:10.1136/jech.43.4.311 PMID:2693574

Pan, Y., Zhang, M., Chen, Z., Zhou, M., & Zhang, Z. (2016, June). An ARIMA based model for forecasting the patient number of epidemic disease. In *Service Systems and Service Management (ICSSSM), 2016 13th International Conference on* (pp. 1-4). IEEE.

Papp, J. R., Abrams, A. J., Nash, E., Katz, A. R., Kirkcaldy, R. D., O'Connor, N. P., O'Brien, P. S., Harauchi, D. H., Maningas, E. V., Soge, O. O., Kersh, E. N., Komeya, A., Tomas, J. E., Wasserman, G. M., Kunimoto, G. Y., Trees, D. L., & Whelen, A. C. (2017). Azithromycin Resistance and Decreased Ceftriaxone Susceptibility in *Neisseria gonorrhoeae*, Hawaii, USA. *Emerging Infectious Diseases, 23*(5), 830–832. doi:10.3201/eid2305.170088 PMID:28418303

Paraskevis, D., Kostaki, E. G., Magiorkinis, G., Panayiotakopoulos, G., Sourvinos, G., & Tsiodras, S. (2020). Full-genome evolutionary analysis of the novel corona virus (2019-nCoV) rejects the hypothesis of emergence as a result of a recent recombination event. *Infection, Genetics and Evolution, 79*, 104212. doi:10.1016/j.meegid.2020.104212 PMID:32004758

Parra, A., Ponte, C., Cenjor, C., García-Olmos, M., Giménez, M. J., Aguilar, L., & Soriano, F. (2004). In vivo activity of amoxicillin/clavulanic acid and erythromycin in experimental otitis media caused by Streptococcus pneumoniae plus Haemophilus influenzae. *International Journal of Antimicrobial Agents, 23*(1), 25–31. doi:10.1016/j.ijantimicag.2003.05.016 PMID:14732310

Pasieka, A. E., Ota, F., Ryan, A., Ashton, F. E., Wallace, R., Perusse, C., & Diena, B. B. (1976). The goat mammary gland as a model infection site for *Neisseria gonorrhoeae. The British Journal of Venereal Diseases, 52*(3), 170–171. doi:10.1136ti.52.3.170 PMID:819088

Patel, A. L., Chaudhry, U., Sachdev, D., Sachdeva, P. N., Bala, M., & Saluja, D. (2011). An insight into the drug resistance profile & mechanism of drug resistance in *Neisseria gonorrhoeae. The Indian Journal of Medical Research, 134*(4), 419–431. PMID:22089602

Patrone, J. B., & Stein, D. C. (2007). Effect of gonococcal lipooligosaccharide variation on human monocytic cytokine profile. *BMC Microbiology, 7*(1), 7. doi:10.1186/1471-2180-7-7 PMID:17257430

Patton, M. E., Kidd, S., Llata, E., Stenger, M., Braxton, J., Asbel, L., Bernstein, K., Gratzer, B., Jespersen, M., Kerani, R., Mettenbrink, C., Mohamed, M., Pathela, P., Schumacher, C., Stirland, A., Stover, J., Tabidze, I., Kirkcaldy, R. D., & Weinstock, H. (2014). Extragenital gonorrhea and chlamydia testing and infection among men who have sex with men—STD Surveillance Network, United States, 2010-2012. *Nephrology, Dialysis, Transplantation, 58*(11), 1564–1570. doi:10.1093/cid/ciu184 PMID:24647015

Peterson, J. W. (1996). Bacterial Pathogenesis. In S. Baron (Ed.), *Medical Microbiology* (4th ed.). University of Texas Medical Branch at Galveston. Available from https://www.ncbi.nlm.nih.gov/books/NBK8526/

Pierce, W. A. Jr, Leong, J. K., & Hough, D. M. (1975). Strain-specific virulence-associated antigen of *Neisseria gonorrhoeae. Infection and Immunity, 11*(5), 898–903. doi:10.1128/IAI.11.5.898-903.1975 PMID:804445

Pinchuk, G. E., Ammons, C., Culley, D. E., Li, S. W., McLean, J. S., Romine, M. F., Nealson, K. H., Fredrickson, J. K., & Beliaev, A. S. (2008). Utilization of DNA as a Sole Source of Phosphorus, Carbon, and Energy by *Shewanella* spp.: Ecological and Physiological Implications for Dissimilatory Metal Reduction. *Applied and Environmental Microbiology, 74*(4), 1198–1208. doi:10.1128/AEM.02026-07 PMID:18156329

Plant, L., Sundqvist, J., Zughaier, S., Lövkvist, L., Stephens, D. S., & Jonsson, A. B. (2006). Lipooligosaccharide structure contributes to multiple steps in the virulence of Neisseria meningitidis. *Infection and Immunity, 74*(2), 1360–1367. doi:10.1128/IAI.74.2.1360-1367.2006 PMID:16428785

Pohlner J, Halter R, Beyreuther K & Meyer TF. (1987).Gene structure and extracellular secretion of *Neisseria gonorrhoeae* IgA protease. *Nature, 325*(6103), 458-62.

Polgreen, P. M., Chen, Y., Pennock, D. M., & Nelson, F. D. (2008). Using internet searches for influenza surveillance. *Clinical Infectious Diseases*, *47*(11), 1443–1448. doi:10.1086/593098 PMID:18954267

Potter, A. J., Kidd, S. P., Edwards, J. L., Falsetta, M. L., Apicella, M. A., Jennings, M. P., & McEwan, A. G. (2009). Thioredoxin reductase is essential for protection of *Neisseria gonorrhoeae* against killing by nitric oxide and for bacterial growth during interaction with cervical epithelial cells. *The Journal of Infectious Diseases*, *199*(2), 227–235. doi:10.1086/595737 PMID:19032106

Poutanen, S. M., Low, D. E., Henry, B., Finkelstein, S., Rose, D., Green, K., Tellier, R., Draker, R., Adachi, D., Ayers, M., Chan, A. K., Skowronski, D. M., Salit, I., Simor, A. E., Slutsky, A. S., Doyle, P. W., Krajden, M., Petric, M., Brunham, R. C., & McGeer, A. J. (2003). Identification of severe acute respiratory syndrome in Canada. *The New England Journal of Medicine*, *348*(20), 1995–2005. doi:10.1056/NEJMoa030634 PMID:12671061

Pryor, J. H., Martin, M. T., Whitney, C. G., Turco, J. H., Baumgartner, Y. Y., & Zegans, M. E. (2002). Rapid response to a conjunctivitis outbreak: The use of technology to leverage information. *Journal of American College Health*, *50*(6), 267–271. doi:10.1080/07448480209603444 PMID:12701651

Purdy, M. A., Harrison, T. J., Jameel, S., Meng, X. J., Okamoto, H., Van der Poel, W., & Smith, D. B.Ictv Report Consortium. (2017). ICTV Virus Taxonomy Profile: Hepeviridae. *The Journal of General Virology*, *98*(11), 2645–2646. doi:10.1099/jgv.0.000940 PMID:29022866

Quillin, S. J., & Seifert, H. S. (2018). *Neisseria gonorrhoeae* host adaptation and pathogenesis. *Nature Reviews. Microbiology*, *16*(4), 226–240. doi:10.1038/nrmicro.2017.169 PMID:29430011

Rahal, A., Kumar, A., Singh, V., Yadav, B., Tiwari, R., Chakraborty, S., & Dhama, K. (2014). Oxidative stress, prooxidants, and antioxidants: The interplay. *BioMed Research International*, *2014*, 761264. doi:10.1155/2014/761264 PMID:24587990

Raupach, J. C., & Hundy, R. L. (2003). An outbreak of Campylobacter jejune infection among conference delegates. *Communicable Diseases Intelligence*, *27*, 380–383. PMID:14510066

Rein, D. B., Stevens, G. A., Theaker, J., Wittenborn, J. S., & Wiersma, S. T. (2012). The global burden of hepatitis E virus genotypes 1 and 2 in 2005. *Hepatology (Baltimore, Md.)*, *55*(4), 988–997. doi:10.1002/hep.25505 PMID:22121109

Riou, J., & Althaus, C. L. (2020). Pattern of early human-to-human transmission of Wuhan 2019 novel coronavirus (2019-nCoV), December 2019 to January 2020. *Eurosurveillance*, *25*(4), 2000058. doi:10.2807/1560-7917.ES.2020.25.4.2000058 PMID:32019669

Rippa, V., Santini, L., Lo Surdo, P., Cantini, F., Veggi, D., Gentile, M. A., Grassi, E., Iannello, G., Brunelli, B., Ferlicca, F., Palmieri, E., Pallaoro, M., Aricò, B., Banci, L., Pizza, M., & Scarselli, M. (2015). Molecular Engineering of Ghfp, the Gonococcal Orthologue of Neisseria meningitidis Factor H Binding Protein. *Clinical and Vaccine Immunology; CVI*, *22*(7), 769–777. doi:10.1128/CVI.00794-14 PMID:25947148

Ritter, J. L., & Genco, C. A. (2018). *Neisseria gonorrhoeae*-Induced Inflammatory Pyroptosis in Human Macrophages is Dependent on Intracellular Gonococci and Lipooligosaccharide. *Journal of Cell Death*, *11*, 1179066017750902. doi:10.1177/1179066017750902 PMID:29434478

Ronpirin, C., Jerse, A. E., & Cornelissen, C. N. (2001). Gonococcal genes encoding transferrin-binding proteins A and B are arranged in a bicistronic operon but are subject to differential expression. *Infection and Immunity*, *69*(10), 6336–6347. doi:10.1128/IAI.69.10.6336-6347.2001 PMID:11553578

Ropp, P. A., Hu, M., Olesky, M., & Nicholas, R. A. (2002). Mutations in ponA, the gene encoding penicillin-binding protein 1, and a novel locus, penC, are required for high-level chromosomally mediated penicillin resistance in *Neisseria gonorrhoeae. Antimicrobial Agents and Chemotherapy*, *46*(3), 769–777. doi:10.1128/AAC.46.3.769-777.2002 PMID:11850260

Roth, R. I., Yamasaki, R., Mandrell, R. E., & Griffiss, J. M. (1992). Ability of gonococcal and meningococcal lipooligosaccharides to clot Limulus amebocyte lysate. *Infection and Immunity*, *60*(3), 762–767. doi:10.1128/IAI.60.3.762-767.1992 PMID:1541549

Rouphael, N. G., & Stephens, D. S. (2012). Neisseria meningitidis: Biology, microbiology, and epidemiology. *Methods in Molecular Biology (Clifton, N.J.)*, *799*, 1–20. doi:10.1007/978-1-61779-346-2_1 PMID:21993636

Rubin, G. J., & Wessely, S. (2020). The psychological effects of quarantining a city. *British Medical Journal*, 368.

Saginur, R., Clecner, B., Portnoy, J., & Mendelson, J. (1982). Superoxol(catalase)test for identification of *Neisseria gonorrhoeae. Journal of Clinical Microbiology*, *15*(3), 475–477. doi:10.1128/JCM.15.3.475-477.1982 PMID:6804487

Sahu, D., Pradhan, J., Jayachandran, V., & Khan, N. (2010). Why immunization coverage fails to catch up in India? A community-based analysis. *Child: Care, Health and Development*, *36*(3), 332–339. doi:10.1111/j.1365-2214.2009.01003.x PMID:19735269

Satterwhite, C. L., Torrone, E., Meites, E., Dunne, E. F., Mahajan, R., Ocfemia, M. C., Su, J., Xu, F., & Weinstock, H. (2013). Sexually transmitted infections among US women and men: Prevalence and incidence estimates, 2008. *Sexually Transmitted Diseases*, *40*(3), 187–193. doi:10.1097/OLQ.0b013e318286bb53 PMID:23403598

Savarino, A., Boelaert, J. R., Cassone, A., Majori, G., & Cauda, R. (2003). Effects of chloroquine on viral infections: An old drug against today's diseases? *The Lancet. Infectious Diseases*, *3*(11), 722–727. doi:10.1016/S1473-3099(03)00806-5 PMID:14592603

Scheenstra, M. R. (2010). *Antiphagocytosis - a bacterial mechanism to inhibit phagocytosis* (Unpublished master thesis). Department of Immunology, UMC Utrecht, Netherlands.

Scheuerpflug, I., Rudel, T., Ryll, R., Pandit, J., & Meyer, T. F. (1999). Roles of PilC and PilE proteins in pilus-mediated adherence of *Neisseria gonorrhoeae* and Neisseria meningitidis to human erythrocytes and endothelial and epithelial cells. *Infection and Immunity*, *67*(2), 834–843. doi:10.1128/IAI.67.2.834-843.1999 PMID:9916098

Schmidt, H., & Hensel, M. (2004). Pathogenicity islands in bacterial pathogenesis. *Clinical Microbiology Reviews*, *17*(1), 14–56. doi:10.1128/CMR.17.1.14-56.2004 PMID:14726454

Schulte, P. A., Ehrenberg, R. L., & Singal, M. (1987). Investigation of occupational cancer clusters: Theory and practice. *American Journal of Public Health*, *77*(1), 52–56. doi:10.2105/AJPH.77.1.52 PMID:3789238

Sharma, A., Gulbahce, N., Pevzner, S. J., Menche, J., Ladenvall, C., Folkersen, L., & Barabasi, A. L. (2013). Network-based analysis of genome wide association data provides novel candidate genes for lipid and lipoprotein traits. *Molecular & Cellular Proteomics*, *12*(11), 3398–3408. doi:10.1074/mcp.M112.024851 PMID:23882023

Shields, P., & Cathcart, L. (2013). *Oxidase Test Protocol*. American Society for Microbiology.

Shikongo, A. The Namibian newspaper. (2020). *Hepatitis-E continues to spread*. Retrieved: https://www.namibian.com.na/198938/archive-read/Hepatitis-E-continues-to-spread

Shim, B. S. (2011). Current concepts in bacterial sexually transmitted diseases. *Korean Journal of Urology*, *52*(9), 589–597. doi:10.4111/kju.2011.52.9.589 PMID:22025952

Simons, M. P., Nauseef, W. M., & Apicella, M. A. (2005). Interactions of *Neisseria gonorrhoeae* with adherent polymorphonuclear leukocytes. *Infection and Immunity*, *73*(4), 1971–1977. doi:10.1128/IAI.73.4.1971-1977.2005 PMID:15784537

Singh, R., Perera, S. R., Katselis, G. S., Chumala, P., Martin, I., Kusalik, A., Mitzel, K. M., & Dillon, J.-A. R. (2019). A β-lactamase-producing plasmid from *Neisseria gonorrhoeae* carrying a unique 6 bp deletion in bla_{TEM-1} encoding a truncated 24 kDa TEM-1 penicillinase that hydrolyses ampicillin slowly. *The Journal of Antimicrobial Chemotherapy*, *74*(10), 2904–2912. doi:10.1093/jac/dkz306 PMID:31335939

Smith, D. B., Izopet, J., Nicot, F., Simmonds, P., Jameel, S., Meng, X. J., Norder, H., Okamoto, H., van der Poel, W. H. M., Reuter, G., & Purdy, M. A. (2020). Update: Proposed reference sequences for subtypes of hepatitis E virus (species Orthohepevirus A). *The Journal of General Virology*, *101*(7), 692–698. doi:10.1099/jgv.0.001435 PMID:32469300

Smith, D. B., Simmonds, P., Jameel, S., Emerson, S. U., Harrison, T. J., Meng, X.-J., Okamoto, H., Van der Poel, W. H. M., & Purdy, M. A.Members Of The International Committee On The Taxonomy Of Viruses Study Group. (2014). Consensus proposals for classification of the family Hepeviridae. *The Journal of General Virology*, *95*(Pt 10), 2223–2232. doi:10.1099/vir.0.068429-0 PMID:24989172

Smith, J. C., Mailman, T., & Macdonald, N. E. (2013). How to get and get rid of gonorrhea. *Advances in Experimental Medicine and Biology*, *764*, 219–239. doi:10.1007/978-1-4614-4726-9_19 PMID:23654071

Soler-García, A. A., & Jerse, A. E. (2007). *Neisseria gonorrhoeae* catalase is not required for experimental genital tract infection despite the induction of a localized neutrophil response. *Infection and Immunity*, *75*(5), 2225–2233. doi:10.1128/IAI.01513-06 PMID:17296753

Song, W., Condron, S., Mocca, B. T., Veit, S. J., Hill, D., Abbas, A., & Jerse, A. E. (2008). Local and humoral immune responses against primary and repeat *Neisseria gonorrhoeae* genital tract infections of 17beta-estradiol-treated mice. *Vaccine*, *26*(45), 5741–5751. doi:10.1016/j.vaccinc.2008.08.020 PMID:18762223

Song, W., Ma, L., Chen, R., & Stein, D. C. (2000). Role of lipooligosaccharide in Opa-independent invasion of *Neisseria gonorrhoeae* into human epithelial cells. *The Journal of Experimental Medicine*, *191*(6), 949–960. doi:10.1084/jem.191.6.949 PMID:10727457

Song, Z., Xu, Y., Bao, L., Zhang, L., Yu, P., Qu, Y., Zhu, H., Zhao, W., Han, Y., & Qin, C. (2019). From SARS to MERS, thrusting coronaviruses into the spotlight. *Viruses*, *11*(1), E59. doi:10.3390/v11010059 PMID:30646565

Speers-Roesch, B., & Ballantyne, J. S. (2005). Activities of antioxidant enzymes and cytochrome c oxidase in liver of Arctic and temperate teleosts. *Comparative Biochemistry and Physiology*, *140*(4), 487–494. doi:10.1016/j.cbpb.2005.02.014 PMID:15936709

Spencer, S. E., Valentin-Bon, I. E., Whaley, K., & Jerse, A. E. (2004). Inhibition of *Neisseria gonorrhoeae*Genital Tract Infection by Leading-Candidate Topical Microbicides in a Mouse Model. *The Journal of Infectious Diseases*, *189*(3), 410–419. doi:10.1086/381125 PMID:14745698

Spinosa, M. R., Progida, C., Talà, A., Cogli, L., Alifano, P., & Bucci, C. (2007). The Neisseria meningitidis capsule is important for intracellular survival in human cells. *Infection and Immunity*, *75*(7), 3594–3603. doi:10.1128/IAI.01945-06 PMID:17470547

Stein, D. C., LeVan, A., Hardy, B., Wang, L. C., Zimmerman, L., & Song, W. (2015). Expression of Opacity Proteins Interferes with the Transmigration of *Neisseria gonorrhoeae*across Polarized Epithelial Cells. *PLoS One*, *10*(8), e0134342. doi:10.1371/journal.pone.0134342 PMID:26244560

Strauss, B. H., Serruys, P. W., de Scheerder, I. K., Tijssen, J. G., Bertrand, M. E., Puel, J., Meier, B., Kaufmann, U., Stauffer, J. C., & Rickards, A. F. (1991). Relative risk analysis of angiographic predictors of restenosis within the coronary Wallstent. *Circulation, 84*(4), 1636–1643. doi:10.1161/01.CIR.84.4.1636 PMID:1914103

Streeter, P. R., & Corbeil, L. B. (1981). Gonococcal infection in endotoxin-resistant and endotoxin-susceptible mice. *Infection and Immunity, 32*(1), 105–110. doi:10.1128/IAI.32.1.105-110.1981 PMID:6783547

Suppawittaya, P., Yiemphat, P., & Yasri, P. (2020). Effects of social distancing, self-quarantine and self-isolation during the COVID-19 pandemic on people's well-being and how to cope with it. *International Journal of Science and HealthCare Research, 5*(2).

Swanepoel, D. W., Hugo, R., & Louw, B. (2006). Infant hearing screening at immunization clinics in South Africa. *International Journal of Pediatric Otorhinolaryngology, 70*(7), 1241–1249. doi:10.1016/j.ijporl.2006.01.002 PMID:16483673

Swanson, J., Robbins, K., Barrera, O., Corwin, D., Boslego, J., Ciak, J., Blake, M., & Koomey, J. M. (1987). Gonococcal pilin variants in experimental gonorrhea. *The Journal of Experimental Medicine, 165*(5), 1344–1357. doi:10.1084/jem.165.5.1344 PMID:3106555

Taylor-Robinson, D., Whytock, S., Green, C. J., & Carney, F. E. Jr. (1974). Effect of *Neisseria gonorrhoeae* on human and rabbit oviducts. *The British Journal of Venereal Diseases, 50*(4), 279–288. doi:10.1136ti.50.4.279 PMID:4213729

Thacker, N., & Shendurnikar, N. (2004). Current status of polio eradication and future prospects. *Indian Journal of Pediatrics, 71*(3), 241–245. doi:10.1007/BF02724277 PMID:15080411

Tian, S., Hu, W., Niu, L., Liu, H., Xu, H., & Xiao, S. Y. (2020). *Pulmonary pathology of Early-phase 2019 Novel Coronavirus (COVID-19) pneumonia in two patients with lung cancer.* doi:10.1016/j.jtho.2020.02.010

Tomori, O. (2011). From smallpox eradication to the future of global health: Innovations, application and lessons for future eradication and control initiatives. *Vaccine, 29*, D145–D148. doi:10.1016/j.vaccine.2011.09.003 PMID:22185830

Trimble, M. J., Mlynárčik, P., Kolář, M., & Hancock, R. E. (2016). Polymyxin: Alternative Mechanisms of Action and Resistance. *Cold Spring Harbor Perspectives in Medicine, 6*(10), a025288. doi:10.1101/cshperspect.a025288 PMID:27503996

Tugwell, B. D., Lee, L. E., Gillette, H., Lorber, E. M., Hedberg, K., & Cieslak, P. R. (2004). Chickenpox outbreak in a highly vaccinated school population. *Pediatrics, 113*(3), 455–459. doi:10.1542/peds.113.3.455 PMID:14993534

Turanalp, M. E., & Can, T. (2008). Discovering functional interaction patterns in protein-protein interaction networks. *BMC Bioinformatics, 9*(1), 276. doi:10.1186/1471-2105-9-276 PMID:18547430

Turner, S. M., Moir, J. W., Griffiths, L., Overton, T. W., Smith, H., & Cole, J. A. (2005). Mutational and biochemical analysis of cytochrome c′, a nitric oxide-binding lipoprotein important for adaptation of *Neisseria gonorrhoeae* to oxygen-limited growth. *The Biochemical Journal, 388*(Pt 2), 545–553. doi:10.1042/BJ20041766 PMID:15689189

Tzeng, Y. L., Datta, A., Kolli, V. K., Carlson, R. W., & Stephens, D. S. (2002). Endotoxin of Neisseria meningitidis composed only of intact lipid A: Inactivation of the meningococcal 3-deoxy-D-manno-octulosonic acid transferase. *Journal of Bacteriology, 184*(9), 2379–2388. doi:10.1128/JB.184.9.2379-2388.2002 PMID:11948150

Unemo, M., Ballard, R., Ison, C., Lewis, D., Ndowa, F., & Peeling, R. (2013). Laboratory Diagnosis of Sexually Transmitted Infections, including human immunodeficiency virus. *World Health Organisation Manual*. Available at: https://www.who.int/reproductivehealth/publications/rtis/9789241505840/en/

Unemo, M., Del Rio, C., & Shafer, W. M. (2016). Antimicrobial Resistance Expressed by *Neisseria gonorrhoeae*: A Major Global Public Health Problem in the 21st Century. *Microbiology Spectrum, 4*(3), doi:10.1128/microbiolspec

Unemo, M., Golparian, D., Skogen, V., Olsen, A. O., Moi, H., Syversen, G., & Hjelmevoll, S. O. (2013). *Neisseria gonorrhoeae* strain with high-level resistance to spectinomycin due to a novel resistance mechanism (mutated ribosomal protein S5) verified in Norway. *Antimicrobial Agents and Chemotherapy*, *57*(2), 1057–1061. doi:10.1128/AAC.01775-12 PMID:23183436

Unemo, M., & Shafer, W. M. (2014). Antimicrobial resistance in *Neisseria gonorrhoeae* in the 21st century: Past, evolution, and future. *Clinical Microbiology Reviews*, *27*(3), 587–613. doi:10.1128/CMR.00010-14 PMID:24982323

UNICEF's strategy for health (2016-2030). (n.d.). Available: https://www.unicef.org/health

Uribe-Querol, E., & Rosales, C. (2017). Control of Phagocytosis by Microbial Pathogens. *Frontiers in Immunology*, *8*, 1368. doi:10.3389/fimmu.2017.01368 PMID:29114249

Usharani, J., & Iyakutti, K. (2013). A genetic algorithm based on cosine similarity for relevant document retrieval. *International Journal of Engineering Research & Technology (Ahmedabad)*, *2*(2), 1–13.

Vaccine India. (n.d.). Available: https://www.vaccineindia.org/

van Tong, H., Hoan, N.X., Wang, B., Wedemeyer, H., Bock, C.T., & Velavan, T.P. (2016). Hepatitis E Virus Mutations: Functional and Clinical Relevance. *EBioMedicine Journal, 11*, 41-42. doi:10.1016/j.ebiom.2016.07.039

Vashishtha, V. M., Kumar, A., John, T. J., & Nayak, N. C. (2007a). Cassia occidentalis poisoning as the probable cause of hepatomyoencephalopathy in children in western Uttar Pradesh. *The Indian Journal of Medical Research, 125*, 756–762. PMID:17704552

Vashishtha, V. M., Kumar, A., John, T. J., & Nayak, N. C. (2007b). Cassia occidentalis poisoning causes fatal coma in children in western Uttar Pradesh. *Indian Pediatrics*, *44*, 522–525. PMID:17684305

Vashishtha, V. M., Nayak, N. C., John, T. J., & Kumar, A. (2007). Recurrent annual outbreaks of a hepato-myoencephalopathy syndrome in children in western Uttar Pradesh, India. *The Indian Journal of Medical Research*, *125*, 523–533. PMID:17598938

Velasquez, L., García, K., Morales, F., Heckels, J. E., Orihuela, P., Rodas, P. I., Christodoulides, M., & Cardenas, H. (2012). *Neisseria gonorrhoeae* pilus attenuates cytokine response of human fallopian tube explants. *Journal of Biomedicine & Biotechnology*, *491298*, 1–7. Advance online publication. doi:10.1155/2012/491298 PMID:22318778

Vermassen, A., Leroy, S., Talon, R., Provot, C., Popowska, M., & Desvaux, M. (2019). Cell Wall Hydrolases in Bacteria: Insight on the Diversity of Cell Wall Amidases, Glycosidases and Peptidases Toward Peptidoglycan. *Frontiers in Microbiology*, *10*, 331. doi:10.3389/fmicb.2019.00331 PMID:30873139

Vidal, M., Cusick, M. E., & Barabási, A. L. (2011). Interactome networks and human disease. *Cell*, *144*(6), 986–998. doi:10.1016/j.cell.2011.02.016 PMID:21414488

Vijay, H. M., Lavergne, G., Ashton, F. E., Ryan, A., & Diena, B. B. (1977). Homocytotropic antibodies (IgE) to *Neisseria gonorrhoeae* in the rat and a cross-reactivity of heterologous gonococcal strains. *The British Journal of Venereal Diseases*, *53*(2), 106–108. doi:10.1136ti.53.2.106 PMID:66964

Vincent, M. J., Bergeron, E., Benjannet, S., Erickson, B. R., Rollin, P. E., Ksiazek, T. G., Seidah, N. G., & Nichol, S. T. (2005). Chloroquine is a potent inhibitor of SARS coronavirus infection and spread. *Virology Journal*, *2*(1), 69. doi:10.1186/1743-422X-2-69 PMID:16115318

Vos, T., Allen, C., Arora, M., Barber, R. M., Bhutta, Z. A., & Brown, A. (2016). Global, regional, and national incidence, prevalence, and years lived with disability for 310 diseases and injuries, 1990-2015: A systematic analysis for the Global Burden of Disease Study 2015. *The Lancet, 388*(10053), 1545–1602. (16)31678-6 doi:10.1016/S0140-6736

Walls, A. C., Park, Y. J., Tortorici, M. A., Wall, A., McGuire, A. T., & Veesler, D. (2020). *Structure, function, and antigenicity of the SARS-CoV-2 spike glycoprotein*. doi:10.1016/j.cell.2020.02.058

Wang, D., Hu, B., Hu, C., Zhu, F., Liu, X., & Zhang, J. (n.d.). Clinical characteristics of 138 hospitalized patients with 2019 novel coronavirus-infected pneumonia in Wuhan, China. Academic Press.

Wang, D., Hu, B., Hu, C., Zhu, F., Liu, X., Zhang, J., Wang, B., Xiang, H., Cheng, Z., Xiong, Y., Zhao, Y., Li, Y., Wang, X., & Peng, Z. (2020). Clinical Characteristics of 138 Hospitalized Patients With 2019 Novel Coronavirus–Infected Pneumonia in Wuhan, China. *Journal of the American Medical Association*, *323*(11), 1061. Advance online publication. doi:10.1001/jama.2020.1585

Wang, X., Gulbahce, N., & Yu, H. (2011). Network-based methods for human disease gene prediction. *Briefings in Functional Genomics*, *10*(5), 280–293. doi:10.1093/bfgp/elr024 PMID:21764832

Weel, J. F., Hopman, C. T., & van Putten, J. P. (1991). In situ expression and localization of *Neisseria gonorrhoeae* opacity proteins in infected epithelial cells: Apparent role of Opa proteins in cellular invasion. *The Journal of Experimental Medicine*, *173*(6), 1395–1405. doi:10.1084/jem.173.6.1395 PMID:1903430

Wenham, C., Smith, J., & Morgan, R. (2020). Gender and C-W Group, COVID-19: The gendered impacts of the outbreak. *Journal*, *395*, 846–848. PMID:32151325

Weyand, N. J., Wertheimer, A. M., Hobbs, T. R., Sisko, J. L., Taku, N. A., Gregston, L. D., Clary, S., Higashi, D. L., Biais, N., Brown, L. M., Planer, S. L., Legasse, A. W., Axthelm, M. K., Wong, S. W., & So, M. (2013). Neisseria infection of rhesus macaques as a model to study colonization, transmission, persistence, and horizontal gene transfer. *Proceedings of the National Academy of Sciences of the United States of America*, *110*(8), 3059–3064. doi:10.1073/pnas.1217420110 PMID:23382234

Weyler, L., Engelbrecht, M., Mata Forsberg, M., Brehwens, K., Vare, D., Vielfort, K., Wojcik, A., & Aro, H. (2014). Restriction endonucleases from invasive *Neisseria gonorrhoeae* cause double-strand breaks and distort mitosis in epithelial cells during infection. *PLoS One*, *9*(12), e114208. doi:10.1371/journal.pone.0114208 PMID:25460012

WHO. (2014). *Waterborne outbreaks of hepatitis E: recognition, investigation and control technical report*. Retrieved: https://apps.who.int/iris/bitstream/handle/10665/129448/9789241507608_eng.pdf;jsessionid=500CBD02380CD28F6956B10FCABEC63B?sequence=1

WHO. (2016). *Report on the 9th Global Conference for Health Promotion: All for Health, Health for All*. https://www.who.int/healthpromotion/conferences/9gchp/shanghai-conference-report/en/

WHO. (2017). *Global hepatitis report*. Retrieved https://apps.who.int/iris/bitstream/handle/10665/255016/9789241565455eng.pdf?sequence=1

WHO. (2018). *Hepatitis E-Namibia. Emergencies preparedness, response*. Retrieved: https://www.who.int/csr/don/15-january-2018-hepatitis-e-namibia/en/

WHO. (2020). *Coronavirus disease (COVID-2019) situation reports*. https:// www.who.int/emergencies/diseases/novel-coronavirus-2019/situationreports

WHO. (2020a). *Hepatitis E*. Retrieved: https://www.who.int/news-room/fact-sheets/detail/hepatitis-e

WHO. (2020b). *Hepatitis*. Retrieved: http://www.emro.who.int/health-topics/hepatitis/index.html

Wilson, K., Atkinson, K. M., & Westeinde, J. (2015). Apps for immunization: Leveraging mobile devices to place the individual at the center of care. *Human Vaccines & Immunotherapeutics*, *11*(10), 2395–2399. doi:10.1080/21645515.2015.1057362 PMID:26110351

Wira, C. R., Ghosh, M., Smith, J. M., Shen, L., Connor, R. I., Sundstrom, P., Frechette, G. M., Hill, E. T., & Fahey, J. V. (2011). Epithelial cell secretions from the human female reproductive tract inhibit sexually transmitted pathogens and Candida albicans but not Lactobacillus. *Mucosal Immunology*, *4*(3), 335–342. doi:10.1038/mi.2010.72 PMID:21048705

Wong, K. H., Arko, R. J., Schalla, W. O., & Steurer, F. J. (1979). Immunological and serological diversity of *Neisseria gonorrhoeae*: Identification of new immunotypes and highly protective strains. *Infection and Immunity*, *23*(3), 717–722. doi:10.1128/IAI.23.3.717-722.1979 PMID:88414

Woods, C. R. (2005). Gonococcal Infections in Neonates and Young Children. *Seminars in Pediatric Infectious Diseases*, *16*(4), 258–270. doi:10.1053/j.spid.2005.06.006 PMID:16210106

Workowski, K. A., Bolan, G. A., & Centers for Disease Control and Prevention. (2015). Sexually transmitted diseases treatment guidelines, 2015. *MMWR. Recommendations and reports: Morbidity and mortality weekly report. Recommendations and reports, 64*(RR-03), 1–137.

World Health Organisation. (2009). *Newborn and infants hearing screening: current issues and guiding principles for action.* Retrieved on the May 14, 2018 from https://www.who.int/blindness/publications/Newborn_and_Infant_Hearing_Screening_Report.pdf

World Health Organization (WHO). (n.d.). Available: http://www.who.int

World Health Organization. (2018a). *Addressing the rising prevalence of hearing loss.* http://apps.who.int/iris/bitstream/handle/10665/260336/9789241550260-eng. pdf?sequence=1&ua=1

World Health Organization. (2018b). *Deafness and hearing loss—Key facts.* https://www.who.int/mediacentre/factsheets/fs300/en/

World Health Organization. (2018c). *Prevention of blindness and deafness—Estimates: Global estimates on prevalence of hearing loss* [Embedded powerpoint presentation]. https://www.who.int/pbd/deafness/estimates/en/

World Health Organization. (2020). *Mental health and psychosocial considerations during the COVID-19 outbreak.* Accessed online: https://www.who. int/docs/default-source/coronaviruse/mental-health-considerations.pdf

Wu, F., Zhao, S., Yu, B., Chen, Y. M., Wang, W., Song, Z. G., Hu, Y., Tao, Z.-W., Tian, J.-H., Pei, Y.-Y., Yuan, M.-L., Zhang, Y.-L., Dai, F.-H., Liu, Y., Wang, Q.-M., Zheng, J.-J., Xu, L., Holmes, E. C., & Zhang, Y.-Z. (2020). A new coronavirus associated with human respiratory disease in China. *Nature*, *579*(7798), 265–269. Advance online publication. doi:10.103841586-020-2008-3 PMID:32015508

Xiong, M., Lan, L., Feng, T., Zhao, G., Wang, F., Hong, F., Wu, X., Zhang, C., Wen, L., Liu, A., Best, J. M. C., & Tang, W. (2016). Analysis of the sex ratio of reported gonorrhoea incidence in Shenzhen, China. *BMJ Open*, *6*(3), e009629. doi:10.1136/bmjopen-2015-009629 PMID:26975933

Xu, Z., Shi, L., Wang, Y., Zhang, J., Huang, L., Zhang, C., Liu, S., Zhao, P., Liu, H., Zhu, L., Tai, Y., Bai, C., Gao, T., Song, J., Xia, P., Dong, J., Zhao, J., & Wang, F. S. (2020). Pathological findings of COVID-19 associated with acute respiratory distress syndrome. *Journal*, *8*(4), 420–422. doi:10.1016/S2213-2600(20)30076-X PMID:32085846

Yahmed, M A B., Bounenni, M. A., Chelly, Z., & Jlassi, A. (2013, April). A new mobile health application for an ubiquitous information system. In *6th Joint IFIP Wireless and Mobile Networking Conference (WMNC)* (pp. 1-4). IEEE.

Yu, L., Wang, B., Ma, X., & Gao, L. (2016). The extraction of drug-disease correlations based on module distance in incomplete human interactome. *BMC Systems Biology*, *10*(4), 111. doi:10.118612918-016-0364-2 PMID:28155709

Zhang, W., Du, R. H., Li, B., Zheng, X. S., Yang, X. L., Hu, B., Wang, Y.-Y., Xiao, G.-F., Yan, B., Shi, Z.-L., & Zhou, P. (2020). Molecular and serological investigation of 2019-nCoV infected patients: Implication of multiple shedding routes. *Emerging Microbes & Infections*, *9*(1), 386–389. doi:10.1080/22221751.2020.1729071 PMID:32065057

Zheng, M., Gao, Y., Wang, G., Song, G., Liu, S., Sun, D., Xu, Y., & Tian, Z. (2020). Functional exhaustion of antiviral lymphocytes in COVID-19 patients. *Cellular & Molecular Immunology*, *17*(5), 533–535. Advance online publication. doi:10.103841423-020-0402-2 PMID:32203188

Zhou, J., & Fu, B. Q. (2018). The research on gene-disease association based on text-mining of PubMed. *BMC Bioinformatics*, *19*(1), 37. doi:10.118612859-018-2048-y PMID:29415654

Zhou, P., Yang, X. L., Wang, X. G., Hu, B., Zhang, L., Zhang, W., Si, H.-R., Zhu, Y., Li, B., Huang, C.-L., Chen, H.-D., Chen, J., Luo, Y., Guo, H., Jiang, R.-D., Liu, M.-Q., Chen, Y., Shen, X.-R., Wang, X., ... Shi, Z.-L. (2020). A pneumonia outbreak associated with a new coronavirus of probable bat origin. *Nature*, *588*(7836), E6. Advance online publication. doi:10.103841586-020-2951-z PMID:32015507

Zumla, A., Chan, J., Azhar, E., Hui, D., & Yuen, K. (2016). Coronaviruses - drug discovery and therapeutic options. *Nature Reviews. Drug Discovery*, *15*(5), 327–347. doi:10.1038/nrd.2015.37 PMID:26868298

Related References

To continue our tradition of advancing information science and technology research, we have compiled a list of recommended IGI Global readings. These references will provide additional information and guidance to further enrich your knowledge and assist you with your own research and future publications.

Abu Seman, S. A., & Ramayah, T. (2017). Are We Ready to App?: A Study on mHealth Apps, Its Future, and Trends in Malaysia Context. In J. Pelet (Ed.), *Mobile Platforms, Design, and Apps for Social Commerce* (pp. 69–83). Hershey, PA: IGI Global. doi:10.4018/978-1-5225-2469-4.ch005

Aggarwal, S., & Azad, V. (2017). A Hybrid System Based on FMM and MLP to Diagnose Heart Disease. In S. Bhattacharyya, S. Dc, I. Pan, & P. Dutta (Eds.), *Intelligent Multidimensional Data Clustering and Analysis* (pp. 293–325). Hershey, PA: IGI Global. doi:10.4018/978-1-5225-1776-4.ch011

Akaichi, J., & Mhadhbi, L. (2016). A Clinical Decision Support System: Ontology-Driven Approach for Effective Emergency Management. In J. Moon & M. Galea (Eds.), *Improving Health Management through Clinical Decision Support Systems* (pp. 270–294). Hershey, PA: IGI Global. doi:10.4018/978-1-4666-9432-3.ch013

Akerkar, R. (2016). Towards an Intelligent Integrated Approach for Clinical Decision Support. In A. Aggarwal (Ed.), *Managing Big Data Integration in the Public Sector* (pp. 187–205). Hershey, PA: IGI Global. doi:10.4018/978-1-4666-9649-5.ch011

Al-Busaidi, S. S. (2018). Interdisciplinary Relationships Between Medicine and Social Sciences. In M. Al-Suqri, A. Al-Kindi, S. AlKindi, & N. Saleem (Eds.), *Promoting Interdisciplinarity in Knowledge Generation and Problem Solving* (pp. 124–137). Hershey, PA: IGI Global. doi:10.4018/978-1-5225-3878-3.ch009

Al Kareh, T., & Thoumy, M. (2018). The Impact of Health Information Digitization on the Physiotherapist-Patient Relationship: A Pilot Study of the Lebanese Community. *International Journal of Healthcare Information Systems and Informatics, 13*(2), 29–53. doi:10.4018/IJHISI.2018040103

Alenzuela, R. (2017). Research, Leadership, and Resource-Sharing Initiatives: The Role of Local Library Consortia in Access to Medical Information. In S. Ram (Ed.), *Library and Information Services for Bioinformatics Education and Research* (pp. 199–211). Hershey, PA: IGI Global. doi:10.4018/978-1-5225-1871-6.ch012

Ameri, H., Alizadeh, S., & Noughabi, E. A. (2017). Application of Data Mining Techniques in Clinical Decision Making: A Literature Review and Classification. In E. Noughabi, B. Raahemi, A. Albadvi, & B. Far (Eds.), *Handbook of Research on Data Science for Effective Healthcare Practice and Administration* (pp. 257–295). Hershey, PA: IGI Global. doi:10.4018/978-1-5225-2515-8.ch012

Anand, S. (2017). Medical Image Enhancement Using Edge Information-Based Methods. In B. Singh (Ed.), *Computational Tools and Techniques for Biomedical Signal Processing* (pp. 123–148). Hershey, PA: IGI Global. doi:10.4018/978-1-5225-0660-7.ch006

Angjellari-Dajci, F., Sapienza, C., Lawless, W. F., & Kavanagh, K. (2016). Human Capital Accumulation in Medical Simulated Learning Environments: A Framework for Economic Evaluation. In M. Russ (Ed.), *Quantitative Multidisciplinary Approaches in Human Capital and Asset Management* (pp. 65–88). Hershey, PA: IGI Global. doi:10.4018/978-1-4666-9652-5.ch004

Anil, M., Ayyildiz-Tamis, D., Tasdemir, S., Sendemir-Urkmez, A., & Gulce-Iz, S. (2016). Bioinspired Materials and Biocompatibility. In M. Bououdina (Ed.), *Emerging Research on Bioinspired Materials Engineering* (pp. 294–322). Hershey, PA: IGI Global. doi:10.4018/978-1-4666-9811-6.ch011

Anton, J. L., Soriano, J. V., Martinez, M. I., & Garcia, F. B. (2018). Comprehensive E-Learning Appraisal System. In M. Khosrow-Pour, D.B.A. (Ed.), Encyclopedia of Information Science and Technology, Fourth Edition (pp. 5787-5799). Hershey, PA: IGI Global. doi:10.4018/978-1-5225-2255-3.ch503

Arabi, M. (2016). Redesigning the Organizational Structure to Reach Efficiency: The Case of Ministry of Health and Medical Education of Iran. In R. Gholipour & K. Rouzbehani (Eds.), *Social, Economic, and Political Perspectives on Public Health Policy-Making* (pp. 257–294). Hershey, PA: IGI Global. doi:10.4018/978-1-4666-9944-1.ch012

Assis-Hassid, S., Heart, T., Reychav, I., & Pliskin, J. S. (2016). Modelling Factors Affecting Patient-Doctor-Computer Communication in Primary Care. *International Journal of Reliable and Quality E-Healthcare*, *5*(1), 1–17. doi:10.4018/IJRQEH.2016010101

Atzori, B., Hoffman, H. G., Vagnoli, L., Messeri, A., & Grotto, R. L. (2018). Virtual Reality as Distraction Technique for Pain Management in Children and Adolescents. In M. Khosrow-Pour, D.B.A. (Ed.), Encyclopedia of Information Science and Technology, Fourth Edition (pp. 5955-5965). Hershey, PA: IGI Global. doi:10.4018/978-1-5225-2255-3.ch518

Audibert, M., Mathonnat, J., Pélissier, A., & Huang, X. X. (2018). The Impact of the New Rural Cooperative Medical Scheme on Township Hospitals' Utilization and Income Structure in Weifang Prefecture, China. In I. Management Association (Ed.), Health Economics and Healthcare Reform: Breakthroughs in Research and Practice (pp. 109-121). Hershey, PA: IGI Global. doi:10.4018/978-1-5225-3168-5.ch007

Ayyachamy, S. (2016). Analysis and Comparison of Developed 2D Medical Image Database Design using Registration Scheme, Retrieval Scheme, and Bag-of-Visual-Words. In N. Dey & A. Ashour (Eds.), *Classification and Clustering in Biomedical Signal Processing* (pp. 149–168). Hershey, PA: IGI Global. doi:10.4018/978-1-5225-0140-4.ch007

Babalola, A. C. (2016). Literacy and Decision Making on Health Issues among Married Women in Southwest Nigeria. In V. Wang (Ed.), *Handbook of Research on Advancing Health Education through Technology* (pp. 191–212). Hershey, PA: IGI Global. doi:10.4018/978-1-4666-9494-1.ch009

Babu, A., & Ayyappan, S. (2017). A Methodological Evaluation of Crypto-Watermarking System for Medical Images. In C. Bhatt & S. Peddoju (Eds.), *Cloud Computing Systems and Applications in Healthcare* (pp. 189–217). Hershey, PA: IGI Global. doi:10.4018/978-1-5225-1002-4.ch010

Bakke, A. (2017). Ethos in E-Health: From Informational to Interactive Websites. In M. Folk & S. Apostel (Eds.), *Establishing and Evaluating Digital Ethos and Online Credibility* (pp. 85–103). Hershey, PA: IGI Global. doi:10.4018/978-1-5225-1072-7.ch005

Bali, S. (2018). Enhancing the Reach of Health Care Through Telemedicine: Status and New Possibilities in Developing Countries. In U. Pandey & V. Indrakanti (Eds.), *Open and Distance Learning Initiatives for Sustainable Development* (pp. 339–354). Hershey, PA: IGI Global. doi:10.4018/978-1-5225-2621-6.ch019

Barrett, T. E. (2018). Essentials for Education and Training for Tomorrow's Physicians. In C. Smith (Ed.), *Exploring the Pressures of Medical Education From a Mental Health and Wellness Perspective* (pp. 230–252). Hershey, PA: IGI Global. doi:10.4018/978-1-5225-2811-1.ch010

Barrett, T. J. (2016). Knowledge in Action: Fostering Health Education through Technology. In V. Wang (Ed.), *Handbook of Research on Advancing Health Education through Technology* (pp. 39–62). Hershey, PA: IGI Global. doi:10.4018/978-1-4666-9494-1.ch003

Berrahal, S., & Boudriga, N. (2017). The Risks of Wearable Technologies to Individuals and Organizations. In A. Marrington, D. Kerr, & J. Gammack (Eds.), *Managing Security Issues and the Hidden Dangers of Wearable Technologies* (pp. 18–46). Hershey, PA: IGI Global. doi:10.4018/978-1-5225-1016-1.ch002

Bhagat, A. P., & Atique, M. (2016). Medical Image Mining Using Fuzzy Connectedness Image Segmentation: Efficient Retrieval of Patients' Stored Images. In W. Karâa & N. Dey (Eds.), *Biomedical Image Analysis and Mining Techniques for Improved Health Outcomes* (pp. 184–209). Hershey, PA: IGI Global. doi:10.4018/978-1-4666-8811-7.ch009

Bhargava, P. (2018). Blended Learning: An Effective Application to Clinical Teaching. In S. Tang & C. Lim (Eds.), *Preparing the Next Generation of Teachers for 21st Century Education* (pp. 302–320). Hershey, PA: IGI Global. doi:10.4018/978-1-5225-4080-9.ch018

Binh, N. T., & Tuyet, V. T. (2016). The Combination of Adaptive Filters to Improve the Quality of Medical Images in New Wavelet Domain. In N. Dey & A. Ashour (Eds.), *Classification and Clustering in Biomedical Signal Processing* (pp. 46–76). Hershey, PA: IGI Global. doi:10.4018/978-1-5225-0140-4.ch003

Bird, J. L. (2017). Writing Healing Narratives. In V. Bryan & J. Bird (Eds.), *Healthcare Community Synergism between Patients, Practitioners, and Researchers* (pp. 1–28). Hershey, PA: IGI Global. doi:10.4018/978-1-5225-0640-9.ch001

Bottrighi, A., Leonardi, G., Piovesan, L., & Terenziani, P. (2016). Knowledge-Based Support to the Treatment of Exceptions in Computer Interpretable Clinical Guidelines. *International Journal of Knowledge-Based Organizations*, *6*(3), 1–27. doi:10.4018/IJKBO.2016070101

Bougoulias, K., Kouris, I., Prasinos, M., Giokas, K., & Koutsouris, D. (2017). Ob/Gyn EMR Software: A Solution for Obstetricians and Gynecologists. In A. Moumtzoglou (Ed.), *Design, Development, and Integration of Reliable Electronic Healthcare Platforms* (pp. 101–111). Hershey, PA: IGI Global. doi:10.4018/978-1-5225-1724-5.ch006

Bouslimi, R., Ayadi, M. G., & Akaichi, J. (2018). Medical Image Retrieval in Healthcare Social Networks. *International Journal of Healthcare Information Systems and Informatics*, *13*(2), 13–28. doi:10.4018/IJHISI.2018040102

Bouzaabia, O., Bouzaabia, R., & Mejri, K. (2017). Role of Internet in the Development of Medical Tourism Service in Tunisia. In A. Capatina & E. Rancati (Eds.), *Key Challenges and Opportunities in Web Entrepreneurship* (pp. 211–241). Hershey, PA: IGI Global. doi:10.4018/978-1-5225-2466-3.ch009

Briz-Ponce, L., Juanes-Méndez, J. A., & García-Peñalvo, F. J. (2016). The Role of Gender in Technology Acceptance for Medical Education. In M. Cruz-Cunha, I. Miranda, R. Martinho, & R. Rijo (Eds.), *Encyclopedia of E-Health and Telemedicine* (pp. 1013–1027). Hershey, PA: IGI Global. doi:10.4018/978-1-4666-9978-6.ch079

Briz-Ponce, L., Juanes-Méndez, J. A., & García-Peñalvo, F. J. (2016). A Research Contribution to the Analysis of Mobile Devices in Higher Education from Medical Students' Point of View. In L. Briz-Ponce, J. Juanes-Méndez, & F. García-Peñalvo (Eds.), *Handbook of Research on Mobile Devices and Applications in Higher Education Settings* (pp. 196–221). Hershey, PA: IGI Global. doi:10.4018/978-1-5225-0256-2.ch009

Brown-Jackson, K. L. (2018). Telemedicine and Telehealth: Academics Engaging the Community in a Call to Action. In S. Burton (Ed.), *Engaged Scholarship and Civic Responsibility in Higher Education* (pp. 166–193). Hershey, PA: IGI Global. doi:10.4018/978-1-5225-3649-9.ch008

Bwalya, K. J. (2017). Next Wave of Tele-Medicine: Virtual Presence of Medical Personnel. In K. Moahi, K. Bwalya, & P. Sebina (Eds.), *Health Information Systems and the Advancement of Medical Practice in Developing Countries* (pp. 168–180). Hershey, PA: IGI Global. doi:10.4018/978-1-5225-2262-1.ch010

Carlton, E. L., Holsinger, J. W. Jr, & Anunobi, N. (2016). Physician Engagement with Health Information Technology: Implications for Practice and Professionalism. *International Journal of Computers in Clinical Practice*, *1*(2), 51–73. doi:10.4018/IJCCP.2016070103

Castillo-Page, L., Eliason, J., Conrad, S. S., & Nivet, M. A. (2016). Diversity in Undergraduate Medical Education: An Examination of Organizational Culture and Climate in Medical Schools. In C. Scott & J. Sims (Eds.), *Developing Workforce Diversity Programs, Curriculum, and Degrees in Higher Education* (pp. 304–326). Hershey, PA: IGI Global. doi:10.4018/978-1-5225-0209-8.ch016

Cebeci, H. I., & Hiziroglu, A. (2016). Review of Business Intelligence and Intelligent Systems in Healthcare Domain. In N. Celebi (Ed.), *Intelligent Techniques for Data Analysis in Diverse Settings* (pp. 192–206). Hershey, PA: IGI Global. doi:10.4018/978-1-5225-0075-9.ch009

Celik, G. (2018). Determining Headache Diseases With Genetic Algorithm. In U. Kose, G. Guraksin, & O. Deperlioglu (Eds.), *Nature-Inspired Intelligent Techniques for Solving Biomedical Engineering Problems* (pp. 249–262). Hershey, PA: IGI Global. doi:10.4018/978-1-5225-4769-3.ch012

Chakraborty, C., Gupta, B., & Ghosh, S. K. (2016). Mobile Telemedicine Systems for Remote Patient's Chronic Wound Monitoring. In A. Moumtzoglou (Ed.), *M-Health Innovations for Patient-Centered Care* (pp. 213–239). Hershey, PA: IGI Global. doi:10.4018/978-1-4666-9861-1.ch011

Chakraborty, S., Chatterjee, S., Ashour, A. S., Mali, K., & Dey, N. (2018). Intelligent Computing in Medical Imaging: A Study. In N. Dey (Ed.), *Advancements in Applied Metaheuristic Computing* (pp. 143–163). Hershey, PA: IGI Global. doi:10.4018/978-1-5225-4151-6.ch006

Chavez, A., & Kovarik, C. (2017). Open Source Technology for Medical Practice in Developing Countries. In K. Moahi, K. Bwalya, & P. Sebina (Eds.), *Health Information Systems and the Advancement of Medical Practice in Developing Countries* (pp. 33–59). Hershey, PA: IGI Global. doi:10.4018/978-1-5225-2262-1.ch003

Chen, E. T. (2016). Examining the Influence of Information Technology on Modern Health Care. In P. Manolitzas, E. Grigoroudis, N. Matsatsinis, & D. Yannacopoulos (Eds.), *Effective Methods for Modern Healthcare Service Quality and Evaluation* (pp. 110–136). Hershey, PA: IGI Global. doi:10.4018/978-1-4666-9961-8.ch006

Chin, S. (2016). Surviving Sandy: Recovering Collections after a Natural Disaster. In E. Decker & J. Townes (Eds.), *Handbook of Research on Disaster Management and Contingency Planning in Modern Libraries* (pp. 366–388). Hershey, PA: IGI Global. doi:10.4018/978-1-4666-8624-3.ch016

Chojnacki, M., & Wójcik, A. (2016). Security and the Role of New Technologies and Innovation in Medical Ethics. In A. Rosiek & K. Leksowski (Eds.), *Organizational Culture and Ethics in Modern Medicine* (pp. 52–77). Hershey, PA: IGI Global. doi:10.4018/978-1-4666-9658-7.ch003

Cılız, N., Yıldırım, H., & Temizel, Ş. (2016). Structure Development for Effective Medical Waste and Hazardous Waste Management System. In U. Akkucuk (Ed.), *Handbook of Research on Waste Management Techniques for Sustainability* (pp. 303–327). Hershey, PA: IGI Global. doi:10.4018/978-1-4666-9723-2.ch016

Ciufudean, C. (2018). Innovative Formalism for Biological Data Analysis. In M. Khosrow-Pour, D.B.A. (Ed.), Encyclopedia of Information Science and Technology, Fourth Edition (pp. 1814-1824). Hershey, PA: IGI Global. doi:10.4018/978-1-5225-2255-3.ch158

Ciufudean, C., & Ciufudean, O. (2016). Tele-Monitoring for Medical Diagnosis Availability. In M. Cruz-Cunha, I. Miranda, R. Martinho, & R. Rijo (Eds.), *Encyclopedia of E-Health and Telemedicine* (pp. 401–411). Hershey, PA: IGI Global. doi:10.4018/978-1-4666-9978-6.ch032

Colaguori, R., & Danesi, M. (2017). Medical Semiotics: A Revisitation and an Exhortation. *International Journal of Semiotics and Visual Rhetoric*, *1*(1), 11–18. doi:10.4018/IJSVR.2017010102

Cole, A. W., & Salek, T. A. (2017). Adopting a Parasocial Connection to Overcome Professional Kakoethos in Online Health Information. In M. Folk & S. Apostel (Eds.), *Establishing and Evaluating Digital Ethos and Online Credibility* (pp. 104–120). Hershey, PA: IGI Global. doi:10.4018/978-1-5225-1072-7.ch006

Contreras, E. C., & Puente, G. J. (2016). How to Identify Rheumatic Diseases by General Physicians. In T. Gasmelseid (Ed.), *Advancing Pharmaceutical Processes and Tools for Improved Health Outcomes* (pp. 136–166). Hershey, PA: IGI Global. doi:10.4018/978-1-5225-0248-7.ch006

D'Andrea, A., Ferri, F., & Grifoni, P. (2016). RFID Technologies in Healthcare Setting: Applications and Future Perspectives. *International Journal of Computers in Clinical Practice, 1*(1), 15–27. doi:10.4018/IJCCP.2016010102

Damianakis, A., Kallonis, P., Loudos, G., Tsatsos, D., & Tsoukalis, A. (2016). Exploiting 3D Medical Equipment Simulations to Support Biomedical Engineering Academic Courses: Design Methodology and Implementation in a Small Scale National Project. In B. Khan (Ed.), *Revolutionizing Modern Education through Meaningful E-Learning Implementation* (pp. 277–295). Hershey, PA: IGI Global. doi:10.4018/978-1-5225-0466-5.ch015

Demiroz, E. (2016). Principles of Instructional Design for E-Learning and Online Learning Practices: Implications for Medical Education. In V. Wang (Ed.), *Handbook of Research on Advancing Health Education through Technology* (pp. 419–451). Hershey, PA: IGI Global. doi:10.4018/978-1-4666-9494-1.ch018

Deperlioglu, O. (2018). Intelligent Techniques Inspired by Nature and Used in Biomedical Engineering. In U. Kose, G. Guraksin, & O. Deperlioglu (Eds.), *Nature-Inspired Intelligent Techniques for Solving Biomedical Engineering Problems* (pp. 51–77). Hershey, PA: IGI Global. doi:10.4018/978-1-5225-4769-3.ch003

Dey, N., & Ashour, A. S. (2018). Meta-Heuristic Algorithms in Medical Image Segmentation: A Review. In N. Dey (Ed.), *Advancements in Applied Metaheuristic Computing* (pp. 185–203). Hershey, PA: IGI Global. doi:10.4018/978-1-5225-4151-6.ch008

Dey, N., Ashour, A. S., & Althoupety, A. S. (2017). Thermal Imaging in Medical Science. In V. Santhi (Ed.), *Recent Advances in Applied Thermal Imaging for Industrial Applications* (pp. 87–117). Hershey, PA: IGI Global. doi:10.4018/978-1-5225-2423-6.ch004

Di Virgilio, F., Camillo, A. A., & Camillo, I. C. (2017). The Impact of Social Network on Italian Users' Behavioural Intention for the Choice of a Medical Tourist Destination. *International Journal of Tourism and Hospitality Management in the Digital Age, 1*(1), 36–49. doi:10.4018/IJTHMDA.2017010103

Dias, C. M., Ribeiro, A. G., & Furtado, S. F. (2016). An Overview about the Use of Healthcare Applications on Mobile Devices. In M. Cruz-Cunha, I. Miranda, R. Martinho, & R. Rijo (Eds.), *Encyclopedia of E-Health and Telemedicine* (pp. 285–298). Hershey, PA: IGI Global. doi:10.4018/978-1-4666-9978-6.ch024

Dogra, A. K., & Dogra, P. (2017). The Medical Tourism Industry in the BRIC Nations: An Indian Analysis. In M. Dhiman (Ed.), *Opportunities and Challenges for Tourism and Hospitality in the BRIC Nations* (pp. 320–336). Hershey, PA: IGI Global. doi:10.4018/978-1-5225-0708-6.ch020

Drowos, J. L., & Wood, S. K. (2017). Preparing Future Physicians to Adapt to the Changing Health Care System: Promoting Humanism through Curricular Design. In V. Bryan & J. Bird (Eds.), *Healthcare Community Synergism between Patients, Practitioners, and Researchers* (pp. 106–125). Hershey, PA: IGI Global. doi:10.4018/978-1-5225-0640-9.ch006

Dulam, K. (2017). Medical Patents and Impact on Availability and Affordability of Essential Medicines in India. In R. Aggarwal & R. Kaur (Eds.), *Patent Law and Intellectual Property in the Medical Field* (pp. 41–57). Hershey, PA: IGI Global. doi:10.4018/978-1-5225-2414-4.ch003

Dutta, P. (2017). Decision Making in Medical Diagnosis via Distance Measures on Interval Valued Fuzzy Sets. *International Journal of System Dynamics Applications*, *6*(4), 63–83. doi:10.4018/IJSDA.2017100104

Edoh, T. O., Pawar, P. A., Brügge, B., & Teege, G. (2016). A Multidisciplinary Remote Healthcare Delivery System to Increase Health Care Access, Pathology Screening, and Treatment in Developing Countries: The Case of Benin. *International Journal of Healthcare Information Systems and Informatics*, *11*(4), 1–31. doi:10.4018/IJHISI.2016100101

El Guemhioui, K., & Demurjian, S. A. (2017). Semantic Reconciliation of Electronic Health Records Using Semantic Web Technologies. *International Journal of Information Technology and Web Engineering*, *12*(2), 26–48. doi:10.4018/IJITWE.2017040102

Ellouze, N., Rekhis, S., & Boudriga, N. (2016). Forensic Investigation of Digital Crimes in Healthcare Applications. In O. Isafiade & A. Bagula (Eds.), *Data Mining Trends and Applications in Criminal Science and Investigations* (pp. 169–210). Hershey, PA: IGI Global. doi:10.4018/978-1-5225-0463-4.ch007

Eneanya, A. N. (2016). Health Policy Implementation and Its Barriers: The Case Study of US Health System. In R. Gholipour & K. Rouzbehani (Eds.), *Social, Economic, and Political Perspectives on Public Health Policy-Making* (pp. 42–63). Hershey, PA: IGI Global. doi:10.4018/978-1-4666-9944-1.ch003

Entico, G. J. (2016). Knowledge Management and the Medical Health Librarians: A Perception Study. In J. Yap, M. Perez, M. Ayson, & G. Entico (Eds.), *Special Library Administration, Standardization and Technological Integration* (pp. 52–77). Hershey, PA: IGI Global. doi:10.4018/978-1-4666-9542-9.ch003

Ferradji, M. A., & Zidani, A. (2016). Collaborative Environment for Remote Clinical Reasoning Learning. *International Journal of E-Health and Medical Communications*, *7*(4), 62–81. doi:10.4018/IJEHMC.2016100104

Fisher, J. (2018). Sociological Perspectives on Improving Medical Diagnosis Emphasizing CAD. In M. Khosrow-Pour, D.B.A. (Ed.), Encyclopedia of Information Science and Technology, Fourth Edition (pp. 1017-1024). Hershey, PA: IGI Global. doi:10.4018/978-1-5225-2255-3.ch088

Flores, C. D., Respício, A., Coelho, H., Bez, M. R., & Fonseca, J. M. (2016). Simulation for Medical Training. In M. Cruz-Cunha, I. Miranda, R. Martinho, & R. Rijo (Eds.), *Encyclopedia of E-Health and Telemedicine* (pp. 827–842). Hershey, PA: IGI Global. doi:10.4018/978-1-4666-9978-6.ch064

Frank, E. M. (2018). Healthcare Education: Integrating Simulation Technologies. In V. Bryan, A. Musgrove, & J. Powers (Eds.), *Handbook of Research on Human Development in the Digital Age* (pp. 163–182). Hershey, PA: IGI Global. doi:10.4018/978-1-5225-2838-8.ch008

Garner, G. (2018). Foundations for Yoga Practice in Rehabilitation. In S. Telles & N. Singh (Eds.), *Research-Based Perspectives on the Psychophysiology of Yoga* (pp. 263–307). Hershey, PA: IGI Global. doi:10.4018/978-1-5225-2788-6.ch015

Gasmelseid, T. M. (2016). Improving Pharmaceutical Care through the Use of Intelligent Pharmacoinformatics. In T. Gasmelseid (Ed.), *Advancing Pharmaceutical Processes and Tools for Improved Health Outcomes* (pp. 167–188). Hershey, PA: IGI Global. doi:10.4018/978-1-5225-0248-7.ch007

Gavurová, B., Kováč, V., & Šoltés, M. (2018). Medical Equipment and Economic Determinants of Its Structure and Regulation in the Slovak Republic. In M. Khosrow-Pour, D.B.A. (Ed.), Encyclopedia of Information Science and Technology, Fourth Edition (pp. 5841-5852). Hershey, PA: IGI Global. doi:10.4018/978-1-5225-2255-3.ch508

Ge, X., Wang, Q., Huang, K., Law, V., & Thomas, D. C. (2017). Designing Simulated Learning Environments and Facilitating Authentic Learning Experiences in Medical Education. In J. Stefaniak (Ed.), *Advancing Medical Education Through Strategic Instructional Design* (pp. 77–100). Hershey, PA: IGI Global. doi:10.4018/978-1-5225-2098-6.ch004

Gewald, H., & Gewald, C. (2018). Inhibitors of Physicians' Use of Mandatory Hospital Information Systems (HIS). *International Journal of Healthcare Information Systems and Informatics, 13*(1), 29–44. doi:10.4018/IJHISI.2018010103

Ghosh, D., & Dinda, S. (2017). Health Infrastructure and Economic Development in India. In R. Das (Ed.), *Social, Health, and Environmental Infrastructures for Economic Growth* (pp. 99–119). Hershey, PA: IGI Global. doi:10.4018/978-1-5225-2364-2.ch006

Ghosh, K., & Sen, K. C. (2017). The Potential of Crowdsourcing in the Health Care Industry. In N. Wickramasinghe (Ed.), *Handbook of Research on Healthcare Administration and Management* (pp. 418–427). Hershey, PA: IGI Global. doi:10.4018/978-1-5225-0920-2.ch024

Ghrab, S., & Saad, I. (2016). Identifying Crucial Know-How and Knowing-That for Medical Decision Support. *International Journal of Decision Support System Technology, 8*(4), 14–33. doi:10.4018/IJDSST.2016100102

Giokas, K., Tsirmpas, C., Anastasiou, A., Iliopoulou, D., Costarides, V., & Koutsouris, D. (2016). Contemporary Heart Failure Treatment Based on Improved Knowledge and Personalized Care of Comorbidities. In D. Fotiadis (Ed.), *Handbook of Research on Trends in the Diagnosis and Treatment of Chronic Conditions* (pp. 301–314). Hershey, PA: IGI Global. doi:10.4018/978-1-4666-8828-5.ch014

Gopalan, V., Chan, E., & Ho, D. T. (2018). Deliberate Self-Harm and Suicide Ideology in Medical Students. In C. Smith (Ed.), *Exploring the Pressures of Medical Education From a Mental Health and Wellness Perspective* (pp. 122–143). Hershey, PA: IGI Global. doi:10.4018/978-1-5225-2811-1.ch005

Goswami, S., Dey, U., Roy, P., Ashour, A., & Dey, N. (2017). Medical Video Processing: Concept and Applications. In N. Dey, A. Ashour, & P. Patra (Eds.), *Feature Detectors and Motion Detection in Video Processing* (pp. 1–17). Hershey, PA: IGI Global. doi:10.4018/978-1-5225-1025-3.ch001

Goswami, S., Mahanta, K., Goswami, S., Jigdung, T., & Devi, T. P. (2018). Ageing and Cancer: The Epigenetic Basis, Alternative Treatment, and Care. In B. Prasad & S. Akbar (Eds.), *Handbook of Research on Geriatric Health, Treatment, and Care* (pp. 206–235). Hershey, PA: IGI Global. doi:10.4018/978-1-5225-3480-8.ch012

Gouva, M. I. (2017). The Psychological Impact of Medical Error on Patients, Family Members, and Health Professionals. In M. Riga (Ed.), *Impact of Medical Errors and Malpractice on Health Economics, Quality, and Patient Safety* (pp. 171–196). Hershey, PA: IGI Global. doi:10.4018/978-1-5225-2337-6.ch007

Gürcü, M., & Tengilimoğlu, D. (2017). Health Tourism-Based Destination Marketing. In A. Bayraktar & C. Uslay (Eds.), *Strategic Place Branding Methodologies and Theory for Tourist Attraction* (pp. 308–331). Hershey, PA: IGI Global. doi:10.4018/978-1-5225-0579-2.ch015

Gürsel, G. (2016). Mobility in Healthcare: M-Health. In A. Panagopoulos (Ed.), *Handbook of Research on Next Generation Mobile Communication Systems* (pp. 485–511). Hershey, PA: IGI Global. doi:10.4018/978-1-4666-8732-5.ch019

Gürsel, G. (2017). For Better Healthcare Mining Health Data. In S. Bhattacharyya, S. De, I. Pan, & P. Dutta (Eds.), *Intelligent Multidimensional Data Clustering and Analysis* (pp. 135–158). Hershey, PA: IGI Global. doi:10.4018/978-1-5225-1776-4.ch006

Guzman-Lugo, G., Lopez-Martinez, M., Lopez-Ramirez, B., & Avila-Vazquez, D. (2016). City-Driven Approach to Determine Health Services Based on Current User Location and Collaborative Information. *International Journal of Knowledge Society Research, 7*(1), 53–62. doi:10.4018/IJKSR.2016010104

Gyaase, P. O., Darko-Lartey, R., William, H., & Borkloe, F. (2017). Towards an Integrated Electronic Medical Records System for Quality Healthcare in Ghana: An Exploratory Factor Analysis. *International Journal of Computers in Clinical Practice, 2*(2), 38–55. doi:10.4018/IJCCP.2017070103

Handayani, P. W., Sandhyaduhita, P. I., Hidayanto, A. N., Pinem, A. A., Fajrina, H. R., Junus, K. M., ... Ayuningtyas, D. (2016). Integrated Hospital Information System Architecture Design in Indonesia. In T. Iyamu & A. Tatnall (Eds.), *Maximizing Healthcare Delivery and Management through Technology Integration* (pp. 207–236). Hershey, PA: IGI Global. doi:10.4018/978-1-4666-9446-0.ch013

Hanel, P. (2017). Is China Catching Up?: Health-Related Applications of Biotechnology. In T. Bas & J. Zhao (Eds.), *Comparative Approaches to Biotechnology Development and Use in Developed and Emerging Nations* (pp. 465–520). Hershey, PA: IGI Global. doi:10.4018/978-1-5225-1040-6.ch016

Harmsen, C. A., & Royle, R. N. (2016). St. Stephen's Hospital Hervey Bay: Study of Developing a Digital Hospital. In J. Moon & M. Galea (Eds.), *Improving Health Management through Clinical Decision Support Systems* (pp. 127–153). Hershey, PA: IGI Global. doi:10.4018/978-1-4666-9432-3.ch006

Harp, D., Shim, R. S., Johnson, J., Harp, J. A., Wilcox, W. C., & Wilcox, J. K. (2016). Race and Gender Inequalities in Medicine and Biomedical Research. In U. Thomas & J. Drake (Eds.), *Critical Research on Sexism and Racism in STEM Fields* (pp. 115–134). Hershey, PA: IGI Global. doi:10.4018/978-1-5225-0174-9.ch006

Hartman, A., & Brown, S. (2017). Synergism through Therapeutic Visual Arts. In V. Bryan & J. Bird (Eds.), *Healthcare Community Synergism between Patients, Practitioners, and Researchers* (pp. 29–48). Hershey, PA: IGI Global. doi:10.4018/978-1-5225-0640-9.ch002

Hazra, J., Chowdhury, A. R., & Dutta, P. (2016). Cluster Based Medical Image Registration Using Optimized Neural Network. In S. Bhattacharyya, P. Banerjee, D. Majumdar, & P. Dutta (Eds.), *Handbook of Research on Advanced Hybrid Intelligent Techniques and Applications* (pp. 551–581). Hershey, PA: IGI Global. doi:10.4018/978-1-4666-9474-3.ch018

Hung, S., Huang, W., Yen, D. C., Chang, S., & Lu, C. (2016). Effect of Information Service Competence and Contextual Factors on the Effectiveness of Strategic Information Systems Planning in Hospitals. *Journal of Global Information Management, 24*(1), 14–36. doi:10.4018/JGIM.2016010102

Iltchev, P., Śliwczyński, A., Szynkiewicz, P., & Marczak, M. (2016). Mobile Health Applications Assisting Patients with Chronic Diseases: Examples from Asthma Care. In A. Moumtzoglou (Ed.), *M-Health Innovations for Patient-Centered Care* (pp. 170–196). Hershey, PA: IGI Global. doi:10.4018/978-1-4666-9861-1.ch009

Iqbal, S., Ahmad, S., & Willis, I. (2017). Influencing Factors for Adopting Technology Enhanced Learning in the Medical Schools of Punjab, Pakistan. *International Journal of Information and Communication Technology Education, 13*(3), 27–39. doi:10.4018/IJICTE.2017070103

Jagan, J., Dalkiliç, Y., & Samui, P. (2016). Utilization of SVM, LSSVM and GP for Predicting the Medical Waste Generation. In G. Hua (Ed.), *Smart Cities as a Solution for Reducing Urban Waste and Pollution* (pp. 224–251). Hershey, PA: IGI Global. doi:10.4018/978-1-5225-0302-6.ch008

Jagiello, K., Sosnowska, A., Mikolajczyk, A., & Puzyn, T. (2017). Nanomaterials in Medical Devices: Regulations' Review and Future Perspectives. *Journal of Nanotoxicology and Nanomedicine, 2*(2), 1–11. doi:10.4018/JNN.2017070101

Jena, T. K. (2018). Skill Training Process in Medicine Through Distance Mode. In U. Pandey & V. Indrakanti (Eds.), *Optimizing Open and Distance Learning in Higher Education Institutions* (pp. 228–243). Hershey, PA: IGI Global. doi:10.4018/978-1-5225-2624-7.ch010

Jesus, Â., & Gomes, M. J. (2016). Web 2.0 Tools in Biomedical and Pharmaceutical Education: Updated Review and Commentary. In T. Gasmelseid (Ed.), *Advancing Pharmaceutical Processes and Tools for Improved Health Outcomes* (pp. 52–78). Hershey, PA: IGI Global. doi:10.4018/978-1-5225-0248-7.ch003

Joseph, V., & Miller, J. M. (2018). Medical Students' Perceived Stigma in Seeking Care: A Cultural Perspective. In C. Smith (Ed.), *Exploring the Pressures of Medical Education From a Mental Health and Wellness Perspective* (pp. 44–67). Hershey, PA: IGI Global. doi:10.4018/978-1-5225-2811-1.ch002

Joyce, B. L., & Swanberg, S. M. (2017). Using Backward Design for Competency-Based Undergraduate Medical Education. In J. Stefaniak (Ed.), *Advancing Medical Education Through Strategic Instructional Design* (pp. 53–76). Hershey, PA: IGI Global. doi:10.4018/978-1-5225-2098-6.ch003

Kaljo, K., & Jacques, L. (2018). Flipping the Medical School Classroom. In M. Khosrow-Pour, D.B.A. (Ed.), Encyclopedia of Information Science and Technology, Fourth Edition (pp. 5800-5809). Hershey, PA: IGI Global. doi:10.4018/978-1-5225-2255-3.ch504

Karon, R. (2016). Utilisation of Health Information Systems for Service Delivery in the Namibian Environment. In T. Iyamu & A. Tatnall (Eds.), *Maximizing Healthcare Delivery and Management through Technology Integration* (pp. 169–183). Hershey, PA: IGI Global. doi:10.4018/978-1-4666-9446-0.ch011

Kasina, H., Bahubalendruni, M. V., & Botcha, R. (2017). Robots in Medicine: Past, Present and Future. *International Journal of Manufacturing, Materials, and Mechanical Engineering*, *7*(4), 44–64. doi:10.4018/IJMMME.2017100104

Katehakis, D. G. (2018). Electronic Medical Record Implementation Challenges for the National Health System in Greece. *International Journal of Reliable and Quality E-Healthcare*, *7*(1), 16–30. doi:10.4018/IJRQEH.2018010102

Katz, A., & Shtub, A. (2016). Design and Build a Wizard of Oz (WOZ) Telemedicine Simulator Platform. In M. Cruz-Cunha, I. Miranda, R. Martinho, & R. Rijo (Eds.), *Encyclopedia of E-Health and Telemedicine* (pp. 128–141). Hershey, PA: IGI Global. doi:10.4018/978-1-4666-9978-6.ch011

Kaur, P. D., & Sharma, P. (2017). Success Dimensions of ICTs in Healthcare. In B. Singh (Ed.), *Computational Tools and Techniques for Biomedical Signal Processing* (pp. 149–173). Hershey, PA: IGI Global. doi:10.4018/978-1-5225-0660-7.ch007

Kaushik, P. (2018). Comorbidity of Medical and Psychiatric Disorders in Geriatric Population: Treatment and Care. In B. Prasad & S. Akbar (Eds.), *Handbook of Research on Geriatric Health, Treatment, and Care* (pp. 448–474). Hershey, PA: IGI Global. doi:10.4018/978-1-5225-3480-8.ch025

Khachane, M. Y. (2017). Organ-Based Medical Image Classification Using Support Vector Machine. *International Journal of Synthetic Emotions*, *8*(1), 18–30. doi:10.4018/IJSE.2017010102

Kirci, P. (2018). Intelligent Techniques for Analysis of Big Data About Healthcare and Medical Records. In N. Shah & M. Mittal (Eds.), *Handbook of Research on Promoting Business Process Improvement Through Inventory Control Techniques* (pp. 559–582). Hershey, PA: IGI Global. doi:10.4018/978-1-5225-3232-3.ch029

Kldiashvili, E. (2016). Cloud Computing as the Useful Resource for Application of the Medical Information System for Quality Assurance Purposes. *International Journal of Computers in Clinical Practice*, *1*(2), 1–23. doi:10.4018/IJCCP.2016070101

Kldiashvili, E. (2018). Cloud Approach for the Medical Information System: MIS on Cloud. In M. Khosrow-Pour (Ed.), *Incorporating Nature-Inspired Paradigms in Computational Applications* (pp. 238–261). Hershey, PA: IGI Global. doi:10.4018/978-1-5225-5020-4.ch008

Kldiashvili, E., Burduli, A., Ghortlishvili, G., & Sheklashvili, I. (2016). Georgian Experience in Telecytology. In M. Cruz-Cunha, I. Miranda, R. Martinho, & R. Rijo (Eds.), *Encyclopedia of E-Health and Telemedicine* (pp. 62–71). Hershey, PA: IGI Global. doi:10.4018/978-1-4666-9978-6.ch006

Ko, H., Mesicek, L., Choi, J., Choi, J., & Hwang, S. (2018). A Study on Secure Contents Strategies for Applications With DRM on Cloud Computing. *International Journal of Cloud Applications and Computing*, *8*(1), 143–153. doi:10.4018/IJCAC.2018010107

Komendziński, T., Dreszer-Drogorób, J., Mikołajewska, E., Mikołajewski, D., & Bałaj, B. (2016). Interdisciplinary Education for Research and Everyday Clinical Practice: Lessons Learned from InteRDoCTor Project. In A. Rosiek & K. Leksowski (Eds.), *Organizational Culture and Ethics in Modern Medicine* (pp. 78–110). Hershey, PA: IGI Global. doi:10.4018/978-1-4666-9658-7.ch004

Komendziński, T., Mikołajewska, E., & Mikołajewski, D. (2018). Cross-Cultural Decision-Making in Healthcare: Theory and Practical Application in Real Clinical Conditions. In A. Rosiek-Kryszewska & K. Leksowski (Eds.), *Healthcare Administration for Patient Safety and Engagement* (pp. 276–298). Hershey, PA: IGI Global. doi:10.4018/978-1-5225-3946-9.ch015

Konecny, L. T. (2018). Medical School Wellness Initiatives. In C. Smith (Ed.), *Exploring the Pressures of Medical Education From a Mental Health and Wellness Perspective* (pp. 209–228). Hershey, PA: IGI Global. doi:10.4018/978-1-5225-2811-1.ch009

Konieczna, A., & Słomkowski, P. (2016). Confrontation of Human Rights in Daily Clinical Situations. In A. Rosiek & K. Leksowski (Eds.), *Organizational Culture and Ethics in Modern Medicine* (pp. 255–281). Hershey, PA: IGI Global. doi:10.4018/978-1-4666-9658-7.ch011

Kromrei, H., Solomonson, W. L., & Juzych, M. S. (2017). Teaching Residents How to Teach. In J. Stefaniak (Ed.), *Advancing Medical Education Through Strategic Instructional Design* (pp. 164–185). Hershey, PA: IGI Global. doi:10.4018/978-1-5225-2098-6.ch008

Kulkarni, S., Savyanavar, A., Kulkarni, P., Stranieri, A., & Ghorpade, V. (2018). Framework for Integration of Medical Image and Text-Based Report Retrieval to Support Radiological Diagnosis. In M. Kolekar & V. Kumar (Eds.), *Biomedical Signal and Image Processing in Patient Care* (pp. 86–122). Hershey, PA: IGI Global. doi:10.4018/978-1-5225-2829-6.ch006

Kumar, A., & Sarkar, B. K. (2018). Performance Analysis of Nature-Inspired Algorithms-Based Bayesian Prediction Models for Medical Data Sets. In U. Singh, A. Tiwari, & R. Singh (Eds.), *Soft-Computing-Based Nonlinear Control Systems Design* (pp. 134–155). Hershey, PA: IGI Global. doi:10.4018/978-1-5225-3531-7.ch007

Kurtz, R. S. (2016). Fortitude: A Study of African Americans in Surgery in New York City. In U. Thomas & J. Drake (Eds.), *Critical Research on Sexism and Racism in STEM Fields* (pp. 153–169). Hershey, PA: IGI Global. doi:10.4018/978-1-5225-0174-9.ch009

Labbadi, W., & Akaichi, J. (2017). Efficient Algorithm for Answering Fuzzy Medical Requests in Pervasive Healthcare Information Systems. *International Journal of Healthcare Information Systems and Informatics, 12*(2), 46–64. doi:10.4018/IJHISI.2017040103

Lagumdzija, A., & Swing, V. K. (2017). Health, Digitalization, and Individual Empowerment. In F. Topor (Ed.), *Handbook of Research on Individualism and Identity in the Globalized Digital Age* (pp. 380–402). Hershey, PA: IGI Global. doi:10.4018/978-1-5225-0522-8.ch017

Lamey, T. W., & Davidson-Shivers, G. V. (2017). Instructional Strategies and Sequencing. In J. Stefaniak (Ed.), *Advancing Medical Education Through Strategic Instructional Design* (pp. 30–52). Hershey, PA: IGI Global. doi:10.4018/978-1-5225-2098-6.ch002

Leon, G. (2017). The Role of Forensic Medicine in Medical Errors. In M. Riga (Ed.), *Impact of Medical Errors and Malpractice on Health Economics, Quality, and Patient Safety* (pp. 144–170). Hershey, PA: IGI Global. doi:10.4018/978-1-5225-2337-6.ch006

Lidia, B., Federica, G., & Maria, V. E. (2016). The Patient-Centered Medicine as the Theoretical Framework for Patient Engagement. In G. Graffigna (Ed.), *Promoting Patient Engagement and Participation for Effective Healthcare Reform* (pp. 25–39). Hershey, PA: IGI Global. doi:10.4018/978-1-4666-9992-2.ch002

Love, L., & McDowelle, D. (2018). Developing a Comprehensive Wellness Program for Medical Students. In C. Smith (Ed.), *Exploring the Pressures of Medical Education From a Mental Health and Wellness Perspective* (pp. 190–208). Hershey, PA: IGI Global. doi:10.4018/978-1-5225-2811-1.ch008

Lovell, K. L. (2017). Development and Evaluation of Neuroscience Computer-Based Modules for Medical Students: Instructional Design Principles and Effectiveness. In J. Stefaniak (Ed.), *Advancing Medical Education Through Strategic Instructional Design* (pp. 262–276). Hershey, PA: IGI Global. doi:10.4018/978-1-5225-2098-6.ch013

Lubin, R., & Hamlin, M. D. (2018). Medical Student Burnout: A Social Cognitive Learning Perspective on Medical Student Mental Health and Wellness. In C. Smith (Ed.), *Exploring the Pressures of Medical Education From a Mental Health and Wellness Perspective* (pp. 92–121). Hershey, PA: IGI Global. doi:10.4018/978-1-5225-2811-1.ch004

Luk, C. Y. (2018). Moving Towards Universal Health Coverage: Challenges for the Present and Future in China. In B. Fong, A. Ng, & P. Yuen (Eds.), *Sustainable Health and Long-Term Care Solutions for an Aging Population* (pp. 19–45). Hershey, PA: IGI Global. doi:10.4018/978-1-5225-2633-9.ch002

Mahat, M., & Pettigrew, A. (2017). The Regulatory Environment of Non-Profit Higher Education and Research Institutions and Its Implications for Managerial Strategy: The Case of Medical Education and Research. In L. West & A. Worthington (Eds.), *Handbook of Research on Emerging Business Models and Managerial Strategies in the Nonprofit Sector* (pp. 336–351). Hershey, PA: IGI Global. doi:10.4018/978-1-5225-2537-0.ch017

Maitra, I. K., & Bandhyopadhyaay, S. K. (2017). Adaptive Edge Detection Method towards Features Extraction from Diverse Medical Imaging Technologies. In S. Bhattacharyya, S. De, I. Pan, & P. Dutta (Eds.), *Intelligent Multidimensional Data Clustering and Analysis* (pp. 159–192). Hershey, PA: IGI Global. doi:10.4018/978-1-5225-1776-4.ch007

Mangu, V. P. (2017). Mobile Health Care: A Technology View. In C. Bhatt & S. Peddoju (Eds.), *Cloud Computing Systems and Applications in Healthcare* (pp. 1–18). Hershey, PA: IGI Global. doi:10.4018/978-1-5225-1002-4.ch001

Manirabona, A., Fourati, L. C., & Boudjit, S. (2017). Investigation on Healthcare Monitoring Systems: Innovative Services and Applications. *International Journal of E-Health and Medical Communications*, *8*(1), 1–18. doi:10.4018/IJEHMC.2017010101

Mannai, M. M., & Karâa, W. B. (2016). Biomedical Image Processing Overview. In W. Karâa & N. Dey (Eds.), *Biomedical Image Analysis and Mining Techniques for Improved Health Outcomes* (pp. 1–12). Hershey, PA: IGI Global. doi:10.4018/978-1-4666-8811-7.ch001

Manzoor, A. (2016). RFID in Health Care-Building Smart Hospitals for Quality Healthcare. *International Journal of User-Driven Healthcare, 6*(2), 21–45. doi:10.4018/IJUDH.2016070102

Marwan, M., Kartit, A., & Ouahmane, H. (2018). A Framework to Secure Medical Image Storage in Cloud Computing Environment. *Journal of Electronic Commerce in Organizations, 16*(1), 1–16. doi:10.4018/JECO.2018010101

Masoud, M. P., Nejad, M. K., Darebaghi, H., Chavoshi, M., & Farahani, M. (2018). The Decision Support System and Conventional Method of Telephone Triage by Nurses in Emergency Medical Services: A Comparative Investigation. *International Journal of E-Business Research, 14*(1), 77–88. doi:10.4018/IJEBR.2018010105

McDonald, W. G., Martin, M., & Salzberg, L. D. (2018). From Medical Student to Medical Resident: Graduate Medical Education and Mental Health in the United States. In C. Smith (Ed.), *Exploring the Pressures of Medical Education From a Mental Health and Wellness Perspective* (pp. 145–169). Hershey, PA: IGI Global. doi:10.4018/978-1-5225-2811-1.ch006

Medhekar, A. (2017). The Role of Social Media for Knowledge Dissemination in Medical Tourism: A Case of India. In R. Chugh (Ed.), *Harnessing Social Media as a Knowledge Management Tool* (pp. 25–54). Hershey, PA: IGI Global. doi:10.4018/978-1-5225-0495-5.ch002

Medhekar, A., & Haq, F. (2018). Urbanization and New Jobs Creation in Healthcare Services in India: Challenges and Opportunities. In U. Benna & I. Benna (Eds.), *Urbanization and Its Impact on Socio-Economic Growth in Developing Regions* (pp. 198–218). Hershey, PA: IGI Global. doi:10.4018/978-1-5225-2659-9.ch010

Mehta, G., Dutta, M. K., & Kim, P. S. (2016). An Efficient and Lossless Cryptosystem for Security in Tele-Ophthalmology Applications Using Chaotic Theory. *International Journal of E-Health and Medical Communications, 7*(4), 28–47. doi:10.4018/IJEHMC.2016100102

Mehta, P. (2017). Framework of Indian Healthcare System and its Challenges: An Insight. In V. Bryan & J. Bird (Eds.), *Healthcare Community Synergism between Patients, Practitioners, and Researchers* (pp. 247–271). Hershey, PA: IGI Global. doi:10.4018/978-1-5225-0640-9.ch011

Metelmann, B., & Metelmann, C. (2016). M-Health in Prehospital Emergency Medicine: Experiences from the EU funded Project LiveCity. In A. Moumtzoglou (Ed.), *M-Health Innovations for Patient-Centered Care* (pp. 197–212). Hershey, PA: IGI Global. doi:10.4018/978-1-4666-9861-1.ch010

Mi, M. (2017). Informal Learning in Medical Education. In J. Stefaniak (Ed.), *Advancing Medical Education Through Strategic Instructional Design* (pp. 225–244). Hershey, PA: IGI Global. doi:10.4018/978-1-5225-2098-6.ch011

Miglioretti, M., Mariani, F., & Vecchio, L. (2016). Could Patient Engagement Promote a Health System Free From Malpractice Litigation Risk? In G. Graffigna (Ed.), *Promoting Patient Engagement and Participation for Effective Healthcare Reform* (pp. 240–264). Hershey, PA: IGI Global. doi:10.4018/978-1-4666-9992-2.ch012

Misra, S. C., & Bisui, S. (2016). Feasibility of Large Scale Implementation of Personalized Medicine in the Current Scenario. *International Journal of E-Health and Medical Communications, 7*(2), 30–49. doi:10.4018/IJEHMC.2016040103

Misra, S. C., Bisui, S., & Fantazy, K. (2016). Identifying Critical Changes in Adoption of Personalized Medicine (PM) in Healthcare Management. *International Journal of E-Health and Medical Communications, 7*(3), 1–15. doi:10.4018/IJEHMC.2016070101

Mohammadian, M., Hatzinakos, D., Spachos, P., & Jentzsh, R. (2016). An Intelligent and Secure Framework for Wireless Information Technology in Healthcare for User and Data Classification in Hospitals. In V. Wang (Ed.), *Handbook of Research on Advancing Health Education through Technology* (pp. 452–479). Hershey, PA: IGI Global. doi:10.4018/978-1-4666-9494-1.ch019

Mokeddem, S., & Atmani, B. (2016). Assessment of Clinical Decision Support Systems for Predicting Coronary Heart Disease. *International Journal of Operations Research and Information Systems, 7*(3), 57–73. doi:10.4018/IJORIS.2016070104

Mokrzycka, A., & Kowalska-Bobko, I. (2016). Public Health Legislation and Patient's Rights: Health2020 Strategy, European Perspective. In A. Rosiek & K. Leksowski (Eds.), *Organizational Culture and Ethics in Modern Medicine* (pp. 298–322). Hershey, PA: IGI Global. doi:10.4018/978-1-4666-9658-7.ch013

Moon, J. D., & Galea, M. P. (2016). Overview of Clinical Decision Support Systems in Healthcare. In J. Moon & M. Galea (Eds.), *Improving Health Management through Clinical Decision Support Systems* (pp. 1–27). Hershey, PA: IGI Global. doi:10.4018/978-1-4666-9432-3.ch001

Mosadeghrad, A. M., & Woldemichael, A. (2017). Application of Quality Management in Promoting Patient Safety and Preventing Medical Errors. In M. Riga (Ed.), *Impact of Medical Errors and Malpractice on Health Economics, Quality, and Patient Safety* (pp. 91–112). Hershey, PA: IGI Global. doi:10.4018/978-1-5225-2337-6.ch004

Moumtzoglou, A. (2017). Digital Medicine: The Quality Standpoint. In A. Moumtzoglou (Ed.), *Design, Development, and Integration of Reliable Electronic Healthcare Platforms* (pp. 179–195). Hershey, PA: IGI Global. doi:10.4018/978-1-5225-1724-5.ch011

Moumtzoglou, A., & Pouliakis, A. (2018). Population Health Management and the Science of Individuality. *International Journal of Reliable and Quality E-Healthcare, 7*(2), 1–26. doi:10.4018/IJRQEH.2018040101

Mpofu, C. (2016). International Medical Experiences Outbound New Zealand: An Economic and Medical Workforce Strategy. In D. Velliaris & D. Coleman-George (Eds.), *Handbook of Research on Study Abroad Programs and Outbound Mobility* (pp. 446–469). Hershey, PA: IGI Global. doi:10.4018/978-1-5225-0169-5.ch018

Mukhtar, W. F., & Abuelyaman, E. S. (2017). Opportunities and Challenges of Big Data in Healthcare. In N. Wickramasinghe (Ed.), *Handbook of Research on Healthcare Administration and Management* (pp. 47–58). Hershey, PA: IGI Global. doi:10.4018/978-1-5225-0920-2.ch004

Munugala, S., Brar, G. K., Syed, A., Mohammad, A., & Halgamuge, M. N. (2018). The Much Needed Security and Data Reforms of Cloud Computing in Medical Data Storage. In M. Lytras & P. Papadopoulou (Eds.), *Applying Big Data Analytics in Bioinformatics and Medicine* (pp. 99–113). Hershey, PA: IGI Global. doi:10.4018/978-1-5225-2607-0.ch005

Narasimhamurthy, A. (2016). An Overview of Machine Learning in Medical Image Analysis: Trends in Health Informatics. In N. Dey & A. Ashour (Eds.), *Classification and Clustering in Biomedical Signal Processing* (pp. 23–45). Hershey, PA: IGI Global. doi:10.4018/978-1-5225-0140-4.ch002

Ngara, R. (2017). Multiple Voices, Multiple Paths: Towards Dialogue between Western and Indigenous Medical Knowledge Systems. In P. Ngulube (Ed.), *Handbook of Research on Theoretical Perspectives on Indigenous Knowledge Systems in Developing Countries* (pp. 332–358). Hershey, PA: IGI Global. doi:10.4018/978-1-5225-0833-5.ch015

O'Connor, Y., & Heavin, C. (2018). Defining and Characterising the Landscape of eHealth. In M. Khosrow-Pour, D.B.A. (Ed.), Encyclopedia of Information Science and Technology, Fourth Edition (pp. 5864-5875). Hershey, PA: IGI Global. doi:10.4018/978-1-5225-2255-3.ch510

Ochonogor, W. C., & Okite-Amughoro, F. A. (2018). Building an Effective Digital Library in a University Teaching Hospital (UTH) in Nigeria. In A. Tella & T. Kwanya (Eds.), *Handbook of Research on Managing Intellectual Property in Digital Libraries* (pp. 184–204). Hershey, PA: IGI Global. doi:10.4018/978-1-5225-3093-0.ch010

Olaniran, B. A. (2016). ICTs, E-health, and Multidisciplinary Healthcare Teams: Promises and Challenges. *International Journal of Privacy and Health Information Management*, *4*(2), 62–75. doi:10.4018/IJPHIM.2016070105

Olaniran, B. A. (2016). ICT Use and Multidisciplinary Healthcare Teams in the Age of e-Health. *International Journal of Reliable and Quality E-Healthcare*, *5*(1), 18–31. doi:10.4018/IJRQEH.2016010102

Olivares, S. L., Cruz, A. G., Cabrera, M. V., Regalado, A. I., & García, J. E. (2017). An Assessment Study of Quality Model for Medical Schools in Mexico. In S. Mukerji & P. Tripathi (Eds.), *Handbook of Research on Administration, Policy, and Leadership in Higher Education* (pp. 404–439). Hershey, PA: IGI Global. doi:10.4018/978-1-5225-0672-0.ch016

Omidoyin, E. O., Opeke, R. O., & Osagbemi, G. K. (2016). Utilization Pattern and Privacy Issues in the use of Health Records for Research Practice by Doctors: Selected Nigerian Teaching Hospitals as Case Study. *International Journal of Privacy and Health Information Management*, *4*(1), 1–11. doi:10.4018/IJPHIM.2016010101

Omoruyi, E. A., & Omidele, F. (2018). Resident Physician and Medical Academic Faculty Burnout: A Review of Current Literature. In C. Smith (Ed.), *Exploring the Pressures of Medical Education From a Mental Health and Wellness Perspective* (pp. 171–189). Hershey, PA: IGI Global. doi:10.4018/978-1-5225-2811-1.ch007

Osop, H., & Sahama, T. (2016). Data-Driven and Practice-Based Evidence: Design and Development of Efficient and Effective Clinical Decision Support System. In J. Moon & M. Galea (Eds.), *Improving Health Management through Clinical Decision Support Systems* (pp. 295–328). Hershey, PA: IGI Global. doi:10.4018/978-1-4666-9432-3.ch014

Ossowski, R., & Izdebski, P. (2016). Ethical Aspects of Talking to a Patient. In A. Rosiek & K. Leksowski (Eds.), *Organizational Culture and Ethics in Modern Medicine* (pp. 203–235). Hershey, PA: IGI Global. doi:10.4018/978-1-4666-9658-7.ch009

Pandian, P. S. (2016). An Overview of Telemedicine Technologies for Healthcare Applications. *International Journal of Biomedical and Clinical Engineering*, *5*(2), 29–52. doi:10.4018/IJBCE.2016070103

Papadopoulou, P., Lytras, M., & Marouli, C. (2018). Bioinformatics as Applied to Medicine: Challenges Faced Moving from Big Data to Smart Data to Wise Data. In M. Lytras & P. Papadopoulou (Eds.), *Applying Big Data Analytics in Bioinformatics and Medicine* (pp. 1–25). Hershey, PA: IGI Global. doi:10.4018/978-1-5225-2607-0.ch001

Paraskou, A., & George, B. P. (2018). An Overview of Reproductive Tourism. In *Legal and Economic Considerations Surrounding Reproductive Tourism: Emerging Research and Opportunities* (pp. 1–17). Hershey, PA: IGI Global. doi:10.4018/978-1-5225-2694-0.ch001

Park, S., & Moon, J. (2016). Strategic Approach towards Clinical Information Security. In J. Moon & M. Galea (Eds.), *Improving Health Management through Clinical Decision Support Systems* (pp. 329–359). Hershey, PA: IGI Global. doi:10.4018/978-1-4666-9432-3.ch015

Pereira, D., Castro, A., Gomes, P., Areias, J. C., Reis, Z. S., Coimbra, M. T., & Cruz-Correia, R. (2016). Digital Auscultation: Challenges and Perspectives. In M. Cruz-Cunha, I. Miranda, R. Martinho, & R. Rijo (Eds.), *Encyclopedia of E-Health and Telemedicine* (pp. 910–927). Hershey, PA: IGI Global. doi:10.4018/978-1-4666-9978-6.ch070

Peters, R. A., & Cruz, M. (2016). The States as Generators of Incremental Change in American Health Care Policy: 1935 to 1965. In R. Gholipour & K. Rouzbehani (Eds.), *Social, Economic, and Political Perspectives on Public Health Policy-Making* (pp. 86–114). Hershey, PA: IGI Global. doi:10.4018/978-1-4666-9944-1.ch005

Phuritsabam, B., & Devi, A. B. (2017). Information Seeking Behavior of Medical Scientists at Jawaharlal Nehru Institute of Medical Science: A Study. In S. Ram (Ed.), *Library and Information Services for Bioinformatics Education and Research* (pp. 177–187). Hershey, PA: IGI Global. doi:10.4018/978-1-5225-1871-6.ch010

Pieczka, B. (2018). Management of Risk and Adverse Events in Medical Entities. In A. Rosiek-Kryszewska & K. Leksowski (Eds.), *Healthcare Administration for Patient Safety and Engagement* (pp. 31–46). Hershey, PA: IGI Global. doi:10.4018/978-1-5225-3946-9.ch003

Poduval, J. (2016). Curriculum Development. In *Optimizing Medicine Residency Training Programs* (pp. 45–102). Hershey, PA: IGI Global. doi:10.4018/978-1-4666-9527-6.ch003

Poduval, J. (2016). Ethics and Professionalism. In *Optimizing Medicine Residency Training Programs* (pp. 103–133). Hershey, PA: IGI Global. doi:10.4018/978-1-4666-9527-6.ch004

Poduval, J. (2016). Management Skills and Leadership. In *Optimizing Medicine Residency Training Programs* (pp. 182–205). Hershey, PA: IGI Global. doi:10.4018/978-1-4666-9527-6.ch008

Poduval, J. (2016). Medicine Residency Training. In *Optimizing Medicine Residency Training Programs* (pp. 1–27). Hershey, PA: IGI Global. doi:10.4018/978-1-4666-9527-6.ch001

Poduval, J. (2016). Personal Issues. In *Optimizing Medicine Residency Training Programs* (pp. 206–221). Hershey, PA: IGI Global. doi:10.4018/978-1-4666-9527-6.ch009

Poduval, J. (2017). Medical Errors: Impact on Health Care Quality. In M. Riga (Ed.), *Impact of Medical Errors and Malpractice on Health Economics, Quality, and Patient Safety* (pp. 33–60). Hershey, PA: IGI Global. doi:10.4018/978-1-5225-2337-6.ch002

Politis, D., Stagiopoulos, P., Aidona, S., Kyriafinis, G., & Constantinidis, I. (2018). Autonomous Learning and Skill Accreditation: A Paradigm for Medical Studies. In A. Kumar (Ed.), *Optimizing Student Engagement in Online Learning Environments* (pp. 266–296). Hershey, PA: IGI Global. doi:10.4018/978-1-5225-3634-5.ch012

Pomares-Quimbaya, A., Gonzalez, R. A., Quintero, S., Muñoz, O. M., Bohórquez, W. R., García, O. M., & Londoño, D. (2016). A Review of Existing Applications and Techniques for Narrative Text Analysis in Electronic Medical Records. In M. Cruz-Cunha, I. Miranda, R. Martinho, & R. Rijo (Eds.), *Encyclopedia of E-Health and Telemedicine* (pp. 796–811). Hershey, PA: IGI Global. doi:10.4018/978-1-4666-9978-6.ch062

Pomares-Quimbaya, A., González, R. A., Sierra, A., Daza, J. C., Muñoz, O., García, A., ... Bohórquez, W. R. (2017). ICT for Enabling the Quality Evaluation of Health Care Services: A Case Study in a General Hospital. In A. Moumtzoglou (Ed.), *Design, Development, and Integration of Reliable Electronic Healthcare Platforms* (pp. 196–210). Hershey, PA: IGI Global. doi:10.4018/978-1-5225-1724-5.ch012

Pouliakis, A., Margari, N., Karakitsou, E., Archondakis, S., & Karakitsos, P. (2018). Emerging Technologies Serving Cytopathology: Big Data, the Cloud, and Mobile Computing. In I. El Naqa (Ed.), *Emerging Developments and Practices in Oncology* (pp. 114–152). Hershey, PA: IGI Global. doi:10.4018/978-1-5225-3085-5.ch005

Queirós, A., Silva, A. G., Ferreira, A., Caravau, H., Cerqueira, M., & Rocha, N. P. (2016). Assessing Mobile Applications Considered Medical Devices. In M. Cruz-Cunha, I. Miranda, R. Martinho, & R. Rijo (Eds.), *Encyclopedia of E-Health and Telemedicine* (pp. 111–127). Hershey, PA: IGI Global. doi:10.4018/978-1-4666-9978-6.ch010

Raffaeli, L., Spinsante, S., & Gambi, E. (2016). Integrated Smart TV-Based Personal e-Health System. *International Journal of E-Health and Medical Communications, 7*(1), 48–64. doi:10.4018/IJEHMC.2016010103

Rai, A., Kothari, R., & Singh, D. P. (2017). Assessment of Available Technologies for Hospital Waste Management: A Need for Society. In R. Singh, A. Singh, & V. Srivastava (Eds.), *Environmental Issues Surrounding Human Overpopulation* (pp. 172–188). Hershey, PA: IGI Global. doi:10.4018/978-1-5225-1683-5.ch010

Ramamoorthy, S., & Sivasubramaniam, R. (2018). Image Processing Including Medical Liver Imaging: Medical Image Processing from Big Data Perspective, Ultrasound Liver Images, Challenges. In M. Lytras & P. Papadopoulou (Eds.), *Applying Big Data Analytics in Bioinformatics and Medicine* (pp. 380–392). Hershey, PA: IGI Global. doi:10.4018/978-1-5225-2607-0.ch016

Rathor, G. P., & Gupta, S. K. (2017). Improving Multimodality Image Fusion through Integrate AFL and Wavelet Transform. In V. Tiwari, B. Tiwari, R. Thakur, & S. Gupta (Eds.), *Pattern and Data Analysis in Healthcare Settings* (pp. 143–157). Hershey, PA: IGI Global. doi:10.4018/978-1-5225-0536-5.ch008

Rawat, D. B., & Bhattacharya, S. (2016). Wireless Body Area Network for Healthcare Applications. In N. Meghanathan (Ed.), *Advanced Methods for Complex Network Analysis* (pp. 343–358). Hershey, PA: IGI Global. doi:10.4018/978-1-4666-9964-9.ch014

Rea, P. M. (2016). Advances in Anatomical and Medical Visualisation. In M. Pinheiro & D. Simões (Eds.), *Handbook of Research on Engaging Digital Natives in Higher Education Settings* (pp. 244–264). Hershey, PA: IGI Global. doi:10.4018/978-1-5225-0039-1.ch011

Rexhepi, H., & Persson, A. (2017). Challenges to Implementing IT Support for Evidence Based Practice Among Nurses and Assistant Nurses: A Qualitative Study. *Journal of Electronic Commerce in Organizations, 15*(2), 61–76. doi:10.4018/JECO.2017040105

Reychav, I., & Azuri, J. (2016). Including Elderly Patients in Decision Making via Electronic Health Literacy. In M. Cruz-Cunha, I. Miranda, R. Martinho, & R. Rijo (Eds.), *Encyclopedia of E-Health and Telemedicine* (pp. 241–249). Hershey, PA: IGI Global. doi:10.4018/978-1-4666-9978-6.ch020

Richards, D., & Caldwell, P. H. (2016). Gamification to Improve Adherence to Clinical Treatment Advice: Improving Adherence to Clinical Treatment. In D. Novák, B. Tulu, & H. Brendryen (Eds.), *Handbook of Research on Holistic Perspectives in Gamification for Clinical Practice* (pp. 47–77). Hershey, PA: IGI Global. doi:10.4018/978-1-4666-9522-1.ch004

Rissman, B. (2016). Medical Conditions Associated with NLD. In B. Rissman (Ed.), *Medical and Educational Perspectives on Nonverbal Learning Disability in Children and Young Adults* (pp. 27–66). Hershey, PA: IGI Global. doi:10.4018/978-1-4666-9539-9.ch002

Rosiek, A. (2018). The Assessment of Actions of the Environment and the Impact of Preventive Medicine for Public Health in Poland. In A. Rosiek-Kryszewska & K. Leksowski (Eds.), *Healthcare Administration for Patient Safety and Engagement* (pp. 106–119). Hershey, PA: IGI Global. doi:10.4018/978-1-5225-3946-9.ch006

Rosiek, A., Leksowski, K., Goch, A., Rosiek-Kryszewska, A., & Leksowski, Ł. (2016). Medical Treatment and Difficult Ethical Decisions in Interdisciplinary Hospital Teams. In A. Rosiek & K. Leksowski (Eds.), *Organizational Culture and Ethics in Modern Medicine* (pp. 121–153). Hershey, PA: IGI Global. doi:10.4018/978-1-4666-9658-7.ch006

Rosiek, A., & Rosiek-Kryszewska, A. (2018). Managed Healthcare: Doctor Life Satisfaction and Its Impact on the Process of Communicating With the Patient. In A. Rosiek-Kryszewska & K. Leksowski (Eds.), *Healthcare Administration for Patient Safety and Engagement* (pp. 244–261). Hershey, PA: IGI Global. doi:10.4018/978-1-5225-3946-9.ch013

Rosiek-Kryszewska, A., Leksowski, Ł., Rosiek, A., Leksowski, K., & Goch, A. (2016). Clinical Communication in the Aspect of Development of New Technologies and E-Health in the Doctor-Patient Relationship. In A. Rosiek & K. Leksowski (Eds.), *Organizational Culture and Ethics in Modern Medicine* (pp. 18–51). Hershey, PA: IGI Global. doi:10.4018/978-1-4666-9658-7.ch002

Rosiek-Kryszewska, A., & Rosiek, A. (2018). The Involvement of the Patient and his Perspective Evaluation of the Quality of Healthcare. In A. Rosiek-Kryszewska & K. Leksowski (Eds.), *Healthcare Administration for Patient Safety and Engagement* (pp. 121–144). Hershey, PA: IGI Global. doi:10.4018/978-1-5225-3946-9.ch007

Rosiek-Kryszewska, A., & Rosiek, A. (2018). The Impact of Management and Leadership Roles in Building Competitive Healthcare Units. In A. Rosiek-Kryszewska & K. Leksowski (Eds.), *Healthcare Administration for Patient Safety and Engagement* (pp. 13–30). Hershey, PA: IGI Global. doi:10.4018/978-1-5225-3946-9.ch002

Roşu, S. M., Păvăloiu, I. B., Dragoi, G., Apostol, C. G., & Munteanu, D. (2016). Telemedicine Based on LMDS in the Urban/Metropolitan Area: A Romanian Case Study. In M. Cruz-Cunha, I. Miranda, R. Martinho, & R. Rijo (Eds.), *Encyclopedia of E-Health and Telemedicine* (pp. 96–109). Hershey, PA: IGI Global. doi:10.4018/978-1-4666-9978-6.ch009

Rouzbehani, K. (2017). Health Policy Implementation: Moving Beyond Its Barriers in United States. In N. Wickramasinghe (Ed.), *Handbook of Research on Healthcare Administration and Management* (pp. 541–552). Hershey, PA: IGI Global. doi:10.4018/978-1-5225-0920-2.ch032

Ruiz, I. M., Cohen, D. S., & Marco, Á. M. (2016). ISO/IEEE11073 Family of Standards: Trends and Applications on E-Health Monitoring. In M. Cruz-Cunha, I. Miranda, R. Martinho, & R. Rijo (Eds.), *Encyclopedia of E-Health and Telemedicine* (pp. 646–660). Hershey, PA: IGI Global. doi:10.4018/978-1-4666-9978-6.ch050

Sam, S. (2017). Mobile Phones and Expanding Human Capabilities in Plural Health Systems. In K. Moahi, K. Bwalya, & P. Sebina (Eds.), *Health Information Systems and the Advancement of Medical Practice in Developing Countries* (pp. 93–114). Hershey, PA: IGI Global. doi:10.4018/978-1-5225-2262-1.ch006

Sankaranarayanan, S., & Ganesan, S. (2016). Applications of Intelligent Agents in Health Sector-A Review. *International Journal of E-Health and Medical Communications*, *7*(1), 1–30. doi:10.4018/IJEHMC.2016010101

Santos-Trigo, M., Suaste, E., & Figuerola, P. (2018). Technology Design and Routes for Tool Appropriation in Medical Practices. In M. Khosrow-Pour, D.B.A. (Ed.), Encyclopedia of Information Science and Technology, Fourth Edition (pp. 3794-3804). Hershey, PA: IGI Global. doi:10.4018/978-1-5225-2255-3.ch329

Sarivougioukas, J., Vagelatos, A., Parsopoulos, K. E., & Lagaris, I. E. (2018). Home UbiHealth. In M. Khosrow-Pour, D.B.A. (Ed.), Encyclopedia of Information Science and Technology, Fourth Edition (pp. 7765-7774). Hershey, PA: IGI Global. doi:10.4018/978-1-5225-2255-3.ch675

Sarkar, B. K. (2017). Big Data and Healthcare Data: A Survey. *International Journal of Knowledge-Based Organizations*, *7*(4), 50–77. doi:10.4018/IJKBO.2017100104

Saxena, K., & Banodha, U. (2017). An Essence of the SOA on Healthcare. In R. Bhadoria, N. Chaudhari, G. Tomar, & S. Singh (Eds.), *Exploring Enterprise Service Bus in the Service-Oriented Architecture Paradigm* (pp. 283–304). Hershey, PA: IGI Global. doi:10.4018/978-1-5225-2157-0.ch018

Schmeida, M., & McNeal, R. (2016). Consulting Online Healthcare Information: E-Caregivers as Knowledgeable Decision Makers. *International Journal of Computers in Clinical Practice*, *1*(1), 42–52. doi:10.4018/IJCCP.2016010104

Sen, K., & Ghosh, K. (2018). Incorporating Global Medical Knowledge to Solve Healthcare Problems: A Framework for a Crowdsourcing System. *International Journal of Healthcare Information Systems and Informatics*, *13*(1), 1–14. doi:10.4018/IJHISI.2018010101

Shakdher, A., & Pandey, K. (2017). REDAlert+: Medical/Fire Emergency and Warning System using Android Devices. *International Journal of E-Health and Medical Communications*, *8*(1), 37–51. doi:10.4018/IJEHMC.2017010103

Shekarian, E., Abdul-Rashid, S. H., & Olugu, E. U. (2017). An Integrated Fuzzy VIKOR Method for Performance Management in Healthcare. In M. Tavana, K. Szabat, & K. Puranam (Eds.), *Organizational Productivity and Performance Measurements Using Predictive Modeling and Analytics* (pp. 40–61). Hershey, PA: IGI Global. doi:10.4018/978-1-5225-0654-6.ch003

Shi, J., Erdem, E., & Liu, H. (2016). Expanding Role of Telephone Systems in Healthcare: Developments and Opportunities. In A. Dwivedi (Ed.), *Reshaping Medical Practice and Care with Health Information Systems* (pp. 87–131). Hershey, PA: IGI Global. doi:10.4018/978-1-4666-9870-3.ch004

Shijina, V., & John, S. J. (2017). Multiple Relations and its Application in Medical Diagnosis. *International Journal of Fuzzy System Applications*, *6*(4), 47–62. doi:10.4018/IJFSA.2017100104

Shipley, N., & Chakraborty, J. (2018). Big Data and mHealth: Increasing the Usability of Healthcare Through the Customization of Pinterest – Literary Perspective. In J. Machado, A. Abelha, M. Santos, & F. Portela (Eds.), *Next-Generation Mobile and Pervasive Healthcare Solutions* (pp. 46–66). Hershey, PA: IGI Global. doi:10.4018/978-1-5225-2851-7.ch004

Singh, A., & Dutta, M. K. (2017). A Reversible Data Hiding Scheme for Efficient Management of Tele-Ophthalmological Data. *International Journal of E-Health and Medical Communications*, *8*(3), 38–54. doi:10.4018/IJEHMC.2017070103

Sivaji, A., Radjo, H. K., Amin, M., & Abu Hashim, M. A. (2016). Design of a Hospital Interactive Wayfinding System: Designing for Malaysian Users. In N. Mohamed, T. Mantoro, M. Ayu, & M. Mahmud (Eds.), *Critical Socio-Technical Issues Surrounding Mobile Computing* (pp. 88–123). Hershey, PA: IGI Global. doi:10.4018/978-1-4666-9438-5.ch005

Skourti, P. K., & Pavlakis, A. (2017). The Second Victim Phenomenon: The Way Out. In M. Riga (Ed.), *Impact of Medical Errors and Malpractice on Health Economics, Quality, and Patient Safety* (pp. 197–222). Hershey, PA: IGI Global. doi:10.4018/978-1-5225-2337-6.ch008

Smith, C. R. (2018). Medical Students' Quest Towards the Long White Coat: Impact on Mental Health and Well-Being. In C. Smith (Ed.), *Exploring the Pressures of Medical Education From a Mental Health and Wellness Perspective* (pp. 1–42). Hershey, PA: IGI Global. doi:10.4018/978-1-5225-2811-1.ch001

Smith, S. I., & Dandignac, M. (2018). Perfectionism: Addressing Lofty Expectations in Medical School. In C. Smith (Ed.), *Exploring the Pressures of Medical Education From a Mental Health and Wellness Perspective* (pp. 68–91). Hershey, PA: IGI Global. doi:10.4018/978-1-5225-2811-1.ch003

Sobrinho, Á. A., Dias da Silva, L., Perkusich, A., Cunha, P., Pinheiro, M. E., & Melo de Medeiros, L. (2016). Towards Medical Systems to Aid the Detection and Treatment of Chronic Diseases. In D. Fotiadis (Ed.), *Handbook of Research on Trends in the Diagnosis and Treatment of Chronic Conditions* (pp. 50–69). Hershey, PA: IGI Global. doi:10.4018/978-1-4666-8828-5.ch003

Soczywko, J., & Rutkowska, D. (2018). The Patient/Provider Relationship in Emergency Medicine: Organization, Communication, and Understanding. In A. Rosiek-Kryszewska & K. Leksowski (Eds.), *Healthcare Administration for Patient Safety and Engagement* (pp. 74–105). Hershey, PA: IGI Global. doi:10.4018/978-1-5225-3946-9.ch005

Sołtysik-Piorunkiewicz, A., Furmankiewicz, M., & Ziuziański, P. (2016). Web Healthcare Applications in Poland: Trends, Standards, Barriers and Possibilities of Implementation and Usage of E-Health Systems. In I. Deliyannis, P. Kostagiolas, & C. Banou (Eds.), *Experimental Multimedia Systems for Interactivity and Strategic Innovation* (pp. 258–283). Hershey, PA: IGI Global. doi:10.4018/978-1-4666-8659-5.ch013

Soni, P. (2018). Implications of HIPAA and Subsequent Regulations on Information Technology. In M. Gupta, R. Sharman, J. Walp, & P. Mulgund (Eds.), *Information Technology Risk Management and Compliance in Modern Organizations* (pp. 71–98). Hershey, PA: IGI Global. doi:10.4018/978-1-5225-2604-9.ch004

Spinelli, R., & Benevolo, C. (2016). From Healthcare Services to E-Health Applications: A Delivery System-Based Taxonomy. In A. Dwivedi (Ed.), *Reshaping Medical Practice and Care with Health Information Systems* (pp. 205–245). Hershey, PA: IGI Global. doi:10.4018/978-1-4666-9870-3.ch007

Srivastava, A., & Aggarwal, A. K. (2018). Medical Image Fusion in Spatial and Transform Domain: A Comparative Analysis. In M. Anwar, A. Khosla, & R. Kapoor (Eds.), *Handbook of Research on Advanced Concepts in Real-Time Image and Video Processing* (pp. 281–300). Hershey, PA: IGI Global. doi:10.4018/978-1-5225-2848-7.ch011

Srivastava, S. K., & Roy, S. N. (2018). Recommendation System: A Potential Tool for Achieving Pervasive Health Care. In J. Machado, A. Abelha, M. Santos, & F. Portela (Eds.), *Next-Generation Mobile and Pervasive Healthcare Solutions* (pp. 111–127). Hershey, PA: IGI Global. doi:10.4018/978-1-5225-2851-7.ch008

Stancu, A. (2016). Correlations and Patterns of Food and Health Consumer Expenditure. In A. Jean-Vasile (Ed.), *Food Science, Production, and Engineering in Contemporary Economies* (pp. 44–101). Hershey, PA: IGI Global. doi:10.4018/978-1-5225-0341-5.ch003

Stanimirovic, D. (2017). Digitalization of Death Certification Model: Transformation Issues and Implementation Concerns. In S. Saeed, Y. Bamarouf, T. Ramayah, & S. Iqbal (Eds.), *Design Solutions for User-Centric Information Systems* (pp. 22–43). Hershey, PA: IGI Global. doi:10.4018/978-1-5225-1944-7.ch002

Stavros, A., Vavoulidis, E., & Nasioutziki, M. (2016). The Use of Mobile Health Applications for Quality Control and Accreditational Purposes in a Cytopathology Laboratory. In A. Moumtzoglou (Ed.), *M-Health Innovations for Patient-Centered Care* (pp. 262–283). Hershey, PA: IGI Global. doi:10.4018/978-1-4666-9861-1.ch013

Sukkird, V., & Shirahada, K. (2018). E-Health Service Model for Asian Developing Countries: A Case of Emergency Medical Service for Elderly People in Thailand. In M. Khosrow-Pour (Ed.), *Optimizing Current Practices in E-Services and Mobile Applications* (pp. 214–232). Hershey, PA: IGI Global. doi:10.4018/978-1-5225-5026-6.ch011

Sygit, B., & Wąsik, D. (2016). Patients' Rights and Medical Personnel Duties in the Field of Hospital Care. In A. Rosiek & K. Leksowski (Eds.), *Organizational Culture and Ethics in Modern Medicine* (pp. 282–297). Hershey, PA: IGI Global. doi:10.4018/978-1-4666-9658-7.ch012

Sygit, B., & Wąsik, D. (2016). The Idea of Human Rights in Conditions of Hospital Treatment. In A. Rosiek & K. Leksowski (Eds.), *Organizational Culture and Ethics in Modern Medicine* (pp. 236–254). Hershey, PA: IGI Global. doi:10.4018/978-1-4666-9658-7.ch010

Talbot, T. B. (2017). Making Lifelike Medical Games in the Age of Virtual Reality: An Update on "Playing Games with Biology" from 2013. In B. Dubbels (Ed.), *Transforming Gaming and Computer Simulation Technologies across Industries* (pp. 103–119). Hershey, PA: IGI Global. doi:10.4018/978-1-5225-1817-4.ch006

Tamposis, I., Pouliakis, A., Fezoulidis, I., & Karakitsos, P. (2016). Mobile Platforms Supporting Health Professionals: Need, Technical Requirements, and Applications. In A. Moumtzoglou (Ed.), *M-Health Innovations for Patient-Centered Care* (pp. 91–114). Hershey, PA: IGI Global. doi:10.4018/978-1-4666-9861-1.ch005

Tiago, M. T., Tiago, F., Amaral, F. E., & Silva, S. (2016). Healthy 3.0: Healthcare Digital Dimensions. In A. Dwivedi (Ed.), *Reshaping Medical Practice and Care with Health Information Systems* (pp. 287–322). Hershey, PA: IGI Global. doi:10.4018/978-1-4666-9870-3.ch010

Tripathy, B. (2016). Application of Rough Set Based Models in Medical Diagnosis. In S. Dash & B. Subudhi (Eds.), *Handbook of Research on Computational Intelligence Applications in Bioinformatics* (pp. 144–168). Hershey, PA: IGI Global. doi:10.4018/978-1-5225-0427-6.ch008

Turcu, C. E., & Turcu, C. O. (2017). Social Internet of Things in Healthcare: From Things to Social Things in Internet of Things. In C. Reis & M. Maximiano (Eds.), *Internet of Things and Advanced Application in Healthcare* (pp. 266–295). Hershey, PA: IGI Global. doi:10.4018/978-1-5225-1820-4.ch010

Unwin, D. W., Sanzogni, L., & Sandhu, K. (2017). Developing and Measuring the Business Case for Health Information Technology. In K. Moahi, K. Bwalya, & P. Sebina (Eds.), *Health Information Systems and the Advancement of Medical Practice in Developing Countries* (pp. 262–290). Hershey, PA: IGI Global. doi:10.4018/978-1-5225-2262-1.ch015

Urooj, S., & Singh, S. P. (2016). Wavelet Transform-Based Soft Computational Techniques and Applications in Medical Imaging. In P. Saxena, D. Singh, & M. Pant (Eds.), *Problem Solving and Uncertainty Modeling through Optimization and Soft Computing Applications* (pp. 339–363). Hershey, PA: IGI Global. doi:10.4018/978-1-4666-9885-7.ch016

Vasant, P. (2018). A General Medical Diagnosis System Formed by Artificial Neural Networks and Swarm Intelligence Techniques. In U. Kose, G. Guraksin, & O. Deperlioglu (Eds.), *Nature-Inspired Intelligent Techniques for Solving Biomedical Engineering Problems* (pp. 130–145). Hershey, PA: IGI Global. doi:10.4018/978-1-5225-4769-3.ch006

Waegemann, C. P. (2016). mHealth: History, Analysis, and Implementation. In A. Moumtzoglou (Ed.), M-Health Innovations for Patient-Centered Care (pp. 1-19). Hershey, PA: IGI Global. doi:10.4018/978-1-4666-9861-1.ch001

Watfa, M. K., Majeed, H., & Salahuddin, T. (2016). Computer Based E-Healthcare Clinical Systems: A Comprehensive Survey. *International Journal of Privacy and Health Information Management*, *4*(1), 50–69. doi:10.4018/IJPHIM.2016010104

Wietholter, J. P., Coetzee, R., Nardella, B., Kincaid, S. E., & Slain, D. (2016). International Healthcare Experiences: Caring While Learning and Learning While Caring. In D. Velliaris & D. Coleman-George (Eds.), *Handbook of Research on Study Abroad Programs and Outbound Mobility* (pp. 470–496). Hershey, PA: IGI Global. doi:10.4018/978-1-5225-0169-5.ch019

Witzke, K., & Specht, O. (2017). M-Health Telemedicine and Telepresence in Oral and Maxillofacial Surgery: An Innovative Prehospital Healthcare Concept in Structurally Weak Areas. *International Journal of Reliable and Quality E-Healthcare*, *6*(4), 37–48. doi:10.4018/IJRQEH.2017100105

Wójcik, A., & Chojnacki, M. (2016). Behavior and Ethical Problems in the Functioning of the Operating Theater (Case Study). In A. Rosiek & K. Leksowski (Eds.), *Organizational Culture and Ethics in Modern Medicine* (pp. 154–179). Hershey, PA: IGI Global. doi:10.4018/978-1-4666-9658-7.ch007

Wolk, K., & Marasek, K. P. (2016). Translation of Medical Texts using Neural Networks. *International Journal of Reliable and Quality E-Healthcare*, *5*(4), 51–66. doi:10.4018/IJRQEH.2016100104

Wong, A. K., & Lo, M. F. (2018). Using Pervasive Computing for Sustainable Healthcare in an Aging Population. In B. Fong, A. Ng, & P. Yuen (Eds.), *Sustainable Health and Long-Term Care Solutions for an Aging Population* (pp. 187–202). Hershey, PA: IGI Global. doi:10.4018/978-1-5225-2633-9.ch010

Wu, W., Martin, B. C., & Ni, C. (2017). A Systematic Review of Competency-Based Education Effort in the Health Professions: Seeking Order Out of Chaos. In K. Rasmussen, P. Northrup, & R. Colson (Eds.), *Handbook of Research on Competency-Based Education in University Settings* (pp. 352–378). Hershey, PA: IGI Global. doi:10.4018/978-1-5225-0932-5.ch018

Yadav, N., Aliasgari, M., & Poellabauer, C. (2016). Mobile Healthcare in an Increasingly Connected Developing World. *International Journal of Privacy and Health Information Management*, *4*(2), 76–97. doi:10.4018/IJPHIM.2016070106

Yadav, S., Ekbal, A., Saha, S., Pathak, P. S., & Bhattacharyya, P. (2017). Patient Data De-Identification: A Conditional Random-Field-Based Supervised Approach. In S. Saha, A. Mandal, A. Narasimhamurthy, S. V, & S. Sangam (Eds.), Handbook of Research on Applied Cybernetics and Systems Science (pp. 234-253). Hershey, PA: IGI Global. doi:10.4018/978-1-5225-2498-4.ch011

Yu, B., Wijesekera, D., & Costa, P. C. (2017). Informed Consent in Healthcare: A Study Case of Genetic Services. In A. Moumtzoglou (Ed.), *Design, Development, and Integration of Reliable Electronic Healthcare Platforms* (pp. 211–242). Hershey, PA: IGI Global. doi:10.4018/978-1-5225-1724-5.ch013

Yu, B., Wijesekera, D., & Costa, P. C. (2017). Informed Consent in Electronic Medical Record Systems. In I. Management Association (Ed.), Healthcare Ethics and Training: Concepts, Methodologies, Tools, and Applications (pp. 1029-1049). Hershey, PA: IGI Global. doi:10.4018/978-1-5225-2237-9.ch049

Yu, M., Li, J., & Wang, W. (2017). Creative Life Experience among Students in Medical Education. In C. Zhou (Ed.), *Handbook of Research on Creative Problem-Solving Skill Development in Higher Education* (pp. 158–184). Hershey, PA: IGI Global. doi:10.4018/978-1-5225-0643-0.ch008

Zarour, K. (2017). Towards a Telehomecare in Algeria: Case of Diabetes Measurement and Remote Monitoring. *International Journal of E-Health and Medical Communications*, *8*(4), 61–80. doi:10.4018/IJEHMC.2017100104

Zavyalova, Y. V., Korzun, D. G., Meigal, A. Y., & Borodin, A. V. (2017). Towards the Development of Smart Spaces-Based Socio-Cyber-Medicine Systems. *International Journal of Embedded and Real-Time Communication Systems*, *8*(1), 45–63. doi:10.4018/IJERTCS.2017010104

Zeinali, A. A. (2018). Word Formation Study in Developing Naming Guidelines in the Translation of English Medical Terms Into Persian. In M. Khosrow-Pour, D.B.A. (Ed.), Encyclopedia of Information Science and Technology, Fourth Edition (pp. 5136-5147). Hershey, PA: IGI Global. doi:10.4018/978-1-5225-2255-3.ch446

Ziminski, T. B., Demurjian, S. A., Sanzi, E., & Agresta, T. (2016). Toward Integrating Healthcare Data and Systems: A Study of Architectural Alternatives. In T. Iyamu & A. Tatnall (Eds.), *Maximizing Healthcare Delivery and Management through Technology Integration* (pp. 270–304). Hershey, PA: IGI Global. doi:10.4018/978-1-4666-9446-0.ch016

Ziminski, T. B., Demurjian, S. A., Sanzi, E., Baihan, M., & Agresta, T. (2016). An Architectural Solution for Health Information Exchange. *International Journal of User-Driven Healthcare*, *6*(1), 65–103. doi:10.4018/IJUDH.2016010104

Zineldin, M., & Vasicheva, V. (2018). Reducing Medical Errors and Increasing Patient Safety: TRM and 5 Q's Approaches for Better Quality of Life. In *Technological Tools for Value-Based Sustainable Relationships in Health: Emerging Research and Opportunities* (pp. 87–115). Hershey, PA: IGI Global. doi:10.4018/978-1-5225-4091-5.ch005

About the Contributors

Simon George Taukeni is an academic, book editor, and researcher. His research interest mainly is in field of psychology and public health.

* * *

Ameen Abdullateef is a researcher in University of Ilorin. He has vast experience in research writing, research methodology and business analysis.

Shivam Agrawal is a curious person who enjoys figuring out the building blocks of the world, and rearranging them to build something even better. My career is developing software, but my life is adventuring. Currently he is building infrastructure at Darwinbox Solutions Pvt. Ltd., and is volunteering in his free time.

Daniel Ashipala is a senior lecturer at the University of Namibia, in the department of General Nursing. His research interest is in nursing education, family health, mental health, and public health.

Suma Dawn, PhD, received her B.E degree in Information Technology from Sardar Vallabhbhai Patel Institute of Technology, Vasad, Gujarat University, Gujarat, India, in 2002; M.Tech. in Computer Science and Engineering from Kalyani University, West Bengal, India in 2005; and Ph.D. from Jaypee Institute of Information Technology, Noida, Uttar Pradesh, India in 2015. She joined Jaypee Institute of Information Technology in 2006 where she is currently an Assistant Professor (Senior Grade) in the Department of Computer Science & Engg. and Information Technology. She has more than 15 years of teaching experience. She has taught subjects like Advanced Computer Graphics, 3D Graphics and Animation, Computer Graphics, Algorithmic Bioinformatics, Computer Games, Image Processing, Multimedia Content and Animation Design, Multimedia Computing, Multimedia Systems, Data Structures, Cryptography, Computer Programming, DBMS, and Fundamentals of Algorithm. She has also been an integral part of Multimedia Labs for Photoshop, Illustrator and Flash, Gaming and Web Technology Labs. Her research interests include HCI & Computer Vision, Image Processing & Computer Graphics, Bioinformatics, Brain-Computer Interface, Data Structures & Algorithms, Pattern Recognition, IoT and Agriculture. She has been an integral part and organizer of the International Conference of Contemporary Computing since its inception in 2008 (to date), participated in some of the International conferences of repute such as ACM's Compute (in 2011), ICGVIP (in 2014), and other. She has published a few papers in International journals too. She has guided more than 120 project theses for postgraduates and graduates. Currently, she has 3 Ph.D. scholars working under her.

Rachel J. Freeman is a Senior Lecturer in the Department of Social Work and Lead of UNAM Cares at the University of Namibia (UNAM). She is a UNAM Social Work Alumni and holds a Master of Arts Degree in Social Behaviour Studies in Sociology (Cum Laude) from the University of South Africa (UNISA, 2011). She holds a Doctorate of Philosophy Degree (PhD) in Sociology from (UNISA, 2018). She is an Honorary Senior Research Fellow at Cardiff University. Dr Freeman is a passionate educationalist, who finds pleasure in transforming minds through education, research and community service, tasks she professionally undertake. She received the University of Namibia's Faculty of Humanities and Social Sciences Meritorius Award (2016) in recognition for outstanding service and performance in the areas of teaching, research and community services. She is inspire by the motto of Dr Nelson Mandela: "Education is the most powerful weapon, which can be used to change the world". Currently, she serves on the President of Namibia's COVID-19 National Health Emergency Management Coordination Task Force. She serves on the COVID-19 Social Mobilization, Risk Communication and Community Engagement pillar as well as, the Mental Health and Psychosocial Support Pillar. She serves as Vice-Chairperson of the Namibia National Palliative Care Task Force. She is the International Exchange Coordinator for the social work Staff and Student Mobility programmes between USA, UK and other European universities in the UNAM Social Work Department. She conducts research and publishes on Palliative care, Hepatitis E aspects of community behaviour and practices; alcohol and substance abuse; combating gender-based violence; HIV and AIDS and promoting social justice and human rights. Dr Freeman has 19 publications in peer-reviewed journals. Her presentation for today will provide an Update of Namibia's different Strategies employed in Response to COVID-19, looking at the outbreak of the COVID-19 pandemic in Namibia, Government's Policy & Programme Responses to COVID-19 Pandemic, Namibia's Strategies in response to COVID-19, the Challenges experienced as well as, Lessons learned and suggesting Recommendations in Strengthening current and future pandemic responses.

Sucharithra Ganesh, B.Tech (Biotechnology), BS Abdur Rahman Crescent Institute of Science and Technology, Chennai, Tamil Nadu, India is an active young researcher. Her areas of interests include cancer biology, nanotechnology and microbiology. She has worked in the preparation and evaluation of anticancer and antimicrobial activities of nano-fibers, nano-particles and nano-emulsions.

Abdussalaam Iyanda Ismail was born in Nigeria. He completed his first degree in Bachelor of Science in Industrial and Labor Relations (ILR) from Olabisi Onabanjo University, Ogun State, Nigeria. He completed his master degree and Ph.D from Universiti Utara Malaysia. Currently, he is an assistant professor of Management at University of Fujairah, Fujairah UAE. He has interest in human resource management, industrial relations, strategic management, and research methodology.

Joel Medusalem is a registered nurse with hands-on experience in emergency nursing and with an interest in nursing education and research.

Md. Musfikur Rahman has been working as a Research Investigator in Maternal and Child Health Division in icddr,b Dhaka, Bangladesh. icddr,b is a Bangladesh-based international health research institute that strives to solve key public health problems through high-quality scientific research and innovation. Mr. Rahman has obtained Master of Public Health degree recently. He has completed his MSS and BSS degree in Anthropology from the University of Rajshahi respectively in 2005 and 2004. He has several journal publications in the field of qualitative social research.

Pothuraju Rajarajeswari, Working as professor and Deputy HOD in KLUniversity in the department of Computer science and Engineering is awarded PhD (Computer Science and Engineering) from Acharya Nagarjuna University and M.Tech [CSE], from JNTU Kakinada. She has 19 years of experience in Teaching computer subjects for B.tech and MCA , MTech Post Graduate Students. She is FIETE ["fellow" in the Institution of Electronics and Telecommunication Engineers], member in MACM, MISTE, MIACSIT, MIAENG. She has published more than 40 Research papers in reputed international journals. Her research interests include Bioinformatics, Data Mining, Artificial Intelligence.

Peddarapu Ramakrishna is Research Scholar of Computer Science at the Koneru Lakshmaiah Education Foundation (KL Deemed to be University), Vaddeswaram, Andhra Pradesh,India since July 2019. He received his B.Tech. and M.Tech degrees in Computer Science and Engineering from JNTU University (JNTUH), Hyderabad, in 2004 and 2010, respectively. His research interests include Machine Learning, Artificial Intelligence and Deep Learning. Currently he is doing his research in the area of Bio-technology. He is a member of the CSI and ISTE. And he is working as Asst. Professor in Dept. of Computer Science and Engineering at VNR Vignana Jyothi Institute of Engineering and Technology, Bachupally, Hyderabad, Telangana.He is having 15 years of teaching experience.

Nestor Tomas is a lecturer in the department of General Nursing at the University of Namibia. His research interest includes nursing education, public health, health economics, and reproductive health.

Md. Nasir Uddin, Ph.D., is a professional who has been working in the field of research and analysis at a department of Prime Minister Office, Dhaka, Bangladesh. He has obtained his Ph.D., MSS and BSS degree in Anthropology from the University of Rajshahi respectively in 2015, 2005 and 2004. He has eight journals and two books chapter publications in the field of qualitative social research. He is an international member of The South Asian Network for Development and Environmental Economics (SANDEE), Author AID & INASP (the International Network for the Availability of Scientific Publications), Open Researcher and Contributor ID (ORCID), Researchgate.net and Amnesty International.

Nurudeen Opeyemi Wahab is a researcher in the department of business administration at Olabisi Onabanjo University, Ago-iwoye, Ogun State. He had vast experience in research writings, data gathering and analysis.

Index

M

O

P

Q

R

S

T

U

V

W

Z

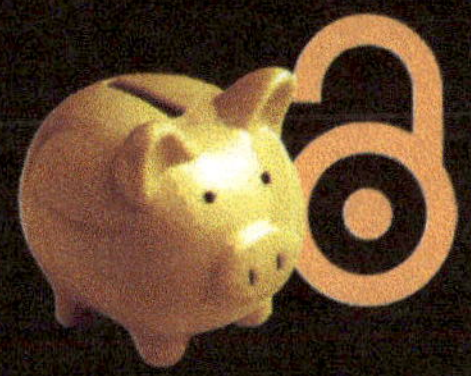

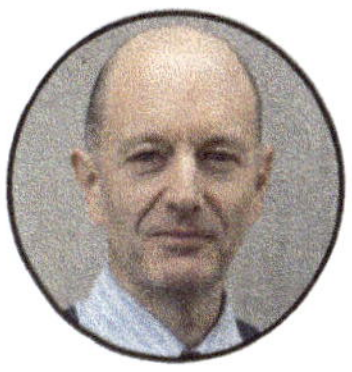

www.ingramcontent.com/pod-product-compliance
Lightning Source LLC
LaVergne TN
LVHW060306011026
849161LV00011B/2781